Osteoporosis

Diagnosis and Management

EDITED BY

Dale W. Stovall MD

Chair and Residency Program Director
Department of Obstetrics and Gynecology
Riverside Regional Medical Center
Newport News, VA;
Clinical Professor, Department of Internal Medicine
University of Virginia Health System
Charlottesville, VA, USA

WILEY Blackwell

Registered office: John Wiley & Sons, Ltd, The Atrium, Southern Gate, Chichester,
West Sussex, PO19 8SQ, UK

Editorial offices: 9600 Garsington Road, Oxford, OX4 2DQ, UK
The Atrium, Southern Gate, Chichester, West Sussex, PO19 8SQ, UK
111 River Street, Hoboken, NJ 07030-5774, USA

For details of our global editorial offices, for customer services and for information about how to
apply for permission to reuse the copyright material in this book please see our website at
www.wiley.com/wiley-blackwell

Library of Congress Cataloging-in-Publication Data

Osteoporosis (2013)
   Osteoporosis : diagnosis and management / edited by Dale W. Stovall.
   p. ; cm.
   Includes bibliographical references and index.
   ISBN 978-1-119-96891-7 (hardback : alk. paper) – ISBN 978-1-118-31632-0 (ePDF) –
ISBN 978-1-118-31631-3 (ePub) – ISBN 978-1-118-31630-6 (Mobi) – ISBN 978-1-118-31629-0
   I. Stovall, Dale W., editor of compilation.   II. Title.
   [DNLM: 1. Osteoporosis–diagnosis.   2. Osteoporosis–therapy.   3. Risk Factors. WE 250]
   RC931.O73
   616.7′16–dc23

                                                                    2013018952

A catalogue record for this book is available from the British Library.

Wiley also publishes its books in a variety of electronic formats. Some content that appears in print
may not be available in electronic books.

Cover image: iStock, file number #4907160 © Rpsycho
Cover design by Meaden Creative

Set in 9.5/13pt Meridien by Aptara® Inc., New Delhi, India
Printed and bound in Singapore by Markono Print Media Pte Ltd

1   2013

Contents

List of Contributors

Robert A. Adler, MD
Chief, Endocrinology and Metabolism
Hunter Holmes McGuire Veterans Affairs
Medical Center;
Professor of Internal Medicine
Professor of Epidemiology and
Community Health
Virginia Commonwealth University
School of Medicine
Richmond, VA, USA

Diane M. Biskobing, MD
Associate Professor of Medicine
Virginia Commonwealth University
School of Medicine
Richmond, VA, USA

Michael A. Bolognese, MD, FACE
Bethesda Health Research
Bethesda, MD, USA

**Juliet Compston, MD, FRCPath,
FRCP, FMedSci**
Professor of Bone Medicine
Cambridge University Hospitals NHS
Foundation Trust
Cambridge, UK

**Cyrus Cooper, MA, DM, FRCP, FFPH,
FMedSci**
MRC Lifecourse Epidemiology Unit
University of Southampton
University Hospital Southampton
Southampton;
Professor of Musculoskeletal Science
NIHR Musculoskeletal Biomedical
Research Unit
University of Oxford
Oxford, UK

Peter R. Ebeling, MBBS, MD, FRACP
Departments of Medicine (NorthWest
Academic Centre) and Endocrinology
Australian Institute of Musculoskeletal Science
The University of Melbourne
St. Albans, VIC, Australia

Mark Edwards, MB, BSc, MRCP
MRC Lifecourse Epidemiology Unit
University of Southampton
University Hospital Southampton
Southampton, UK

Erik Fink Eriksen, MD, DMSc
Department of Clinical Endocrinology
Oslo University Hospital
Oslo, Norway

Ronald C. Hamdy, MD, FRCP, FACP
Professor of Medicine
Cecile Cox Quillen Chair of Excellence in
Geriatric Medicine
East Tennessee State University
Johnson City, TN, USA

**Nick Harvey, MA, MB, BChir, MRCP,
PhD**
MRC Lifecourse Epidemiology Unit
University of Southampton
University Hospital Southampton
Southampton, UK

Michael F. Holick, PhD, MD
Department of Medicine, Section of
Endocrinology, Nutrition, and Diabetes
Vitamin D, Skin and Bone Research Laboratory
Boston University Medical Center
Boston, MA, USA

E. Michael Lewiecki, MD, FACP, FACE
New Mexico Clinical Research &
Osteoporosis Center, Inc
Albuquerque, NM, USA

Robert Lindsay, MD, PhD
Helen Hayes Hospital;
College of Physicians and Surgeons
Columbia University
New York, NY, USA

Michael R. McClung, MD
Oregon Osteoporosis Center
Portland, OR, USA

Paul D. Miller, MD
Distinguished Clinical Professor of Medicine
University of Colorado Health Sciences Center;
Medical Director
Colorado Center for Bone Research
Lakewood, CO, USA

Rebecca Moon, BM, BSc, MRCPCH
MRC Lifecourse Epidemiology Unit
University of Southampton
University Hospital Southampton
Southampton, UK

John T. Schousboe, MD, PhD
Co-Director, Park Nicollet Osteoporosis Center
Medical Director for Research, Park Nicollet
Institute for Research and Education
Park Nicollet Health Services;
Adjunct Assistant Professor
Division of Health Policy and Management
School of Public Health
University of Minnesota
Minneapolis, MN, USA

Maziar Shabestari, DDS, PhD
Department of Clinical Endocrinology
Oslo University Hospital
Oslo, Norway

Stuart Silverman, MD, FACP, FACR
Rheumatology Division
Cedars-Sinai Medical Center
Los Angeles, CA, USA

James A. Simon, MD, CCD, NCMP, FACOG
Department of Obstetrics and Gynecology
The School of Medicine and Health Sciences
The George Washington University;
Women's Health & Research Consultants®
Washington, DC, USA

Pilar Valenzuela Mazo, MD, NCMP
Department of Obstetrics and Gynecology
Pontificia Universidad Católica de Chile
School of Medicine
Santiago, Chile

Swamy Venuturupalli, MD, FACR
Clinical Chief - Rheumatology Division
Cedars-Sinai Medical Center;
Associate Clinical Professor of Medicine
University of California, Los Angeles
Los Angeles, CA, USA

Nelson B. Watts, MD
Director, Mercy Health Osteoporosis and
Bone Health Services
Cincinnati, OH, USA

Cristiano A. F. Zerbini, MD
Department of Rheumatology
Hospital Heliópolis;
Centro Paulista de Investigação Clinica
São Paulo, Brazil

Preface

Osteoporosis is a highly prevalent disease that increases one's risk for fracture. The disease is primarily defined by the results of a bone mineral density test. However, there are many risk factors for osteoporosis and fracture. Determining which patients are at significant risk for fracture; and therefore, are candidates for intervention can be challenging. The development of the ten year absolute fracture risk assessment tool, FRAX, has greatly enhanced the clinician's ability to select patients for therapy.

Currently, there is no cure for osteoporosis, and treatment is focused on reducing the patient's risk for fracture. Our understanding of the physiology of bone remodeling is on-going. As we learn more about this process, our ability to identify new highly effective, safe therapies will improve. Several treatment options are currently approved and available for the treatment of patients with osteoporosis and low bone mass. The information gained from numerous randomized trials has clarified the benefits of these therapies, and their existence in clinical practice for many years has provided clinicians with additional safety information regarding their use.

This text reviews the epidemiology of this disease, its pathophysiology, and its clinical impact in both women and men. Assessment of fracture risk, secondary causes of osteoporosis, initiation of therapy and follow-up are reviewed. Medical therapies, including the administration of calcium and Vitamin D are reviewed in detail to enhance the clinician's depth of knowledge of these subjects.

The primary aim of this text is to empower the primary care clinician to identify and treat patients with osteoporosis. In addition, this text will supply the primary care provider with in-depth information regarding the mechanisms of action of numerous approved medical therapies, when treatment is indicated, how to select a therapy, and how to manage the disease on an on-going basis. Finally, a look into future medical therapies for this disease is presented.

I am grateful to the authors of this text who have put their time, energy, and significant skill towards comprising a work that we hope will contribute to the improvement of patient care.

Dale W. Stovall, MD
Newport News, VA, USA

CHAPTER 1

Epidemiology and Genetics of Postmenopausal Osteoporosis

Mark Edwards[1], Rebecca Moon[1], Nick Harvey[1] & *Cyrus Cooper[1,2]*

[1]University of Southampton, University Hospital Southampton, Southampton, UK
[2]University of Oxford, Oxford, UK

Introduction

Osteoporosis is a skeletal disease characterized by low bone mass and micro-architectural deterioration of bone tissue with a consequent increase in bone fragility and susceptibility to fracture [1]. The term osteoporosis literally means "porous bone" and refers to a condition in which bone is normally mineralized but reduced in quantity. In 1994, a working group of the World Health Organization (WHO) provided a practical definition of osteoporosis as a bone mineral density (BMD) of greater than 2.5 SD below the young normal mean [2]. Earlier definitions had incorporated fracture and so to provide comparability, the subset of women with osteoporosis who had also suffered one or more fragility fractures were deemed to have severe "established" osteoporosis.

The etiology of osteoporotic fractures is complex. Low bone density is not the only risk factor for fracture and there has been a move towards making an assessment of individualized 10-year absolute fracture risk using the WHO FRAX based on multiple clinical risk factors [3]. Family history, and in particular parental hip fracture, is included in the FRAX tool reflecting the hereditary component of the condition. There is growing recognition of a complex interaction between genetic and environmental factors. Only a small number of specific genes contributing to osteoporosis risk have been consistently identified; however, the investigation of gene-environment interactions with developmental plasticity has yielded promising results, raising the possibility of intervening during fetal development or early life to reduce individual fracture risk and the global burden of this disease. It is estimated that around 200 million women worldwide have osteoporosis with an osteoporotic fracture occurring every 3 seconds [4]. This equates to 1 in 3 women over 50 years of age

---

suffering an osteoporotic fracture [5,6]. Fragility fractures make up 0.83% of the worldwide burden of noncommunicable disease. This figure rises to 1.75% in Europe, where fragility fractures also account for more disability adjusted life years (DALYs) than many other chronic diseases [7]. At present the annual cost of all osteoporotic fractures worldwide is in excess of $17 billion and is expected to rise to $25 billion by 2025 [8]. The cost of treating osteoporotic fractures is also increasing in the UK and expected to rise to over £2 billion by 2020 [9]. This chapter will review the genetic and early environmental factors associated with osteoporosis and describe the demographic, global and secular trends in its epidemiology.

Genetics

Heritability estimates in osteoporosis

Peak bone mass is an important factor in determining BMD in later life. It has been suggested by twin and family studies that between 50% and 85% of the variance in BMD is determined by heritable factors [10–12], including both genetics and shared environmental exposures. These estimates do, however, vary depending on the skeletal site, with lumbar spine BMD demonstrating a greater heritable component than the distal forearm BMD [10, 12, 13]. Several studies have suggested that increasing age also influences the extent to which bone outcomes are determined by heritable factors. It has been shown that the heritable component of BMD is lower in postmenopausal compared with premenopausal women [10, 12], probably reflecting the greater role of additional lifestyle, dietary and disease-related factors occurring in postmenopausal women. Similarly, the heritable component of the rate of change in BMD in postmenopausal women is lower than that for peak bone mass, which occurs much earlier in life [14].

In terms of osteoporotic fractures, it is known that the risk is greater in those with a parent who has suffered a hip fracture. There is, however, less evidence for a significant genetic component to this association. A heritable component has also been found in the determination of femoral neck geometry [15], markers of bone turnover [16], age at menopause [17], and muscle strength [18], all of which confer some susceptibility to osteoporotic fracture. These factors, in addition to the associations with BMD, suggest that there is likely to be a role in fracture prediction; however, due to the size of the effect, it has been difficult to demonstrate in epidemiological studies.

Genetic studies in osteoporosis

Having determined that there is a small, but significant, genetic component to the risk of osteoporosis, different types of genetic investigations have been used to attempt to identify specific genetic loci. Linkage studies are useful in identifying genetic mutations in monogenic disorders and the genes responsible for a number of rare diseases associated with severe osteoporosis, fragility fractures or high bone mass, which result from single gene mutations inherited in classical Mendelian fashion, have been identified through this technique. Osteogenesis imperfecta, for example, is most commonly caused by mutations in the *COL1A1* and *COL1A2* genes resulting in abnormal type 1 collagen formation. Loss of function mutations in the *LRP5* gene, encoding LDL receptor-related protein 5, a key regulator in osteoblastic bone formation, have been implicated in osteoporosis-pseudoglioma syndrome. Conversely gain-of-function mutations in the same gene are associated with familial high bone mass syndrome.

However, postmenopausal osteoporosis has been associated with a large number of common genetic variants each of which imparts only a minor effect. Linkage studies have therefore been of limited success in identifying contributory genes due to the low power to detect these common variants.

Candidate gene association studies (CGAS) and genome wide association studies (GWAS) have successfully identified a number of susceptibility loci. In CGAS, candidate genes are chosen for analysis based on a known role in the regulation of calcium metabolism or bone cell function. Many of the causative genes in monogenic disorders of bone fragility have been investigated. Single nucleotide polymorphisms (SNPs) are common variants which occur in at least 1% of the population. The frequency of these SNPs in candidate genes are compared in unrelated subjects in either a case-control study for categorical outcomes, for example history of an osteoporotic fracture, or as a population study for a quantitative outcome, for example BMD. A number of susceptibility variants have been identified using this method. However, false negative results are not uncommon due to limited power of the studies, and the results of studies in different populations are often conflicting.

With increasing acceptability to undertake genetic studies that are not hypothesis driven, GWAS have been able to clearly and reproducibly identify susceptibility loci for BMD variation. Large numbers (100 000–1 000 000) of common SNPs spread at close intervals across the genome are analyzed rather than focusing on a single candidate gene. A significant observation in the variant site is interpreted to indicate that the corresponding region of the genome contains functional DNA-sequence variants for the disease or trait being studied. These can include sequence variants leading to amino acid alterations in proteins, changes to gene promoter regions or alterations to mRNA degradation. However, a number of potential loci have also been identified, for which the function remains unknown. This might additionally offer the possibility of identifying novel pathways and mechanisms involved in bone formation and the development of osteoporosis.

Due to the large number of tests, GWAS are subject to stringent statistical thresholds. As with CGAS, false negatives are likely. Meta-analysis has been increasingly used to determine the true effects of genetic polymorphisms. The GENOMOS consortium (Genetic Markers of Osteoporosis; www.genomos.eu) was initially formed to undertake prospective meta-analysis of CGAS, and has identified SNP variants in *COL1A1* and *LRP5* associated with femoral and lumbar spine BMD. It has subsequently developed into the GEFOS (Genetic Factors for Osteoporosis; www.gefos.org) consortium which is undertaking meta-analysis of ongoing GWAS, and has identified or confirmed a number of loci associated with lumbar spine or femoral neck BMD [19].

Genes involved in osteoporosis

A number of genes have been identified through CGAS and GWAS as possible candidates for the regulation of bone mass and osteoporotic fracture susceptibility. A substantial number of these can be classified as influencing three biological pathways: the estrogen pathway, the Wnt-ß-catenin signaling pathway and the RANKL-RANK-OPG pathway. These are briefly summarized below.

The estrogen pathway

Estrogen is a well-recognized regulator of skeletal growth, bone mass and bone geometry. Estrogen receptor deficiency and aromatase deficiency are monogenic disorders associated with osteoporosis. Genetic variation at a number of SNPs in the estrogen receptor type 1 gene (*ESR1*) have been associated with many osteoporotic traits and risk factors including BMD [19], age at menopause [20] and postmenopausal bone loss [21].

Wnt-ß-catenin signaling pathway

The Wnt signaling pathway has a key role in many developmental processes. In bone, the activation of this pathway by Wnt binding to LRP5 or LRP6 transmembrane receptors leads to osteoblast differentiation and proliferation, bone mineralization and reduction in apoptosis. Loss of function mutations of *LRP5* result in osteoporosis-pseudoglioma syndrome, but more subtle polymorphisms have been associated with variance in BMD or fracture risk in the normal population. Some of these variants have been confirmed by meta-analysis [19, 22]. Other osteoporosis susceptibility genes affecting the Wnt-ß-catenin signaling pathway have been indentified at genome-wide significance level. These include *SOST* encoding sclerostin, an antagonist of Wnt; *MEF2C*, which may regulate *SOST* expression; *FOXC2*, which activates the signaling pathway; *WLS* encoding a transmembrane protein which promotes Wnt release; and *CTNNB1*, which encodes ß-catenin, a protein involved in the signaling cascade [23].

RANKL-RANK-OPG pathway

RANKL (receptor activator of nuclear factor κB ligand) binds to RANK on osteoclast precursor cells. It stimulates the differentiation of osteoclasts and activates bone resorption. Osteoprotegerin (OPG) has antagonistic actions to RANKL. A number of SNPs in the coding regions and in proximity to the OPG (*TNFRSF11B*), RANK (*TNFRSF11A*) and RANKL (*TN-FRSF11*) genes have been associated with BMD and osteoporotic fracture risk through CGAS and GWAS and subsequently confirmed by meta-analysis [19, 24, 25]. Although the variance in BMD explained by these genes is small, the identification of these associations highlights the importance of this pathway in skeletal maintenance.

Additionally a number of candidate osteoporosis susceptibility genes have been identified from GWAS but their function in bone metabolism is yet to be elucidated; and a number of other candidate genes known to have a role in skeletal maintenance have shown inconsistent association with BMD in CGAS and not yet attained genome-wide significance in meta-analysis, including COL1A1 and the vitamin D receptor gene (*VDR*) [23]. The influence of environmental exposures on the genome might account for these inconsistent findings.

Early life, gene-environment interactions and epigenetics

Despite a large number of potential genetic loci suggested through CGAS and GWAS studies, these polymorphisms can explain only a small proportion (1–3%) of the observed variance in BMD in the population. There is, however, increasing recognition that environmental factors influence osteoporosis risk through alterations in gene expression and epigenetic mechanisms. As a result, the phenotype that develops from a specific genotype varies greatly depending on environmental exposures and it is likely to be the significant role of these epigenetic mechanisms that explains why BMD is highly heritable but only a small proportion is accounted for by genetic variation.

A number of examples of gene–environment interaction in both the fetal and early postnatal phases of life are emerging with regards to one's risk for osteoporosis. For example, in a UK cohort study, no significant associations were identified between either the *VDR* genotype or birthweight and lumbar spine BMD. However, the relationship between lumbar spine BMD and VDR genotype varied according to category of birth weight, and a statistically significant interaction between birth weight and VDR genotype as a determinant of lumbar spine BMD was found [26]. As birth weight reflects fetal nutrition, this finding suggests an interaction between the in utero environment and genetic influences. A similar study also demonstrated a significant interaction between human growth hormone (*GH1*) polymorphisms and weight in infancy, a reflection of early life environment, as determinants of rate of bone loss [27]. In the Framingham Offspring Cohort, genetic variation in the interleukin-6 promoter gene was only associated with hip BMD in a subset of women who were not using estrogen replacement therapy, and in those with an inadequate calcium intake [28], demonstrating gene-environment interactions in later life.

Epigenetics refers to stable alterations in gene expression that arise during development and cell proliferation. These changes are heritable and may persist through several generations, but do not involve DNA mutations [29]. Chemical modifications of the DNA and alterations to proteins associated with DNA loci lead to gene repression or increased gene activity. The most studied of these, and now believed to be a major contributor to gene expression, is DNA methylation. This involves the addition of a methyl group to cytosine at carbon-5 position of CpG dinucleotides. When methylation occurs in the promoter region of a gene, it generally leads to gene repression. The patterns of methylation vary with stages of development, but importantly, during fetal development, maternal and environmental factors can alter the pattern of DNA methylation, and subsequently influence gene expression during adult life.

Although no epigenetic mechanisms for osteoporosis have been fully elucidated in humans, the vitamin D response elements and glucocorticoid receptor are potential targets. Lower maternal 25(OH)-vitamin D concentration during late pregnancy has been associated with reduced bone mass in offspring during the neonatal period and mid-childhood [30, 31]. This is partly mediated by umbilical venous calcium concentration [31]. Expression of the placental calcium transporter (*PMCA3*) also determines fetal skeletal growth [32]. It is therefore possible that epigenetic regulation of the *PMCA3* gene represents the mechanism by which maternal vitamin D status effects offspring bone mass [33].

Environmental influences in childhood

Longitudinal growth in childhood begins to track shortly after birth, progressively increasing along a centile curve. Recent longitudinal studies have shown that tracking also occurs with bone traits from early childhood, through the pubertal growth spurt and into early adulthood [34]. Despite this, bone mineral accrual in childhood and early adult life can be influenced by environmental factors and is of paramount importance in achieving optimum peak bone mass, which has a major effect on the risk of osteoporosis in later life [35]. In this same regard, a Finnish cohort study found directional associations between childhood growth rates and the risk of hip fracture in later life [36]. After adjustment for age and sex, the study demonstrated that a low growth rate between the ages of 7 and 15 years was associated with a significantly greater risk of hip fracture. This risk was also elevated in adults who were born short, but who obtained an average height by 7 years of age. In these children it is hypothesized that the skeletal envelope is forced ahead of the capacity to mineralize, a phenomenon which is accelerated during pubertal growth, and subsequently leads to the increased fracture risk. In adult life, several factors, such as diet, lifestyle, medication and comorbidities, are known to influence the risk of low BMD and fracture; these will be discussed in more detail in Chapter 4: Fracture risk assessment.

Fracture epidemiology

The incidence of fracture is bimodal, with peaks in childhood and in the elderly [37, 38]. Fractures in the young usually occur due to substantial trauma, are less common in females and tend to affect long bones. Bone mass progressively increases through childhood and usually reaches a peak by 30 years at which point the incidence of fracture is low. There is a progressive decline in BMD thereafter causing the prevalence of osteoporosis to increase with age. Rates of osteoporosis are particularly high in older women due mainly to the development of hypoestrogenemia following menopause. The reduction in bone density is associated with an increase in fracture risk; it has been shown that there is an approximate doubling of fracture risk for every standard deviation drop in BMD [39]. As a result, nearly three-quarters of all hip, vertebral and distal forearm fractures occur in those over 65 years of age [40]. Figure 1.1 clearly shows progressive increases in the incidence of hip, vertebral and wrist fractures with age in women with the exact nature of the relationship dependent on the type of fracture. Once an individual has suffered a fracture, their risk of further fracture is greatly increased and one meta-analysis has shown that the risk is up to 86% higher [41]. This may partly explain the clustering of fractures in some individuals.

In 2004 a report from the US Surgeon General highlighted the huge burden of osteoporosis-related fractures [42]. At that time, it was estimated that 10 million Americans over 50 years of age had osteoporosis and that 1.5 million fragility fractures were occurring each year. A study of fractures in Britain showed the population at risk to be a similar proportion to

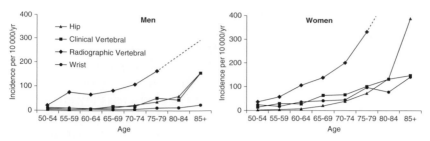

Figure 1.1 Hip, clinical vertebral, radiographic vertebral and wrist fracture incidence by age in men and women.

that in the US [43]. The lifetime risk of a hip fracture for a white woman is 1 in 6 [44]. In Western populations, hip fracture incidence increases exponentially with age with 90% occurring in those over 50 years of age [45]. In this age group, the risk in women is approximately double that in men [46], and as such when combined with greater longevity in females, 75% of hip factures occur in women [47].

Hip fractures commonly lead to chronic pain, disability, reduced mobility and increased levels of dependence [48]. A significant number of individuals subsequently require long-term nursing care and this proportion increases with age. Hip fractures are also attended by an excess risk of mortality in the years immediately post fracture; survival rates at 5 years were found to be 80% of those expected when compared to age and sex matched individuals without a fracture [49]. Globally, it has been estimated that hip fractures account for around 740 000 deaths per year [50]. They also contribute to over a third of the total economic burden of fractures, reflecting their need for hospital inpatient management and the major costs associated with subsequent residential care. As the numbers of hip fractures are rising, it is estimated that by 2050 the worldwide direct and indirect costs will reach $131.5 billion per year [51].

The majority of vertebral fractures occur due to compressive loading associated with lifting, changing position, or are discovered incidentally. Vertebral fractures are not uncommon in postmenopausal women, with a 50-year-old white woman having a 16% lifetime risk of being affected [5]. Figure 1.1 shows an approximately linear increase in clinical vertebral fractures, and an almost exponential increase in radiographic vertebral fractures, with age. Although only about one third of radiographic vertebral deformities come to clinical attention, symptomatic vertebral fractures cause back pain, loss of height, deformity, immobility, and reduced pulmonary function. As with hip fractures they are also attended by an excess mortality [49].

Distal forearm fractures usually occur as a result of a fall on an outstretched hand. Unsurprisingly, there is a peak in the incidence of these fractures in the winter, most likely to represent an increased frequency of falls on icy surfaces [52]. The gender disparity with this type of fracture is marked with an age-adjusted female to male ratio of 4:1 [43]. Although these fractures can lead to significant disability, particularly when they affect the dominant limb, there is no known associated increase in mortality rate.

Geography

Fracture incidence varies greatly across the world. On the whole, regions that are further from the equator have higher rates of fracture. This is thought to be related to less sun exposure resulting in lower levels of vitamin D [53]. However, exceptions to this rule do exist. In countries, such as Iran, where cultural codes encourage covering the majority of the body with clothes, skin exposure to the sun is limited. This practice may explain why, despite being close to the equator, 80% of the population are deficient in vitamin D and high rates of fracture are seen.

In general, fracture rates are similar in all Westernized Caucasian populations such as in Europe, America and Oceania. Within each of these individual regions, however, significant variation can be found. In the US, part of this disparity may be due to ecological factors that have been found to correlate with incidence patterns. These include water fluoride content, urbanization and socioeconomic status. Rates are particularly high in areas with a large proportion of those over the age of 65 years living below the poverty line [54].

In Europe, hip fracture rates are almost seven times lower in parts of southern European than in Scandinavia, and in particular Norway, which has some of the highest rates worldwide [55]. In areas where hip fracture risk is high, this tends to be reflected by increased rates of fragility fractures at other anatomical sites [18, 19]. The EVOS study examined the prevalence of vertebral deformities in countries across Europe. They showed a 3-fold difference in prevalence and again the highest frequencies were to be found in Scandinavia [56].

Moderate variation is seen throughout Asia with the highest rates identified in urbanized countries [57]. Due in part to its vast population, hip fractures arising in Asia account for a significant proportion of the world's burden; recent estimates have put this figure at around 30%. In contrast, fracture rates from populations in Africa appear to be low. However, there is limited data from this region and its validity has been questioned.

Inaccurate case identification may therefore partly explain the low numbers but population demographics may also play a role.

Secular trends

Throughout the world, life expectancy is increasing and the number of elderly people is rising, particularly in developing countries. It is predicted that by the year 2050 there will be more than 1500 million people aged 65 years or over worldwide. Between 1990 and 2000, the incidence of fractures worldwide increased by one-quarter [4], and it has been estimated that the number of hip fractures will rise from 1.66 million in 1990 to over 6 million in 2050 [58]. These estimates assume a constant age-specific hip fracture incidence; however, the secular trends found depend markedly on geographical location (Figure 1.2).

It has been shown that in the majority of Western populations, including Oceania, North America and the UK, age-specific fracture rates rose until

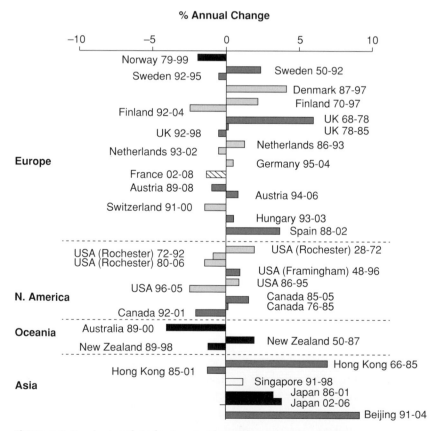

Figure 1.2 Secular trends in fracture incidence throughout the world (*Source*: Cooper C, *et al.* (2011) [61]. With kind permission from Springer Science+Business Media).

around 1980. This might have been caused in part by decreasing levels of physical activity, with less time spent outside, and higher rates of vitamin D insufficiency. Furthermore, during this time, a combination of medical and social factors led to improved survival of the frail elderly (i.e., those at greatest risk of fracture). Since this point, rates have either remained constant or started to decline. This trend may be due to a birth cohort effect, an increase in obesity or a specific improvement in the screening and treatment of osteoporosis. In particular, the introduction of bisphosphonates may have played a role although does not provide a full explanation [59, 60]. These changes are in contrast to rates in the developing world which have not declined.

The combination of disparate regional changes in population demographics and age-specific fracture rates is likely to cause a shift in the geographic distribution of fracture burden towards Asia and the developing world. Consequently, it has been estimated that only around 25% of hip fractures will occur in Europe and North America by 2050 [58].

Conclusion

Osteoporosis and osteoporotic fracture is globally a common condition, representing a huge individual and public health burden and associated with increased mortality. Although the clinical outcomes most frequently occur in females in later life, there is increasing evidence to suggest that environmental factors and gene-environment interactions occurring throughout the lifecourse, including prenatal life, childhood and early adulthood, are implicated in osteoporosis and fracture risk. Further identification of and consideration for these factors are important in reducing the currently increasing global burden of osteoporosis.

Acknowledgements

The authors would like to acknowledge the support of the Medical Research Council of Great Britain; Arthritis Research UK; the International Osteoporosis Foundation; the NIHR Nutrition BRC, University of Southampton and the NIHR Musculoskeletal BRU, University of Oxford.

References

1 Consensus development conference (1993) Diagnosis, prophylaxis, and treatment of osteoporosis. *Am J Med* **94**(6): 646–50.
2 WHO (1994) Assessment of fracture risk and its application to screening for postmenopausal osteoporosis. Report of a WHO Study Group. *World Health Organ Tech Rep Ser* 1994, **843**: 1–129.

3 Kanis JA, Hans D, Cooper C, Baim S, Bilezikian JP, Binkley N, *et al.* (2011) Interpretation and use of FRAX in clinical practice. *Osteoporos Int* **22**(9): 2395–2411.

4 Johnell O, Kanis JA (2006) An estimate of the worldwide prevalence and disability associated with osteoporotic fractures. *Osteoporos Int* **17**(12): 1726–33.

5 Melton LJ, III, Chrischilles EA, Cooper C, Lane AW, Riggs BL (1992) Perspective. How many women have osteoporosis? *J Bone Miner Res* **7**(9): 1005–10.

6 Kanis JA, Johnell O, Oden A, Sembo I, Redlund-Johnell I, Dawson A, *et al.* (2000) Long-term risk of osteoporotic fracture in Malmo. *Osteoporos Int* **11**(8): 669–74.

7 Royal College of Physicians (1989) Fractured neck of femur. Prevention and management. Summary and recommendations of a report of the Royal College of Physicians. *J R Coll Physicians Lond* **23**(1): 8–12.

8 Burge R, Dawson-Hughes B, Solomon DH, Wong JB, King A, Tosteson A (2007) Incidence and economic burden of osteoporosis-related fractures in the United States, 2005–2025. *J Bone Miner Res* **22**(3): 465–75.

9 Burge RT, Worley D, Johansen A, Bhattacharyya S, Bose U (2001) The cost of osteoporotic fractures in the UK: projections for 2000–2020. *Journal of Medical Economics* **4**: 51–62.

10 Pocock NA, Eisman JA, Hopper JL, Yeates MG, Sambrook PN, Eberl S (1987) Genetic determinants of bone mass in adults. A twin study. *J Clin Invest* **80**(3): 706–10.

11 Krall EA, Dawson-Hughes B (1993) Heritable and life-style determinants of bone mineral density. *J Bone Miner Res* **8**(1): 1–9.

12 Slemenda CW, Christian JC, Williams CJ, Norton JA, Johnston CC, Jr. (1991) Genetic determinants of bone mass in adult women: a reevaluation of the twin model and the potential importance of gene interaction on heritability estimates. *J Bone Miner Res* **6**(6): 561–7.

13 Park JH, Song YM, Sung J, Lee K, Kim YS, Park YS (2012) Genetic influence on bone mineral density in Korean twins and families: the healthy twin study. *Osteoporos Int* **23**(4): 1343–9.

14 Makovey J, Nguyen TV, Naganathan V, Wark JD, Sambrook PN (2007) Genetic effects on bone loss in peri- and postmenopausal women: a longitudinal twin study. *J Bone Miner Res* **22**(11): 1773–80.

15 Arden NK, Baker J, Hogg C, Baan K, Spector TD (1996) The heritability of bone mineral density, ultrasound of the calcaneus and hip axis length: a study of postmenopausal twins. *J Bone Miner Res* **11**(4): 530–4.

16 Hunter D, De LM, Snieder H, MacGregor AJ, Swaminathan R, Thakker RV, *et al.* (2001) Genetic contribution to bone metabolism, calcium excretion, and vitamin D and parathyroid hormone regulation. *J Bone Miner Res* **16**(2): 371–8.

17 Morris DH, Jones ME, Schoemaker MJ, Ashworth A, Swerdlow AJ (2011) Familial concordance for age at natural menopause: results from the Breakthrough Generations Study. *Menopause* **18**(9): 956–61.

18 Arden NK, Spector TD (1997) Genetic influences on muscle strength, lean body mass, and bone mineral density: a twin study. *J Bone Miner Res* **12**(12): 2076–81.

19 Rivadeneira F, Styrkarsdottir U, Estrada K, Halldorsson BV, Hsu YH, Richards JB, *et al.* (2009) Twenty bone-mineral-density loci identified by large-scale meta-analysis of genome-wide association studies. *Nat Genet* **41**(11): 1199–1206.

20 Weel AE, Uitterlinden AG, Westendorp IC, Burger H, Schuit SC, Hofman A, *et al.* (1999) Estrogen receptor polymorphism predicts the onset of natural and surgical menopause. *J Clin Endocrinol Metab* **84**(9): 3146–50.

21 Albagha OM, Pettersson U, Stewart A, McGuigan FE, Macdonald HM, Reid DM, *et al.* (2005) Association of oestrogen receptor alpha gene polymorphisms with postmenopausal bone loss, bone mass, and quantitative ultrasound properties of bone. *J Med Genet* **42**(3): 240–6.

22 van Meurs JB, Trikalinos TA, Ralston SH, Balcells S, Brandi ML, Brixen K, *et al.* (2008) Large-scale analysis of association between LRP5 and LRP6 variants and osteoporosis. *JAMA* **299**(11): 1277–90.

23 Ralston SH, Uitterlinden AG (2010) Genetics of osteoporosis. *Endocr Rev* **31**(5): 629–62.

24 Richards JB, Rivadeneira F, Inouye M, Pastinen TM, Soranzo N, Wilson SG, *et al.* (2008) Bone mineral density, osteoporosis, and osteoporotic fractures: a genome-wide association study. *Lancet* **371**(9623): 1505–12.

25 Richards JB, Kavvoura FK, Rivadeneira F, Styrkarsdottir U, Estrada K, Halldorsson BV, *et al.* (2009) Collaborative meta-analysis: associations of 150 candidate genes with osteoporosis and osteoporotic fracture. *Ann Intern Med* 2009, **151**(8): 528–37.

26 Dennison EM, Arden NK, Keen RW, Syddall H, Day IN, Spector TD, *et al.* (2001) Birthweight, vitamin D receptor genotype and the programming of osteoporosis. *Paediatr Perinat Epidemiol* **15**(3): 211–19.

27 Dennison EM, Syddall HE, Rodriguez S, Voropanov A, Day IN, Cooper C (2004) Polymorphism in the growth hormone gene, weight in infancy, and adult bone mass. *J Clin Endocrinol Metab* **89**(10): 4898–4903.

28 Ferrari SL, Karasik D, Liu J, Karamohamed S, Herbert AG, Cupples LA, *et al.* (2004) Interactions of interleukin-6 promoter polymorphisms with dietary and lifestyle factors and their association with bone mass in men and women from the Framingham Osteoporosis Study. *J Bone Miner Res* **19**(4): 552–9.

29 Jaenisch R, Bird A (2003) Epigenetic regulation of gene expression: how the genome integrates intrinsic and environmental signals. *Nat Genet* **33** Suppl: 245–54.

30 Harvey NC, Javaid MK, Poole JR, Taylor P, Robinson SM, Inskip HM, *et al.* (2008) Paternal skeletal size predicts intrauterine bone mineral accrual. *J Clin Endocrinol Metab* **93**(5): 1676–81.

31 Javaid MK, Crozier SR, Harvey NC, Gale CR, Dennison EM, Boucher BJ, *et al.* (2006) Maternal vitamin D status during pregnancy and childhood bone mass at age 9 years: a longitudinal study. *Lancet* **367**(9504): 36–43.

32 Martin R, Harvey NC, Crozier SR, Poole JR, Javaid MK, Dennison EM, *et al.* (2007) Placental calcium transporter (PMCA3) gene expression predicts intrauterine bone mineral accrual. *Bone* **40**(5): 1203–8.

33 Holroyd C, Harvey N, Dennison E, Cooper C (2012) Epigenetic influences in the developmental origins of osteoporosis. *Osteoporos Int* **23**(2): 401–10.

34 Donaldson LJ, Cook A, Thomson RG (1990) Incidence of fractures in a geographically defined population. *J Epidemiol Community Health* **44**(3): 241–5.

35 Hernandez CJ, Beaupre GS, Carter DR (2003) A theoretical analysis of the relative influences of peak BMD, age-related bone loss and menopause on the development of osteoporosis. *Osteoporos Int* **14**(10): 843–7.

36 Cooper C, Eriksson JG, Forsen T, Osmond C, Tuomilehto J, Barker DJ (2001) Maternal height, childhood growth and risk of hip fracture in later life: a longitudinal study. *Osteoporos Int* **12**(8): 623–9.

37 Garraway WM, Stauffer RN, Kurland LT, O'Fallon WM (1979) Limb fractures in a defined population. I. Frequency and distribution. *Mayo Clin Proc* **54**(11): 701–7.

38 Lancet (authors' names not given) (1990) Fracture patterns revisited. *Lancet* **336**(8726): 1290–1.

39 Marshall D, Johnell O, Wedel H (1996) Meta-analysis of how well measures of bone mineral density predict occurrence of osteoporotic fractures. *BMJ* **312**(7041): 1254–9.

40 Melton LJ, III, Crowson CS, O'Fallon WM (1999) Fracture incidence in Olmsted County, Minnesota: comparison of urban with rural rates and changes in urban rates over time. *Osteoporos Int* **9**(1): 29–37.

41 Kanis JA, Johnell O, de LC, Johansson H, Oden A, Delmas P, *et al.* (2004) A meta-analysis of previous fracture and subsequent fracture risk. *Bone* **35**(2): 375–82.

42 US Department of Health and Human Services (2004) *Bone Health and Osteoporosis: A Report of the Surgeon General.* Rockville, MD.

43 van Staa TP, Dennison EM, Leufkens HG, Cooper C (2001) Epidemiology of fractures in England and Wales. *Bone* **29**(6): 517–22.

44 Cummings SR, Melton LJ (2002) Epidemiology and outcomes of osteoporotic fractures. *Lancet* **359**(9319): 1761–7.

45 Gallagher JC, Melton LJ, Riggs BL, Bergstrath E (1980) Epidemiology of fractures of the proximal femur in Rochester, Minnesota. *Clin Orthop Relat Res* **150**: 163–71.

46 Melton LJ, III (1988) Epidemiology of fractures. In: Riggs BL, Melton LJ, III, eds. *Osteoporosis: Etiology, Diagnosis, and Management.* New York: Raven Press, pp. 133–54.

47 Jordan KM, Cooper C (2002) Epidemiology of osteoporosis. *Best Pract Res Clin Rheumatol* **16**(5): 795–806.

48 Keene GS, Parker MJ, Pryor GA (1993) Mortality and morbidity after hip fractures. *BMJ* **307**(6914): 1248–50.

49 Cooper C, Atkinson EJ, Jacobsen SJ, O'Fallon WM, Melton LJ, III (1993) Population-based study of survival after osteoporotic fractures. *Am J Epidemiol* **137**(9): 1001–5.

50 Johnell O, Kanis JA (2004) An estimate of the worldwide prevalence, mortality and disability associated with hip fracture. *Osteoporos Int* **15**(11): 897–902.

51 Johnell O (1997) The socioeconomic burden of fractures: today and in the 21st century. *Am J Med* **103**(2A): 20S–5S.

52 Jacobsen SJ, Sargent DJ, Atkinson EJ, O'Fallon WM, Melton LJ, III (1999) Contribution of weather to the seasonality of distal forearm fractures: a population-based study in Rochester, Minnesota. *Osteoporos Int* **9**(3): 254–9.

53 Pfeifer M, Minne HW (1999) Vitamin D and hip fracture. *Trends Endocrinol Metab* **10**(10): 417–20.

54 Jacobsen SJ, Goldberg J, Miles TP, Brody JA, Stiers W, Rimm AA (1990) Regional variation in the incidence of hip fracture. US white women aged 65 years and older. *JAMA* **264**(4): 500–2.

55 Johnell O, Gullberg B, Allander E, Kanis JA (1992) The apparent incidence of hip fracture in Europe: a study of national register sources. *MEDOS Study Group. Osteoporos Int* **2**(6): 298–302.

56 O'Neill TW, Felsenberg D, Varlow J, Cooper C, Kanis JA, Silman AJ (1996) The prevalence of vertebral deformity in European men and women: the European Vertebral Osteoporosis Study. *J Bone Miner Res* **11**(7): 1010–18.

57 Lau EM, Lee JK, Suriwongpaisal P, Saw SM, Das DS, Khir A, *et al.* (2001) The incidence of hip fracture in four Asian countries: the Asian Osteoporosis Study (AOS). *Osteoporos Int* **12**(3): 239–43.

58 Cooper C, Campion G, Melton LJ, III (1992) Hip fractures in the elderly: a world-wide projection. *Osteoporos Int* **2**(6): 285–9.

59 Leslie WD, O'Donnell S, Jean S, Lagace C, Walsh P, Bancej C, *et al.* (2009) Trends in hip fracture rates in Canada. *JAMA* **302**(8): 883–9.

60 Siris ES, Selby PL, Saag KG, Borgstrom F, Herings RM, Silverman SL (2009) Impact of osteoporosis treatment adherence on fracture rates in North America and Europe. *Am J Med* **122**(2 Suppl): S3–13.

61 Cooper C, Cole ZA, Holroyd CR, Earl SC, Harvey NC, Dennison EM, *et al.* (2011) Secular trends in the incidence of hip and other osteoporotic fractures. *Osteoporos Int* **22**(5): 1277–88.

CHAPTER 2

Osteoporosis in Men

Robert A. Adler

Hunter Holmes McGuire Veterans Affairs Medical Center *and* Virginia Commonwealth University
School of Medicine, Richmond, VA, USA

Introduction

Osteoporosis has finally been recognized as an important condition in men, and increased research in the last 15 years has provided new information about all aspects of male osteoporosis. Nonetheless, the parallel between osteoporosis in men and heart disease in women remains: women have cardiac events 10 years later than men and generally do worse. Men have "bone events" (i.e., fractures) 10 years later than women and generally do worse. Much of what we know about heart disease in women is based on studies in men; much of what we know about osteoporosis in men is based on studies in women. This chapter will review what we have learned by actual studies in men with or at risk for osteoporosis.

Epidemiology

Early in adult life, men actually have more fractures than women, but these are mainly traumatic fractures and are probably related to more risky behavior. As people age, and particularly after the menopause in women, the rate of fracture increases, with men lagging behind women by about 10 years. Based on various populations, a man at age 50 has a risk between 10 and 25% of suffering an osteoporotic fracture [1, 2]. Hip fracture is the most important fragility fracture because it can lead to considerable morbidity and mortality and incurs the greatest costs. About one-fourth of all hip fractures occur in men [3]. As longevity increases in men, the risk for hip fracture will increase. This is illustrated by an interesting new study from Canada [4]. The authors predicted the chance of a hip fracture for women and men at age 50, first without adjustment and then with adjustment for a recent trend towards fewer hip fractures in women and greater longevity in men. The unadjusted rates for women and men were

---

12.1% and 4.6%. When adjusted for the new trends, the rate in women decreased to 8.9%, and the men's rate increased to 6.7% [4].

For certain types of osteoporosis (see below), the rates of fracture are even higher. For example, in patients taking oral glucocorticoid drugs such as prednisone, the fracture rate increases markedly as early as after 3 months of treatment [5]. Men with prostate cancer treated by androgen deprivation therapy (ADT) have up to a 20% fracture risk by 5 years of ADT treatment [6]. After a first fragility fracture, men and women have about the same chance of a subsequent fracture [7]. After a hip fracture, men have about twice the chance of dying, presumably from complications [8, 9], although the exact cause of the increased mortality is not established. Those men who survive a hip fracture are more likely than women to never regain independence. Thus, osteoporosis in men is an important disorder because it is more common than thought and may have a fatal outcome.

Classification and pathophysiology

An osteoporosis classification scheme [10] proposed by Riggs and Melton over 25 years ago remains helpful today. It divides osteoporosis into primary and secondary types and further subdivides primary osteoporosis into two types. The first type of primary osteoporosis (type I osteoporosis) has been called postmenopausal osteoporosis because it affects many more women than men (by a ratio of about 6 to 1) and is associated with the dramatic loss of estrogen that women experience after the menopause. The more metabolically active trabecular bone is lost, leading to fractures in the spine and distal radius, where there is more trabecular than cortical bone. Men do not undergo a similar rapid decline in sex steroids. As will be discussed below, there is a gradual decrease in testosterone with aging. But some men present with vertebral fractures at middle age [11]. There are several potential causes for the man who presents with acute back pain due to a compression fracture. Probably the most common is hypercalciuria [12], and some of these men may have a history of kidney stones. A group of younger men has been identified [13] as having low levels of insulin-like growth factor I (IGF-I) despite normal levels of growth hormone. Such men appear to have low IGF-I levels due to specific alleles from a variable region of the IGF-I gene. Another interesting cause may be decreased bioactive estradiol levels [14]. A group of men and their male family members have been identified in Belgium with this disorder. The cause of the steroid abnormality is unknown but generations have been found to have low bone density or fractures. A few other specific causes have been postulated but not fully proven or widely seen. It is important to note, however, that many men with secondary osteoporosis may present at middle age, including men with hypogonadism. Symptoms may be few, so they may be considered to have primary osteoporosis until evaluation reveals the secondary cause.

Type II primary osteoporosis is associated with ages > 70 years in both sexes and affects both trabecular and cortical bone [10]. Therefore both vertebral and hip fractures occur in such patients. As will be discussed later, there are several validated risk factors gleaned from epidemiologic studies that help determine which aging men are more likely to fracture. Men tend to fracture later in life than women. In general they have larger bones and thus have more to lose after peak bone mass is attained. In addition, bone changes with aging are different in men and women. In women, the spaces between trabeculae increase as the number of trabeculae actually decreases, whereas in men there is just thinning of trabeculae [15]. In a recent study [16], the cortical portion of vertebral bodies (a rim at the exterior) is lost more markedly in women than men. Finally, in long mostly cortical bones, periosteal deposition of bone with aging is greater in men than women [17], increasing bone strength as the bone imperceptibly increases in diameter.

Secondary osteoporosis is particularly important and common in men (Table 2.1). In one study [18] of men referred to an osteoporosis clinic,

Table 2.1 Important secondary causes of osteoporosis or increased fracture risk in men.

Hypogonadism
Glucocorticoid excess (exogenous glucocorticoids or Cushing's syndrome)
Hypercalciuria
Hyperthyroidism
Hyperparathyroidism
Celiac disease (gluten sensitive enteropathy) or other malabsorption syndromes
Gastrointestinal surgery (Bilroth surgery, bariatric surgery)
Alcoholism
Hemochromatosis
Hyperprolactinemia
Multiple myeloma
Medications (in addition to glucocorticoids)
   Gonadotropin-releasing hormone analogs (e.g., leuprolide)
   Androgen receptor blockers (e.g., spironolactone, nilutamide)
   Neuroleptic dopamine antagonists (e.g., phenothiazines, haloperidol)
   Enzyme-inducing anticonvulsants (e.g., phenytoin, carbamazepine)
   Thiazolidinediones (e.g., pioglitazone, rosiglitazone)
   Proton pump inhibitors (e.g., omeprazole)
   Antineoplastics (e.g., cyclophosphamide)
   Antidepressants (e.g., citalopram, sertraline)

further risk factors and other causes of secondary osteoporosis were found even in those men who already carried one secondary osteoporosis diagnosis at referral. Overall, the prevalence of secondary osteoporosis was 75%. A very common cause of secondary osteoporosis is glucocorticoid excess, not due to Cushing's syndrome, but rather to use of prednisone and other pharmacologic glucocorticoids for at least 3 months [5]. In men, chronic obstructive pulmonary disease is probably the most common indication for glucocorticoid therapy [19], as opposed to rheumatologic inflammatory disorders in women [20], although there are also neurologic, oncologic, and dermatologic indications for glucocorticoids. Whatever the indication, glucocorticoids decrease osteoblast function [21], leading to a rapid decrease in bone mass as well as changes in bone quality. The protein matrix of bone and muscle are subjected to the catabolic effects of glucocorticoids [22]. Regardless of other potential mechanisms of increased fracture risk, the result is greatly and quickly increased fracture risk that decreases after the glucocorticoid therapy is discontinued. See Chapter 6 for a detailed review of glucocorticoid-induced osteoporosis.

Some other important causes of secondary osteoporosis [23] include hyperthyroidism, malabsorption (e.g., celiac sprue), alcoholism, hyperparathyroidism, and hypogonadism. A list of some of the most important secondary causes of osteoporosis in men is shown in Table 2.1. Many medications are associated with increased fracture risk such as thiazolidinediones [24], proton pump inhibitors [25], and antidepressants [26]. Antiseizure medications that increase vitamin D catabolism can lead to osteoporosis and/or osteomalacia [27]. Finally, many drugs exert their effect on bone via hypogonadism. For a more complete overview of the medications associated with osteoporosis see Chapter 7.

It is well established that men with organic causes of hypogonadism are at risk for osteoporosis. Hypogonadism due to a testicular cause (primary hypogonadism) may be chromosomal (e.g., Klinefelter's syndrome) or due to orchitis (e.g., mumps), after radiation or trauma, or from drugs (e.g., cyclophosphamide). Secondary hypogonadism may be congenital (e.g., Kallman's syndrome), due to a tumor or its treatment (pituitary or hypothalamic tumors), traumatic brain injury, granulomatous disease (e.g., sarcoidosis) or hemochromatosis. There may be effects at more than one part of the hypothalamo–pituitary–gonadal axis as in severe illness, HIV disorders, and alcohol excess. Several drugs cause hypogonadism. Spironolactone and drugs such as nilutamide and bicalutamide are androgen receptor blockers. Ketoconazole decreases adrenal androgen secretion. Glucocorticoids and opiates decrease pituitary function leading to hypogonadism, whereas dopamine antagonists such as phenothiazines raise the serum prolactin, leading to pituitary gonadotropin suppression. For men with prostate cancer, gonadotropin releasing hormone analogs such as leuprolide are used to suppress gonadotropin secretion, causing profound decreases of testosterone (and estradiol) and putting the patient at high risk for fracture [28, 29]. For the man with a specific cause of hypogonadism, the loss of bone and muscle may be the proximate reason for increased fracture risk. Replacement of testosterone (in those men who do not have a contraindication to replacement) increases bone mineral density [30], but no studies have been large enough to demonstrate that testosterone replacement lowers fracture risk.

In parallel to the decreased bone mass and increased fracture risk of aging, serum testosterone levels fall [31]. Is there any connection? Most studies [32] have failed to find a strong correlation between testosterone (total, free, or bioactive) and fracture risk. However, bioavailable estradiol [33] is more robustly associated with lower bone density in older men. In this way, testosterone serves as a prohormone because most estradiol in men is derived from aromatization of testosterone. Hence, when exogenous testosterone is administered, the patient receives both testosterone and estradiol. In small studies [34] testosterone administration to older men with mildly low serum testosterone levels results in increased muscle and bone without apparent side effects. However, the studies are too small to determine if testosterone leads to lower fracture risk or if there are cardiac or prostate safety issues. Osteoporosis is not considered an indication for therapy for the majority of older men with the lower serum testosterone levels associated with aging. Instead, decreased libido [35] is considered the most specific symptom of hypogonadism, and some men will be candidates for testosterone replacement. For some men with osteoporosis, a case can be made to test for hypogonadism. In the younger man with osteoporosis and hypogonadism, replacement with testosterone will improve bone mineral density. For the older man, measuring serum testosterone should probably be considered only in men who have decreased libido or other symptoms of hypogonadism and who do not have contraindications to testosterone replacement. If the older man has osteoporosis in addition to hypogonadism, there is evidence that he will respond to standard nonhormonal osteoporosis therapy (see below).

Diagnosis and evaluation of men at risk for osteoporosis

There are many unanswered questions about how to identify the men who are likely to suffer an osteoporotic fracture. Similar to the recommendation that all women have a bone mineral density (BMD) test by dual energy x-ray absorptiometry (DXA) by age 65, some organizations [36, 37] have suggested that all men be screened by DXA at age 70.

Table 2.2 Some indications for DXA testing in men.

Fragility fracture
Glucocorticoid therapy (≥5 mg prednisone for ≥ 3 months)
Androgen deprivation therapy for prostate cancer
Hypogonadism
Height loss > 1.5–2 inches from maximum height
Current smoking/chronic obstructive pulmonary disease
Malabsorption
Bariatric or Bilroth surgery
Alcoholism
Use of medication associated with secondary osteoporosis
Hyperparathyroidism
Hypercalciuria/recurrent calcium-containing kidney stones

However, the United States Preventive Services Task Force [38] has concluded that as of now there is insufficient evidence to support such screening. The United States Department of Veterans Affairs [39] has recommended that men at highest risk for fracture be identified and undergo evaluation with DXA. A list of possible indications for DXA is shown in Table 2.2. The three most important indications for DXA are previous fragility fracture, oral glucocorticoid therapy, and androgen deprivation therapy (ADT) for prostate cancer. Men in these three categories are at high risk for fracture. Interestingly, Medicare will support DXA testing in men with a previous fracture or on glucocorticoid therapy, but DXA testing for hypogonadal men, including those on ADT may not be reimbursed.

Further complications arise from technical aspects of DXA in men. The larger bones of men tend to raise the apparent bone mineral density. While there are studies [40] that show that men fracture at a higher BMD than women, there are other studies [41] that suggest that absolute BMD can be used to predict fracture in both sexes. Two consequences of using a female normative database for both genders are that fewer men would be considered eligible for treatment [42] and a group of men known to respond to therapy might be denied fracture-reducing treatment. The latter point is due to the fact that men in the treatment trials were eligible for treatment (and responded) if they had a T-score of −2.5 (osteoporosis) based on a male normative database or had a T-score of −2.0 (low bone mass) plus a previous fragility fracture. Using the female database as a reference for treatment of these patients would exclude a proportion of such men from receiving treatment.

One method to identify those men with the highest risk for fracture is to use fracture risk calculators based on large epidemiologic studies. The most widely used is FRAX [43], established by the World Health

Organization. FRAX uses validated risk factors (age, body mass index, prior fragility fracture, parental hip fracture, glucocorticoid exposure, current smoking, excess alcohol consumption, and rheumatoid arthritis) to predict one's 10-year hip and major osteoporotic fracture risk. These factors may be entered by themselves or with the femoral neck bone density (in absolute terms, g/cm^2) in an online calculation tool (www.shef.ac.uk/FRAX/) that provides the fracture risk. The rationale for this and other risk calculators is that while the patient with osteoporosis (T-score ≤ -2.5) is clearly at higher risk for fracture, there are many more people with low bone mass (T-score between -1 and -2.4) who will fracture. Thus, identifying which men and women with low bone mass are at the highest fracture risk is important, and FRAX is an attempt to quantify risk. Each country or medical entity (or patient) can then determine what risk is acceptable. FRAX does not include falls as a risk factor, but another fracture risk calculator, the Garvan nomogram [44], includes the number of falls, quantifies the number of fractures, but does not use glucocorticoid treatment as a risk factor, nor does it adjust for the competing risk of death (www.fractureriskcalculator.com). Both calculators use femoral neck DXA. It is well recognized that men are more likely to have artifacts (osteophytes, facet sclerosis, DISH syndrome, etc.) that raise the apparent BMD in the spine. It is less well known that arthritis in the hip also can spuriously raise the apparent BMD [45]. Thus, the bigger bones and frequent hip arthritis can make the risk of fracture seem less in men. In one study [46] of men on ADT, there was a large difference between FRAX calculated with or without hip BMD. While one small study [47] suggested that the Garvan score predicted fracture in men better than FRAX, there is a need for much larger validation studies in men to help the clinician decide which patients with low bone mass to treat. See Chapter 4 for a more in-depth review of the use of FRAX and other methods to predict the risk for fracture in women.

There are additional methods to identify men at risk for fracture. It has been known for some time that forearm BMD predicts fracture well in men [48]. In men on ADT, forearm BMD may be the only abnormality found on DXA testing [46, 49]. The International Society for Clinical Densitometry recommends [50] that for those patients in whom the spine or hip DXA cannot be interpreted because of artifacts that the distal 1/3 radius be measured. While the best forearm DXA region of interest is not fully established [51], consideration of a forearm measurement such as distal 1/3 radius is very reasonable, particularly in men on ADT. However, there are no studies that demonstrate that men with osteoporosis only in the forearm respond to therapy. Vertebral compression fracture, identified by spine x-rays or vertebral fracture analysis (a low radiation dose method available on some bone densitometers) is a strong predictor of future fracture [52].

For the patient with osteoporosis by DXA or low bone mass plus high fracture risk by a risk calculator or osteopenia plus a vertebral fracture, there are a few laboratory tests that should be done to assist in management. History and physical examination will provide evidence for many secondary causes of osteoporosis as well as risk factors for fractures, but patients should have measurement of serum calcium (with serum albumin for calculation of corrected serum calcium), a measure of renal function (serum creatinine or estimated glomerular filtration rate), serum 25-hydroxyvitamin D (the best reflection of vitamin D status), and a measure of urinary calcium excretion (preferably a 24-hour urine collection). These tests will provide basic information and may lead to diagnoses such as hyperparathyroidism, malabsorption, hypercalciuria, or vitamin D deficiency. Multiple myeloma can present with spine abnormalities that are similar to osteoporotic compression deformities. For this reason, a complete blood count is a good screening tool because about $3/4$ of multiple myeloma patients are anemic, but more specific testing is necessary: serum and/or urine protein electrophoresis and serum light chain assays [53]. For the patient with suspected hyperthyroidism, serum TSH and Free T4 are recommended. If the patient is at risk for hypogonadism, a fasting morning serum testosterone with concomitant measurements of gonadotropins (LH and FSH) and sometimes prolactin are indicated. A recent review [54] lists more specific tests for many of the secondary causes of osteoporosis.

Treatment of men with osteoporosis

For the man with secondary osteoporosis, treatment of the underlying cause may be helpful. For example, treatment of hyperthyroidism leads to increased BMD [55] and presumably decreased fracture risk. For many other secondary causes of osteoporosis in men, the situation is similar: no fracture outcomes are available. Nonetheless, treatment of the underlying problem is important for the patient's overall health. However, it is likely that many men with secondary osteoporosis will need the same therapy as those with primary osteoporosis.

The first study [56] of a modern osteoporosis drug was that using alendronate in 241 men (mean age 63) with a femoral neck T—score of −2 or worse or with a T-score of −1 plus a fragility fracture (either by history or demonstrated on a vertebral x-ray). The T-scores were based on BMDs in normal young men. All men received supplements of calcium and vitamin D. Compared to men taking placebo, men on alendronate had a 5.3% greater increase in spine BMD at 2 years, as well as a 2.6% greater increase in hip BMD. When spine x-rays at 2 years were compared with baseline x-rays, 7.1% of the placebo group had a new vertebral fracture (by a quantitative method) compared to only 0.8% of the alendronate group. In studies large enough to demonstrate that alendronate decreased clinical fractures, the effects of alendronate in women were similar to those reported in men [57]. Thus, it was concluded that alendronate would likely decrease fracture risk in men to about the same degree, and alendronate was the first drug to be approved by the U.S. Food and Drug Administration (FDA) for treatment of osteoporosis in men. Although a daily (10 mg) preparation was used in this study, the standard treatment with alendronate is a weekly 70 mg tablet. Now that alendronate is available in generic form, it is the most widely prescribed osteoporosis drug for men.

The second FDA approved medication for men with osteoporosis was risedronate. In a two-year trial [58], weekly risedronate (35 mg) was compared with placebo. The DXA criterion for inclusion in the study was a spine T-score ≤ -2.5 and a femoral neck T-score ≤ -1 or a spine T-score ≤ -1 and a femoral neck of ≤ -2, based on a male normative database. At baseline about 1/3 of the men had a vertebral compression fracture. By two years, the spine BMD was 4.5% greater in the risedronate group compared to placebo, and there was about a 2% greater hip bone density improvement in the risedronate group. There were very few new vertebral fractures noted on x-ray in either group. Markers of bone turnover were decreased by risedronate, similar to studies in women. Using the fracture surrogates of bone density increases and bone turnover marker decreases, risedronate was given FDA approval for men. Studies from Japan have demonstrated clinical fracture risk reduction in men given risedronate. For example, men suffering a cerebral vascular accident were randomized to risedronate or placebo [59]; those who received risedronate had fewer hip fractures. Similarly, men with Parkinson's disease treated with risedronate [60] had fewer fractures than those given a placebo. Interestingly, these patients may or may not have had osteoporosis.

The third FDA-approved drug for osteoporosis in men is zoledronic acid (ZA), available as a 5 mg intravenous infusion administered no more often than yearly. The study [61] that led to its approval for men was not placebo controlled. Instead, ZA was compared with the standard therapy, alendronate. Over two years, both drugs increased spine bone density just over 6% and femoral neck about 3%. While there were fewer vertebral fractures in the men that received ZA compared to alendronate, the difference was not statistically significant. In a landmark international study [62], men and women who had suffered a hip fracture were randomized to ZA or placebo. Those who received ZA had fewer subsequent fractures and importantly were less likely to die during the follow-up period. In an observational study of ZA in "real world" conditions [63],

ZA increased BMD more in those men new to bisphosphonate therapy compared to those who had previously taken oral bisphosphonates such as alendronate and risedronate. While ibandronate is FDA-approved for women with osteoporosis and increases BMD in men [64], it does not have FDA approval for men.

All of the bisphosphonates, alendronate, risedronate, ibandronate, and ZA work by decreasing osteoclast (bone resorption) activity, allowing osteoblasts (bone formation) to "catch up." Despite the differences in trabecular bone and cortical bone between men and women, it is assumed that bisphosphonates will have the same effect on fracture risk in men and women. It is highly doubtful that there will ever be a prospective study large enough to demonstrate that bisphosphonates decrease clinical fracture in men. For a more in-depth review of the mechanism of action of bisphosphonates, and their use in women, see Chapter 9.

A newer type of antiresorptive agent is denosumab, which works via the RANK Ligand – RANK (receptor activator of nuclear factor κB) system that stimulates osteoclasts. Denosumab is a humanized monoclonal antibody against RANK Ligand and prevents stimulation of osteoclasts [65]. In women, denosumab appears to be more potent than alendronate in increasing BMD and decreasing bone turnover markers [66]. In the registration trial [67] denosumab decreased clinical fractures in women. There is only one published study [68] of denosumab in men. In this study, men on ADT for prostate cancer were randomized to placebo or denosumab injection every 6 months for 24 months. The men in the study did not necessarily have osteoporosis; the mean and median T-score in the total hip was −0.9, in the normal range, whereas the mean femoral neck T-score was −1.4, mild low bone mass. About one-fifth of the men in this study had a vertebral fracture at baseline x-ray. Another one-fifth of the men in this study had a history of a fragility fracture. At 2 years, the difference in spine BMD between the denosumab group and the placebo control group was 6.6%, where the differences in the hip regions were 2–4%. Forearm BMD is often low in men on ADT, and denosumab increased 1/3 distal radius BMD to about the same extent it increased hip BMD. In this study of 734 men in each group, there were significantly fewer new spine fractures on x-ray in the denosumab group. The FDA approved denosumab for men on ADT for prostate cancer, a high risk group and for men with osteoporosis [6]. See Chapter 10 for a review of denosumab.

As stated above, antiresorptive agents work by decreasing osteoclast activity, allowing osteoblasts to form new bone, although these drugs decrease osteoblast function as well. There is only one FDA-approved anabolic medication for osteoporosis, teriparatide, which consists of the first 34 amino acids of the amino-terminal end of parathyroid hormone. In the registration trial in women [69], teriparatide increased BMD markedly and decreased clinical fractures compared to placebo. In a trial in men [70], teriparatide was given to men with T-scores of −2 or lower (compared with normal young men). Those men who received the FDA-approved dose of 20 micrograms daily for 1 year had a 5.9% increase in spine BMD, and femoral neck BMD increased 1.5%. In a 3.5 year observational follow up study [71] of men in the trial, those who had been treated with teriparatide probably had fewer vertebral fractures than those who had been on placebo during the trial. In a 36-month trial of men and women with glucocorticoid-induced osteoporosis [72], teriparatide increased bone density more and decreased vertebral fracture risk more than alendronate. See Chapter 11 for a complete review of teriparatide.

The choice of treatment in men with osteoporosis may be made on the basis of the studies cited above plus practical reasons. Generic alendronate costs as little as $40 per year, and therefore it is a very reasonable choice for therapy. Risedronate is now available in a monthly dosing regimen, making it very convenient but more expensive. Teriparatide appears to be very potent but can only be given for 2 years, requires a daily subcutaneous injection, and is expensive. Intravenous zoledronic acid (given once yearly) and subcutaneous denosumab (given every 6 months) are both convenient but relatively expensive.

All of these medications improve BMD and are likely to decrease fracture risk. What about side effects? All oral bisphosphonates can cause esophageal irritation, which can be minimized by taking the pills properly, but some patients will have worsening of gastro-esophageal reflux or peptic ulcer disease by the oral bisphosphonate. All bisphosphonates have been associated with osteonecrosis of the jaw, basically exposed bone usually after an invasive dental procedure. The incidence of this side effect is about 1/10 000 to 1/100 000 [73], and new recommendations [74] for avoiding this complication have been published. In a few patients on bisphosphonates, mostly women, atypical subtrochanteric femoral fractures have occurred [75]. The background incidence of such fractures is unknown, and the role of bisphosphonates, specific risk factors, and predictors of such fractures are all obscure. There may be a prodrome of thigh or groin pain to herald these stress-like fractures. Clearly much more must be learned [76] about these fractures. For now, osteoporosis treatment should be assessed at 5 years by DXA. If the patient has had a good response to therapy, then consideration of a "drug holiday" should be made. For those who have not had an adequate response, continued therapy is recommended [77]. The two most common reasons that patients do not respond to therapy are: 1.The patient does not take [78] the treatment (or take it correctly) and 2. The 25-hydroxyvitamin D level is inadequate [79]. It is clear that osteoporosis in both men and women is a chronic disorder and that long-term follow-up of patients is necessary. In addition, long-term surveillance of therapy and long-term treatment studies are needed to provide guidance on managing this disorder. See Appendix for a comparative review of all therapies.

Finally, it is important to remind the clinician that the reason we treat osteoporosis in men is that hip fracture is a fatal disorder. Men ages 75–84 have a 34% chance of dying within 1 year after hip fracture [8]. Many of those who survive never regain independence. Thus, knowing the patient's hip fracture risk and comparing it with the low risk of side effects is important in determining whether a man should be treated and for how long.

References

1 Byberg L, Gedeborg R, Cars T, *et al.* (2012) Prediction of fracture risk in men: a cohort study. *J Bone Miner Res* **27**:797–807.

2 Baim S, Leslie WD (2012) Assessment of fracture risk. *Curr Osteoporos Rep* **10**: 28–41.

3 Burge R, Dawson-Hughes B, Solomon DH, *et al.* (2007) Incidence and economic burden of osteoporosis-related fractures in the United States 2005–2025. *J Bone Miner Res* **22**: 465–75.

4 Hopkins RB, Pullenayegum E, Goeree R, *et al.* (2012) Estimation of the lifetime risk of hip fracture for women and men in Canada. *Osteoporos Int* **23**: 921–7.

5 Van Staa TP, Leufkens HMG, Abenhaim L, *et al.* (2000) Use of oral corticosteroids and risk of fractures. *J Bone Miner Res* **15**: 993–1000.

6 Shahinian VB, Kuo YF, Freeman JL, *et al.* (2005) Risk of fracture after androgen deprivation for prostate cancer. *N Engl J Med* **352**: 154–64.

7 Center JR, Bliuc D, Nguyen TV, *et al.* (2007) Risk of subsequent fracture after low-trauma fracture in men and women. *JAMA* **297**: 387–94.

8 Block JE, Stubbs H (1997) Hip fracture-associated mortality reconsidered. *Calcif Tissue Int* **61**: 84.

9 Bass E, French DD, Bradham DD, *et al.* (2007) Risk-adjusted mortality rates of elderly veterans with hip fractures. *Ann Epidemiol* **17**: 514–19.

10 Riggs BL, Melton LJ III (1986) Involutional osteoporosis. *N Engl J Med* **314**: 1676–86.

11 Adler RA (2005) Fracture syndromes in men. *Adv Osteoporotic Fract Manag* **3**: 112–17.

12 Heilberg IP, Weisinger JR (2006) Bone disease in idiopathic hypercalciuria. *Curr Opin Nephrol Hypertens* **15**: 394–402.

13 Rosen CJ, Kurland ES, Vereault D, *et al.* (1998) Association between serum insulin growth factor-I (IGF-I) and a simple sequence repeat in the IGF-I gene: implications for genetic studies of bone mineral density. *J Clin Endocrinol Metab* **83**: 2286–90.

14 Van Pottelburgh I, Goemaere S, Zmierczak H, *et al.* (2004) Perturbed sex steroid status in men with idiopathic osteoporosis and their sons. *J Clin Endocrinol Metab* **89**: 4949–53.

15 Khosla S, Riggs BL, Atkinson EJ, *et al.* (2006) Effects of sex and age on bone microstructure at the ultradistal radius: a population-based noninvasive in vivo assessment. *J Bone Miner Res* **21**: 124–31.

16 Christiansen BA, Kopperdahl DL, Kiel DP, *et al.* (2011) Mechanical contributions of the cortical and trabecular compartments contribute to differences in age-related

changes in vertebral body strength in men and women assessed by qCT-based finite element analysis. *J Bone Miner Res* **26**: 974–83.

17 Szulc P, Delmas PD (2007) Bone loss in elderly men: increased endosteal bone loss and stable periosteal apposition. The prospective MINOS study. *Osteoporos Int* **18**: 495–503.

18 Ryan CS, Petkov VI, Adler RA (2011) Osteoporosis in men: the value of laboratory testing. *Osteoporos Int* **22**: 1845–53.

19 Adler RA, Hochberg MC (2011) Glucocorticoid-induced osteoporosis in men. *J Endocrinol Invest* **34**: 481–4.

20 Grossman JM, Gordon R, Ranganath VK *et al.* (2010) American College of Rheumatology 2010 recommendations for the prevention and treatment of glucocorticoid-induced osteoporosis. *Arthritis Care Res (Hoboken)* **62**: 1515–26.

21 Weinstein RS (2011) Glucocorticoid-induced bone disease. *N Engl J Med* **365**: 62–70.

22 Adler RA, Curtis J, Weinstein RS, *et al.* (2008) Glucocorticoid-induced osteoporosis. In Marcus R, Feldman D, Nelson DA, Rosen CJ (eds.) *Osteoporosis*, 3rd edn. Elsevier: New York, pp. 1135–66.

23 Fitzpatrick LA (2002) Secondary causes of osteoporosis. *Mayo Clin Proc* **77**: 453–68.

24 Bilik D, McEwen LN, Brown MB, *et al.* (2010) Thiazolidinediones and fractures: evidence from translating research into action for diabetes. *J Clin Endocrinol Metab* **95**: 4560–5.

25 Yu EW, Bauer SR, Bain PA, *et al.* (2011) Proton pump inhibitors and risk of fractures: a meta-analysis of 11 international studies. *Am J Med* **124**: 519–26.

26 Mezuk B, Eaton WW, Golden SH, *et al.* (2008) Depression, antidepressants, and bone mineral density in a population-based cohort. *J Gerontol A Biol Sci Med Sci* **63**: 1410–15.

27 Lee RH, Lyles KW, Colon-Emeric C (2010) A review of the effect of anticonvulsant medications on bone mineral density and fracture risk. *Am J Geriatr Pharmacother* **8**: 34–46.

28 Smith MR (2007) Obesity and sex steroids during gonadotropin-releasing hormone agonist treatment for prostate cancer. *Clin Cancer Res* **13**: 241–5.

29 Adler RA (2011) Management of osteoporosis in men on androgen deprivation therapy. *Maturitas* **68**: 143–7.

30 Behre HM, Kliesch S, Leifke E *et al.* (1997) Long-term effect of testosterone therapy on bone mineral density in hypogonadal men. *J Clin Endocrinol Metab* **82**: 2386–90.

31 Harman SM, Metter EJ, Tobin JD, *et al.* (2001) Longitudinal effects of aging on serum total and free testosterone levels in healthy men. Baltimore longitudinal study of aging. *J Clin Endocrinol Metab* **86**: 724–31.

32 Fink HA, Ewing SK, Ensrud KE, *et al.* (2006) Association of testosterone and estradiol deficiency with osteoporosis and rapid bone loss in older men. *J Clin Endocrinol Metab* **91**: 3908–15.

33 Khosla S, Melton LJ III, Atkinson EJ, *et al.* (1998) Relationship of serum sex steroid levels and bone turnover markers with bone mineral density in men and women: a key role for bioavailable estrogen. *J Clin Endocrinol Metab* **83**: 2266–74.

34 Amory JK, Watts NB, Easley KA, *et al.* (2004) Exogenous testosterone or testosterone plus finasteride increases bone mineral density in older men with low serum testosterone. *J Clin Endocrinol Metab* **89**: 503–10.

35 Wu FC, Tajar A, Beynon JM, *et al.* (2010) Identification of late-onset hypogonadism in middle-aged and elderly men. *N Engl J Med* **363**: 123–35.

36 Lim LS, Hoeksema LJ, Sherin K (2009) ACPM Preventive Practice Committee. Screening for osteoporosis in the adult U.S. population: ACPM position statement on preventive practice. *Am J Prev Med* **36**: 366–75.

37 National Osteoporosis Foundation (2008) *Clinician's Guide to Prevention and Treatment of Osteoporosis*. Washington, DC: National Osteoporosis Foundation.

38 US Preventive Services Task Force (2011) Screening for osteoporosis: US preventive services task force recommendation statement. *Ann Intern Med* **154**: 356–64.

39 Adler RA, Semla T, Cunningham F, *et al.* (2012) The VHA male osteoporosis program: a national model for bone health. *Fed Pract* **29**: 31–7.

40 Selby PL, Davies M, Adams JE (2000) Do men and women fracture bones at similar bone densities? *Osteoporos Int* **11**: 153–7.

41 Kanis JA, Bianchi G, Bilezikian, JP, *et al.* (2011) Towards a diagnostic and therapeutic consensus in male osteoporosis. *Osteoporos Int* **22**: 2789–98.

42 Langsetmo L, Leslie WD, Zhou W, *et al.* (2010) Using the same bone density reference database for men and women provides a simpler estimation of fracture risk. *J Bone Miner Res* **25**: 2108–14.

43 Kanis JA, Johansson H, Oden A, *et al.* (2010) The effects of a FRAX revision for the USA. *Osteoporos Int* **21**: 35–40.

44 Nguyen ND, Frost SA, Center JR, *et al.* (2007) Development of a nomogram for individualizing hip fracture risk in men and women. *Osteoporos Int* **18**: 1109–17.

45 Chaganti RK, Parimi N, Lang T, *et al.* (2010) Bone mineral density and prevalent osteoarthritis of the hip in older men for the Osteoporotic Fractures in Men (MrOS) Study Group. *Osteoporos Int* **21**: 1307–16.

46 Adler RA, Hastings FW, Petkov VI (2010) Treatment thresholds for osteoporosis in men on androgen deprivation therapy: T-score versus FRAX. *Osteoporos Int* **21**: 647–53.

47 Sandhu SK, Nguyen ND, Center JR, *et al.* (2010) Prognosis of fracture evaluation of predictive accuracy of the FRAX algorithm and the Garvan nomogram. *Osteoporos Int* **21**: 863–71.

48 Melton LJ III, Atkinson EJ, O'Connor MK *et al.* (1998) Bone density and fracture risk in men. *J Bone Miner Res* **13**: 195–202.

49 Bruder JM, Ma JZ, Basler JW, *et al.* (2006) Prevalence of osteopenia and osteoporosis by central and peripheral bone mineral density in men with prostate cancer during androgen-deprivation therapy. *Urology* **67**: 152–5.

50 Simonelli C, Adler RA, Blake GM, *et al.* (2008) Dual-energy x-ray absorptiometry technical issues: the 2007 ISCD official positions. *J Clin Densitom* **11**: 109–22.

51 Binkley N, Adler RA (2010) Dual-energy x-ray absorptiometry (DXA) in men. In *Osteoporosis in Men*, 2nd edn. Academic Press: New York, pp. 525–40.

52 Schousboe JT, Vokes T, Broy SB, *et al.* (2008) Vertebral fracture assessment: the 2007 ISCD official positions. *J Clin Densitom* **11**: 92–108.

53 Drake MT (2009) Bone disease in multiple myeloma. *Oncology (Williston Park)* **14** (Suppl 5): 28–32.

54 Adler RA (2012) Laboratory testing for secondary osteoporosis evaluation. *Clin Biochem*, **45**: 894–900.

55 Karga H, Papapetrou PD, Korakovouni A, *et al.* (2004) Bone mineral density in hyperthyroidism. *Clin Endocrinol (Oxf)* **61**: 466–72.

56 Orwoll E, Ettinger M, Weiss S, *et al.* (2000) Alendronate for the treatment of osteoporosis in men. *N Engl J Med* **343**: 604–10.

57 Karpf DB, Shapiro DR, Seeman E, *et al.* (1997) Prevention of nonvertebral fractures by alendronate: a meta-analysis. *JAMA* **277**: 1159–64.

58 Boonen S, Orwoll ES, Wenderoth D *et al.* (2009) Once-weekly risedronate in men with osteoporosis: results of a 2-year, placebo-controlled, double-blind, multicenter study. *J Bone Miner Res* **24**: 719–25.

59 Sato Y, Iwamoto J, Kanoko T, *et al.* (2005) Risedronate sodium therapy for prevention of hip fracture in men 65 years or older after stroke. *Arch Intern Med* **165**: 1743–8.

60 Sato Y, Honda Y, Iwamoto J (2007) Risedronate and ergocalciferol prevent hip fracture in elderly men with Parkinson disease. *Neurology* **68**: 911–15.

61 Orwoll ES, Miller PD, Adachi JD, *et al.* (2010) Efficacy and safety of a once-yearly i.v. infusion of zoledronic acid 5 mg versus once-weekly 70-mg oral alendronate in the treatment of male osteoporosis: a randomized, multicenter, double-blind, active-controlled study. *J Bone Miner Res* **25**: 2239–50.

62 Lyles KW, Colon-Emeric CS, Magaziner JS, *et al.* (2007) Zoledronic acid in reducing clinical fractures and mortality after hip fracture. *N Engl J Med* **357**: 1799–1809.

63 Johnson DA, Williams MI, Petkov VI, *et al.* (2010) Zoledronic acid treatment of osteoporosis: effects in men. *Endocr Pract* **16**: 960–7.

64 Orwoll ES, Binkley NC, Lewiecki EM, *et al.* (2010) Efficacy and safety of monthly ibandronate in men with low bone density. *Bone* **46**: 970–6.

65 Adler RA, Gill RS (2011) Clinical utility of denosumab for treatment of bone loss in men and women. *Clin Interv Aging* **6**: 119–24.

66 Brown JP, Prince RL, Deal C, *et al.* (2009) Comparison of the effect of denosumab and alendronate on BMD and biochemical markers of bone turnover in post-menopausal women with low bone mass: a randomized, blinded, phase 3 trial. *J Bone Miner Res* **24**: 153–61.

67 Cummings SR, San Martin J, McClung MR, *et al.* (2009) Denosumab for prevention of fractures in postmenopausal women with osteoporosis. *N Engl J Med* **361**: 756–65.

68 Smith MR, Egerdie B, Toriz NH, *et al.* (2009) Denosumab in men receiving androgen-deprivation therapy for prostate cancer. *N Engl J Med* **361**: 745–55.

69 Neer RM, Arnaud CD, Zanchetta JR, *et al.* (2001) Effect of parathyroid hormone (1-34) on fractures and bone mineral density in postmenopausal women with osteoporosis. *N Engl J Med* **344**: 1434–41.

70 Orwoll ES, Scheele WH, Paul S, *et al.* (2003) The effect of teriparatide (human parathyroid hormone 1-34) therapy on bone density in men with osteoporosis. *J Bone Miner Res* **18**: 9–17.

71 Kaufman J-M, Orwoll E, Goemaere S, *et al.* (2005) Teriparatide effects on vertebral fractures and bone mineral density in men with osteoporosis: treatment and discontinuation of therapy. *Osteoporos Int* **16**: 510–16.

72 Saag KG, Zanchetta JR, Devogelaer J-P, *et al.* (2009) Effects of teriparatide versus alendronate for treating glucocorticoid-induced osteoporosis. *Arthritis Rheum* **60**: 3346–55.

73 Khosla S, Burr D, Cauley J *et al.* (2007) Bisphosphonate-associated osteonecrosis of the jaw: report of a task force of the American Society for Bone and Mineral Research. *J Bone Miner Res* **22**: 1479–91.

74 Hellstein JW, Adler RA, Edwards B, *et al.* (2011) Managing the care of patients receiving antiresorptive therapy for prevention and treatment of osteoporosis. *JADA* **142**: 1243–51.

75 Shane E, Burr D, Ebeling PR, *et al.* (2010) Atypical subtrochanteric and diaphyseal femoral fractures: report of a task force of the American Society for Bone and Mineral Research. *J Bone Miner Res* **25**: 2267–94.

76 Rizzoli R, Akesson K, Bouxsein M, *et al.* (2011) Subtrochanteric fractures after long-term treatment with bisphosphonates: a European Society on Clinical and Economic Aspects of Osteoporosis and Osteoarthritis and Internal Osteoporosis Foundation Working Group report. *Osteoporos Int* **22**: 983–91.

77 Watts NB, Diab DL (2010) Long-term use of bisphosphonates in osteoporosis. *J Clin Endocrinol Metab* **95**: 1555–65.

78 Hansen KE, Swenson ED, Baltz B, *et al.* (2008) Adherence to alendronate in male veterans. *Osteoporos Int* **19**: 349–56.

79 Carmel AS, Shieh A, Bang H, *et al.* (2012) The 25(OH)D level needed to maintain a favorable bisphosphonate response is >33 ng/ml. *Osteoporos Int*, **23**: 2479–87.

CHAPTER 3

Mechanisms of Bone Remodeling

Maziar Shabestari & Erik Fink Eriksen
Oslo University Hospital, Oslo, Norway

Introduction

Bone histomorphometry has given us great insights into bone physiology and bone remodeling in particular. Dynamic histomorphometry using tetracycline double labeling techniques is unique, because it provides data on in vivo cellular activity of osteoclasts and osteoblasts by using the incorporation of a time marker (tetracycline) at two separate time points. The study of bone remodeling originated with the classical works of Harold Frost 40 years ago [1] and our ever-expanding understanding of this process is the basis for our understanding of osteoporosis and the development of highly effective treatments, that have emerged over the last 20 years.

The bone remodeling cycle

The ability of bone to sustain the loads placed upon it in everyday life depends on constant adaptation to loads (modeling) and repair of mechanical microdamage (remodeling). Both processes are based on the concerted action of resorptive and formative cell populations in order to replace old bone with new bone and thus secure the integrity of the skeleton. Modeling usually results in changes in bone morphology and is especially active during skeletal growth, which is outside the scope of this review. Remodeling happens within the confines of the existing skeleton and bone resorption as well as bone formation are tightly regulated by both local and systemic factors, normally securing a neutral balance between resorption and formation. Perturbations of this regulation causes either severe accelerated bone loss, as seen in osteoporosis, or bone gains as seen in osteopetrotic states, with possible disastrous consequences in terms of increased fracture risk or compression syndromes.

Osteoporosis: Diagnosis and Management, First Edition. Edited by Dale W. Stovall.
© 2013 John Wiley & Sons, Ltd. Published 2013 by John Wiley & Sons, Ltd.

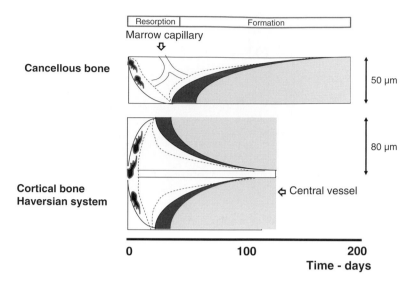

Figure 3.1 Schematic representation of Bone Multicellular Units (BMUs) and their dimensions in cancellous and cortical bone. Broken lines denote the outer limit of Bone Remodeling Compartment associated with the resorptive and formative sites of the BMU. The mean thickness of the structure in cancellous bone is 50 μm and 80 μm in cortical bone equivalent to a mean Haversian system diameter of 160 μm. The blood supply for the BRCs is provided by capillaries either coming from the marrow space as is the case for cancellous BMUs or from the central vessel of Haversian systems in cortical bone. The duration of the remodeling sequence is somewhat longer in cancellous than in cortical bone. The position of marrow cappilaries is hypothetical, as the exact distribution is poorly elucidated. (*Source*: Eriksen EF (2010) [54]. With kind permission from Springer Science+Business Media).

Bone remodeling takes place in what Frost coined the Basic Multicellular Unit (BMU), which comprises the osteoclasts, osteoblasts, and osteocytes within the bone-remodeling cavity (Figure 3.1). In cancellous bone, remodeling occurs on the surface of trabeculae and lasts about 200 days in normal bone [2]. Remodeling is initiated by osteoclastic resorption, which erodes a resorption lacuna, the depth of which varies between 60 um in young individuals and 40 um in older individuals. The resorption period has a median duration of 30–40 days and is followed by bone formation over a period of 150 days (Figure 3.1) [3, 4]. In cortical bone, remodeling proceeds in tunnels with osteoclasts forming and removing damaged bone in the "cutting cones" followed by refilling by osteoblasts in the "closing cone" following the osteoclastic activity [5]. In normal bone the duration of the remodeling cycle in cortical is shorter than in cancellous bone with a median of 120 days [5]. Under normal circumstances the total surface of cancellous bone is completely remodeled every 2 years.

Bone remodeling can be both targeted and nontargeted (stochastic). Nontargeted remodeling involves regulation of overall osteoclastic vigor by hormones like PTH, thyroxine, growth hormone and estrogen. Antiresorptive drugs like estrogens, bisphosphonates or Denosumab also affect nontargeted remodeling via their direct effects on osteoclast function. Targeted remodeling is a response to microdamage in bone and secures removal of damaged bone. Osteocyte death due to microdamage seems to be the primary trigger of targeted osteoclastic resorption [6].

Osteoclast differentiation

The dominating pathway regulating osteoclast differentiation involves binding to the Receptor Activator of Nuclear factor Kappa-B (RANK) on mononuclear osteoclast precursors. This pathway is based on osteoblastic presentation of a ligand for the receptor (RANKL) and binding of this factor to RANK on mononuclear osteoclast precursors [7]. Osteoclast differentiation is also modulated by M-CSF [7]. The promotion of osteoclast differentiation by RANKL is inhibited by the decoy receptor osteoprotegerin (OPG), which is also produced by osteoblasts [7]. Estrogens favor bone formation by increasing OPG and decreasing RANKL expression in osteoblasts. Therefore, postmenopausal bone loss is linked to reduced estrogen levels favoring increased resorption. PTH given as daily injections promote bone anabolism by reducing RANKL and increasing OPG levels. In primary hyperparathyroidism with chronic elevation of circulating PTH levels, however, the opposite pattern is seen with elevated RANKL and reduced OPG levels causing bone loss in conditions like primary hyperparathyroidism. A humanized monoclonal antibody against RANKL (Denosumab) causes more pronounced reduction in osteoclast numbers [8] than bisphosphonates and has demonstrated excellent fracture risk reduction in women with postmenopausal osteoporosis [9].

Osteoblast differentiation

Osteoblasts are derived from precursors of mesenchymal origin and their formation involves differentiation from progenitors into proliferating pre-osteoblasts, bone matrix–producing osteoblasts, and eventually terminally into osteocytes or bone-lining cells. The earliest osteoblastic marker, Runt-related transcription factor 2 (Runx2) is necessary for progenitor cell differentiation along the osteoblast lineage [10] and regulates expression of genes encoding osteocalcin, VEGF, RANKL, sclerostin, and dentin matrix protein 1 [DMP1] [11]. Osterix is another transcription factor necessary for osteoblast differentiation [12]. In addition, a large number of paracrine, autocrine, and endocrine factors affect osteoblast development and maturation. Included are bone morphogenetic proteins (BMPs), growth factors (fibroblast growth factor (FGF) and Insulin like growth factor (IGF), angiogenic factors (vascular endothelial growth factor (VEGF), endothelin), hormones like PTH and prostaglandin agonists, all modulate osteoblast differentiation [13].

Fully differentiated osteoblasts are characterized by coexpression of alkaline phosphatase, type I collagen and a wide variety of noncollagenous matrix proteins (osteocalcin, osteopontin and ostenectin), which are embedded in bone matrix and regulate the subsequent mineralization thereof [14]. Mature osteoblasts also produce RANKL, and PTH-receptor (PTHR1). Terminal differentiation of osteoblasts results in the formation of either osteocytes which become embedded in the mineralized matrix or lining cells, which cover all surfaces of bone. Osteocytes secrete a variety of cell specific proteins including DMP1, fibroblast growth factors (FGF 23) and sclerostin, which control bone formation and phosphate metabolism [15].

Wnts and osteoblast differentiation

The vast majority of steps involved in osteoblast differentiation are associated with activation of Wnt signaling pathways [16]. Wnts are secreted signaling glycoproteins crucial for the development and renewal of many tissues, including bone. Wnt signaling acts via binding to a receptor complex consisting of LDL receptor–related protein 5 (LRP5) or LRP6 and one of ten Frizzled molecules [16]. The canonical Wnt signaling pathway is active in all cells of the osteoblastic lineage, and involves the stabilization of β-catenin and regulation of multiple transcription factors [17]. Wnt/β-catenin signaling is also important for mechanotransduction, fracture healing and osteoclast maturation [18–20]. The activation of canonical Wnt-signaling promotes osteoblast differentiation from mesenchymal progenitors at the expense of adipogenesis and is modulated by Runx2 and osterix [21].

Wnt signaling is currently the prime target for the development of pharmaceuticals for the treatment of osteoporosis and include inhibition of Wnt signaling with agents like Dickopf protein 1 (Dkk1), sclerostin, and Sfrp1 with neutralizing antibodies. As well as inhibition of glycogen synthase kinase 3 β (GSK3 β), which promotes phosphorylation and degradation of β-catenin. One of the most promising approaches so far has been inhibition of the osteocyte protein sclerostin, which exerts tonic inhibition of osteoblast activity [22] and has bone anabolic action in animals as well as humans [23]. Sclerostin is the product of the *SOST* gene, and is mutated and down regulated in patients with van Buchem disease and sclerosteosis [24], both diseases characterized by high bone density. Expression levels of sclerostin are also suppressed in response to mechanical loading and intermittent PTH treatment [25].

Coupling between resorption and formation

In normal bone remodeling the tight coupling of bone resorption to bone formation assures that the amount of resorbed bone is completely replaced in location and amount by new bone. Many of the mechanisms underlying the tight regulation still remain largely elusive, although the last 15 years have increased our knowledge significantly.

The dominating hypothesis years ago was that liberation of growth factors like IGFs and cytokines embedded in bone matrix during bone resorption secured the balance between resorption and formation during bone remodeling [26]. Later work showing that osteoblastic bone formation proceeded in the absence of bone resorption [27] has supplemented this hypothesis. The important role that osteoclasts play in the regulation of bone formation is also corroborated by studies on mice lacking c-fos or M-CSF, which display absence of osteoclasts and defective bone formation [28].

Other systems involved in coupling of bone resorption to bone formation are: the transmembrane proteins, ephrinB2, which are expressed on osteoblasts and EPH receptors B4 (EphB4), which are expressed on osteoclasts [29]. Also the osteoclastic factor sphingosine 1-phosphate (S1P) [30] seems to play a significant role. The interaction of Ephrin and EPH by cell to cell contact promotes osteoblast differentiation and represses osteoclast differentiation. Secretion of S1P by osteoclast seems to recruit osteoblast progenitor cells to sites of bone resorption and stimulates differentiation of these progenitor cells by stimulating EphB4 signaling. This causes a shutdown of bone resorption and initiates the formative phase of bone remodeling in the so called transition phase.

The bone remodeling compartment

Until recently, it was assumed, that local growth factors, cytokines and even nitric oxide (NO) emerged either from cells in the marrow space or vascular cells having free access to the remodeling site without barriers, or were produced by osteoclasts and osteoblasts at the remodeling site. The seminal work by Hauge *et al.* [31], however, demonstrated that the cells in the BMU, even in cancellous bone, were not directly contiguous to the bone marrow, but were covered by a "canopy" of cells comprising the outer lining of a specialized vascular structure with the denuded bone surface as the other delineation. The structure has been demonstrated in cancellous as well as cortical bone (Figure 3.2). Penetrating the canopy, are capillaries presumably serving as a conduit for the cells needed in the BMU. The cells of this structure express an abundance of osteoblastic markers (Table 3.1), similar to the phenotypic characteristics of

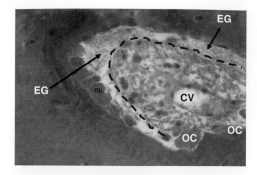

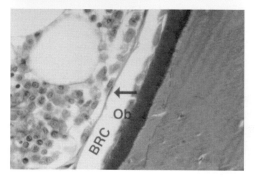

Figure 3.2 Different representations of BRC structures in cortical (upper panel) and trabecular bone (lower panel). In cortical bone the BRC (outer demarcation by the broken line) is filled with erythrocyte ghosts (EG) and is located at the closing cone of the Haversian system situated over osteoblasts (OB). A few osteoclasts (OC) are also seen. CV denotes the central vessel of the Haversian system. In trabecular bone (lower panel) the outer lining of the BRC is clearly discernible, demarcating a vascular structure on top of osteoblasts (OB). (*Sources*: Picture in upper panel courtesy of Pierre Delmas, Lyon, France. Picture in lower panel: Eriksen EF (2010) [54]. With kind permission from Springer Science+Business Media).

Table 3.1 Osteoblastic and endothelial markers detected on cells lining the Bone Remodeling Compartment (BRC) vs. vascular endothelial cells as assessed by immuno- and enzyme histochemical staining.

Antigen	BRC	Vascular Endothelium
VEGF	−	+
Von Willebrand Factor	−	+
CD 34	−	+
Alkaline Phosphatase*	+	−
Osteocalcin	+	−
Osteonectin	+	−
IGF 1,2	+	−
TGF β 1,2,3	+	−
bFGF	+	−
OPG	+	−
RANKL	+	−

bone-lining cells, which cover all cancellous, subendosteal and intracortical bone surfaces.

The BRC concept implies that the all factors liberated from the cells or vessels in the marrow space exert their regulatory role either through diffusion through the outer layer of the BRC, transport via the bloodstream to the interior of the BRC or indirectly via modulation of cell activity in the outer wall of the BRC. The presence of a specific compartment, in which remodeling can proceed without interference from factors liberated in the marrow space, secures the tight local regulation of these interactions. If the access to the marrow space was open, the very high levels of growth factors in the marrow microenvironment might have offset eventual effects by local growth factors, crucial to osteoclast and osteoblast differentiation and the remodeling process.

Angiogenesis is closely associated with bone resorption and formation. Angiogenic factors like VEGF and endothelin regulate osteoclast and osteoblast activity [32]. In addition blood vessels transport circulating osteoblast [33] and osteoclast precursors [34] to sites undergoing active remodeling. The involvement of vascular cells during the initiation of bone resorption is still unresolved, but early adhesion of a blood vessel to bone lining cells at a site of targeted repair may be an early event in the remodeling sequence. Conceivably, osteocyte apoptosis and possible release of osteotropic growth factors and cytokines could be attractants for blood vessels, which would subsequently initiate the formation of a resorptive BRC. Osteocyte/lining cell-BRC link would be useful for conveying signals pertaining to strain and damage to the bone surface. Evidence for a common lineage and close interaction between vascular endothelial cells and bone cells is steadily increasing. Endothelin and VEGF are intimately involved in signaling between vasculature and bone [35]. Osteoblasts as well as osteoclasts express receptors for and also secrete VEGF [36]. Expression of VEGF is closely associated with the early events of bone modeling and remodeling [37], where it promotes osteoblast chemotaxis and differentiation [38].

Canopy cells are connected to lining cells on the quiescent bone surface and the osteocyte network via gap junctions and are therefore involved in the transduction of signals from the osteocyte network to the surface [39] (Figure 3.3). The BRC therefore provides the primary structure translating microdamage and changes in mechanical strain into targeted remodeling by which mechanosensory signals from the osteocyte network are translated into changes in osteoclast and osteoblast activity on trabecular surfaces. Signals from lining cells indicating damage or mechanical strain could be transmitted to the outer lining cell layer of the BRC and trigger osteoclast recruitment. By analogy with remodeling in cortical bone, which is clearly associated with growth of a blood vessel into the remodeling site (5), the presumed ingrowth of a capillary into the BRC

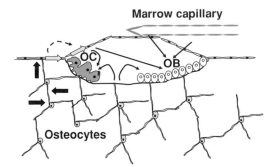

Figure 3.3 Connections between the osteocyte network, lining cells and the BRC. All cells in this network are connected with gap junctions, which may provide a pathway (block arrows), by which signals generated deep within bone may reach the surface and elicit remodeling events by osteoclasts (OC) and osteoblasts (OB) in response to mechanical stimuli. The response may be modulated by factors liberated from the vascular endothelium or marrow capillaries/sinusoids and paracrine factors (broken arrow) liberated from lining cells may also play a role. (*Source*: Eriksen EF (2010) [54]. With kind permission from Springer Science+Business Media).

provides the vascular supply for the cells in the BMU of cancellous bone. It might also provide the necessary osteoclasts and, subsequently, the osteoblasts that are needed for bone remodeling in both cancellous and cortical bone. The BRC would also be a site where hormonal modulation (e.g., estrogen therapy) of the mechanosensory input could take place [40].

The BRC is the most probable structure at which coupling between osteoclasts and osteoblasts occurs. The RANKL/OPG pathway involves presentation of membrane bound RANKL on the osteoblast to the RANK receptor on osteoclast precursors by cell to cell contact. Due to the timing and sequence of bone resorption and bone formation, however, resorption and formation are generally separated in time and space, which makes the needed cell to cell contact between osteoclast precursors and active osteoblasts highly unlikely. Even if soluble RANKL played a major role in this process, it would have no RANK on precursor cells within the BRC to bind to. A more likely cell, which could present RANKL to RANK on osteoclast precursors, would be the lining cell, which expresses both RANKL and OPG [41, 42] (Figure 3.4).

It has always been a challenge to explain how the different cell types are directed to sites in bone, where their specific functions are needed. The BRC also obviates the need for a "postal code" system ensuring that resorptive and formative cells adhere to areas on the bone surface, where they are needed. Bone surfaces are generally covered by lining cells, which would prevent direct contact between bone cells and integrins or other adhesion molecules known to modulate cell activity. The BRC would be

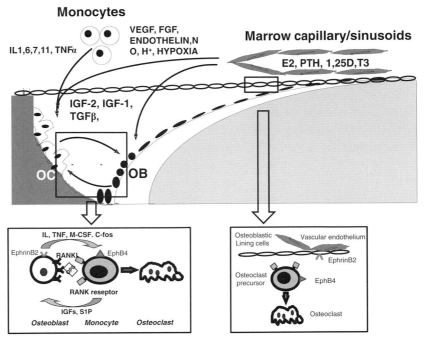

Figure 3.4 Depiction of some of the main local regulatory factors operating at remodeling sites with osteoclasts (OC) and osteoblasts (OB) and their relation to the Bone Remodeling Compartment (BRC). Interleukins (IL), tumor necrosis factors (TNF), transforming growth factors (TGF), colony stimulating factors (CSF), Insulin like growth factors (IGF), fibroblast growth factors (FGF), platelet derived growth factors (PDGF), bone morphogenetic proteins (BMP) are formed by both monocytic cells in the marrow space or circulation, as well as bone cells in the BMU. NFκB- or RANK- ligand (RANKL) and osteoprotegerin (OPG) are formed specifically by osteoblasts. Factors from the marrow space as well as factors liberated by endothelial cells(vascular endothelial growth factor (VEGF), endothelin, nitrogen oxide (NO)) may diffuse to receptors on osteoclasts or osteoblasts. The cellular responses in the BMU are then further modulated by systemic hormones in the circulation (estrogen (E2), parathyroid hormone (PTH), active vitamin D (1,25D), thyroid hormone (T3)). Left lower insert depicts in detail osteoblast-osteoclast interactions inside the BRC and right lower insert depict an alternative, still hypothetical, version of that interaction based on lining cells acting as the osteoblastic component in that interaction. (*Source*: Eriksen EF (2010) [54]. With kind permission from Springer Science+Business Media).

the only place where these cells (circulating osteoclasts as well as circulating osteoblast precursors) would be exposed to these matrix constituents, because the formation of the BRC involves detachment of lining cells from the bone surface.

The BRC may play a crucial role in the spread of bone metastases. It is well established that, apart from entering bone via local ingrowth, tumor cells reach bony surfaces via the circulation. The adhesion of metastatic cells to the bone surface as well as their growth has been shown to be promoted by interaction with bone matrix constituents [43]. The BRC is the only site where such cells in the circulation would come into contact with denuded bone. A recent study demonstrated that the breakdown of the BRC-dome was associated with progression of myeloma supporting this notion [44]. The microenvironment of the BRC is therefore highly conducive to metastatic seeding and the formation of the so-called "vicious cycle," further enabling growth of the bone metastasis [43]. Moreover, the existence of a closed compartment would make vicious cycle formation easier due to absence of interference with cytokine and growth factors from the marrow space. Several large scale studies have established that bisphosphonates reduce the number of skeletal events in breast cancer, prostate cancer and myelomatosis, and IV bisphosphonates are now used routinely in advanced cancer with bone metastases [45]. There is still debate as to how much of the beneficial effects of bisphosphonates in advanced cancer are due to inhibition of angiogenesis or to other, direct antitumor effects. Bisphosphonates, however, could exert their inhibitory effects on bone metastases simply by reducing the number of BRCs and thereby the surface covered by blood vessels and denuded bone available for metastatic seeding.

Bone remodeling in osteoporosis

Changes in bone remodeling during menopause

Loss of ovarian estrogen production leads to an increase in bone turnover by 50–100% after menopause and oophorectomy [46–48]. This increase in the number of sites undergoing active remodeling (i.e., increased activation frequency) coupled with osteoclastic hyperactivity leads to increased resorption depth. These changes result in accelerated, irreversible bone loss, and an increased probability for trabecular perforation [49]. Inversely, estrogen treatment in postmenopausal women reduces bone turnover by 50% and reduces osteoclastic hyperactivity [47, 49] (Figure 3.5). The changes in bone remodeling associated with estrogen loss are associated with changes in the RANK/RANKL/OPG system favoring bone resorption as outlined above, but increased secretion levels of proinflammatory, osteoclast stimulating cytokines, mainly IL-1, IL6 and TNF-α, all known osteoclast stimulators, also play a role [50].

Age dependent bone loss

The aging processes leads to loss of bone after the age of 35. The mechanisms underlying the age dependent bone loss are poorly defined, but several factors have been implicated.

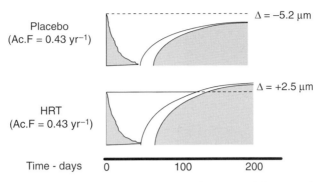

BONE HISTOMORPHOMETRY
Effects of HRT for 2 years on bone remodeling

Placebo
(Ac.F = 0.43 yr^{-1})

$\Delta = -5.2$ µm

HRT
(Ac.F = 0.43 yr^{-1})

$\Delta = +2.5$ µm

Time - days   0   100   200

Figure 3.5 Schematic representation of bone remodeling in early postmenopausal women on hormone replacement therapy (HT) (17β-estradiol (2 mg)/Norethisterone acetate (1 mg)) or placebo (Ca (500 mg) and vitamin D (400 IE)). Women on Ca+D exhibited a negative bone balance at each BMU due to increased erosion depth and impaired bone formation not balancing bone resorption. HT reversed this trend leading to a neutral balance. (*Source*: Eriksen EF, Langdah B, Vesterby A, *et al.* (1999) [49]).

Increased bone resorption

With increasing age, calcium intake and calcium absorption decrease. Age dependent reductions in calcium absorption and reduced production of active vitamin D due to thinning of the skin and reduced sun exposure play important roles in this respect. Reduced calcium absorption leads to secondary hyperparathyroidism, which, on top of the changes in bone remodeling induced by loss of endogenous estrogen secretion, amplifies bone loss. If osteoblastic bone formation was able to keep up with the increased resorptive activity, only bone loss due to spurious perforations of trabeculae would occur. Due to impaired osteoblastic function, however, bone loss is accelerated.

Defective osteoblastic function

Like skin fibroblasts, osteoblasts undergo cellular aging. In long term culture the cells undergo expansion or cumulative population doubling up to 50 populations, but with increasing age collagen synthesis and secretion of other osteotropic factors decreases [51]. This reduction in osteoblast function may explain the osteoblastic insufficiency that has been demonstrated with increasing age and in postmenopausal osteoporosis.

Compared to age-matched women without osteoporotic fractures, osteoporotic females exhibit significant thinner bone structural units (BSU's) [52], while resorption depth in the two groups remains unchanged. Thus, the main difference between osteoporotic women and

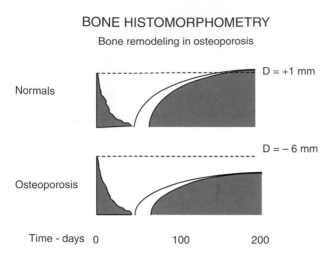

BONE HISTOMORPHOMETRY

Bone remodeling in osteoporosis

Normals

D = +1 mm

D = − 6 mm

Osteoporosis

Time - days   0   100   200

Figure 3.6 Schematic representation of bone remodeling in women mean age 65 years with postmenopausal osteoporosis. Compared to women without osteoporosis and a BMD t-score > 1, who exhibited a neutral balance at each BMU, while impaired bone formation relative to resorption leads to a pronounced negative balance at each BMU in women with osteoporosis. (*Source*: Eriksen EF, Hodgson SF, Eastell R, *et al.* (1990) [52]).

their nonosteoporotic peers is defective bone formation, that is, resorption lacunae dug out by osteoclasts are not completely refilled, which leads to bone loss (Figure 3.6). This loss is further amplified by the increased bone turnover present in most, if not all, patients with severe osteoporosis. This intimate relation between bone turnover and bone loss also explains the pronounced effects of antiresorptive drugs in osteoporosis.

Bone remodeling in secondary osteoporosis

Histomorphometric analyses of bone remodeling in various disease states such as glucocorticoid induced osteoporosis (GIO), thyrotoxicosis, and primary hyperparathyroidism have shown that the main perturbation of remodeling is the induction of a high turnover state. The degree of remodeling imbalance varies between diseases with the most pronounced being present in GIO [53] and thyrotoxicosis [2], while mild cases of primary hyperparathyroidism display no imbalance [2].

Conclusion

Bone remodeling involves tight coupling and regulation of osteoclasts and osteoblasts and is modulated by a wide variety of hormones and osteocyte products secreted in response to mechanical stimulation and microdamage. Bone remodeling occurs in a specialized vascular entity – the BRC.

This specialized compartment provides the structural basis for coupling and local regulation of cellular activity.

Bone remodeling in osteoporosis is primarily characterized by two defects: 1) impaired osteoblastic function and 2) increased bone turnover, which causes accelerated bone loss. Bone loss in secondary osteoporosis associated with glucocorticoid use, thyrotoxicosis or primary hyperparathyroidism is also caused by high turnover and varying degrees of remodeling imbalance.

References

1 Frost HM (1969) Tetracycline-based histological analysis of bone remodeling. *Calcif Tissue Res* **3**: 211–37.

2 Eriksen EF (1986) Normal and pathological remodeling of human trabecular bone: three dimensional reconstruction of the remodeling sequence in normals and in metabolic bone disease. *Endocr Rev* **7**: 379–408.

3 Eriksen EF, Gundersen HJ, Melsen F, Mosekilde L (1984) Reconstruction of the formative site in iliac trabecular bone in 20 normal individuals employing a kinetic model for matrix and mineral apposition. *Metab Bone Dis Relat Res* **5**: 243–52.

4 Eriksen EF, Melsen F, Mosekilde L (1984) Reconstruction of the resorptive site in iliac trabecular bone: a kinetic model for bone resorption in 20 normal individuals. *Metab Bone Dis Relat Res* **5**: 235–42.

5 Agerbaek MO, Eriksen EF, Kragstrup J, *et al.* (1991) A reconstruction of the remodelling cycle in normal human cortical iliac bone. *Bone Miner* **12**: 101–12.

6 Cardoso L, Herman BC, Verborgt O, *et al.* (2009) Osteocyte apoptosis controls activation of intracortical resorption in response to bone fatigue. *J Bone Miner Res* **24**: 597–605.

7 Khosla S (2001) Minireview: the OPG/RANKL/RANK system. *Endocrinology* **142**: 5050–5.

8 Reid IR, Miller PD, Brown JP, *et al.* (2010) Effects of denosumab on bone histomorphometry: the FREEDOM and STAND studies. *J Bone Miner Res* **25**: 2256–65.

9 Cummings SR, San MJ, McClung MR, *et al.* (2009) Denosumab for prevention of fractures in postmenopausal women with osteoporosis. *N Engl J Med* **361**: 756–65.

10 Komori T, Yagi H, Nomura S, *et al.* (1997) Targeted disruption of Cbfa1 results in a complete lack of bone formation owing to maturational arrest of osteoblasts. *Cell* **89**: 755–64.

11 Lian JB, Stein GS, Javed A, *et al.* (2006) Networks and hubs for the transcriptional control of osteoblastogenesis. *Rev Endocr Metab Disord* **7**: 1–16.

12 Nakashima K, Zhou X, Kunkel G, *et al.* (2002) The novel zinc finger-containing transcription factor osterix is required for osteoblast differentiation and bone formation. *Cell* **108**: 17–29.

13 Qin L, Qiu P, Wang L, *et al.* (2003) Gene expression profiles and transcription factors involved in parathyroid hormone signaling in osteoblasts revealed by microarray and bioinformatics. *J Biol Chem* **278**: 19723–31.

14 Murshed M, Harmey D, Millan JL (2005) Unique coexpression in osteoblasts of broadly expressed genes accounts for the spatial restriction of ECM mineralization to bone. *Genes Dev* **19**: 1093–1104.

15 Bonewald L (2006) Osteocytes as multifunctional cells. *J Musculoskelet Neuronal Interact* **6**: 331–3.

16 Westendorf JJ, Kahler RA, Schroeder TM (2004) Wnt signaling in osteoblasts and bone diseases. *Gene* **341**: 19–39.

17 Hens JR, Wilson KM, Dann P, *et al.* (2005) TOPGAL mice show that the canonical Wnt signaling pathway is active during bone development and growth and is activated by mechanical loading in vitro. *J Bone Miner Res* **20**: 1103–13.

18 Robinson JA, Chatterjee-Kishor, *et al.* (2006) Wnt/beta-catenin signaling is a normal physiological response to mechanical loading in bone. *J Biol Chem* **281**: 31720–8.

19 Chen Y, Whetstone HC, Lin AC, *et al.* (2007) Beta-catenin signaling plays a disparate role in different phases of fracture repair: implications for therapy to improve bone healing. *PLoS Med* **4**: e249.

20 Spencer GJ, Utting JC, Etheridge SL, *et al.* (2006) Wnt signalling in osteoblasts regulates expression of the receptor activator of NFkappaB ligand and inhibits osteoclastogenesis in vitro. *J Cell Sci* **119**: 1283–96.

21 Hill TP, Spater D, Taketo MM, *et al.* (2005) Canonical Wnt/beta-catenin signaling prevents osteoblasts from differentiating into chondrocytes. *Dev Cell* **8**: 727–38.

22 van Bezooijen RL, Svensson JP, Eefting D, *et al.* (2007) Wnt but not BMP signaling is involved in the inhibitory action of sclerostin on BMP-stimulated bone formation. *J Bone Miner Res* **22**: 19–28.

23 Padhi D, Jang G, Stouch B, Fang L, *et al.* (2011) Single-dose, placebo-controlled, randomized study of AMG 785, a sclerostin monoclonal antibody. *J Bone Miner Res* **26**(1): 19–26.

24 Balemans W, Ebeling M, Patel N, *et al.* (2001) Increased bone density in sclerosteosis is due to the deficiency of a novel secreted protein (SOST). *Hum Mol Genet* **10**: 537–43.

25 Keller H, Kneissel M (2005) SOST is a target gene for PTH in bone. *Bone* **37**: 148–58.

26 Mohan S, Baylink DJ (1996) Insulin-like growth factor system components and the coupling of bone formation to resorption. *Horm Res* **45** Suppl 1: 59–62.

27 Karsdal MA, Martin TJ, Bollerslev, *et al.* (2007) Are nonresorbing osteoclasts sources of bone anabolic activity? *J Bone Miner Res* **22**: 487–94.

28 Dai XM, Zong XH, Akhter MP, *et al.* (2004) Osteoclast deficiency results in disorganized matrix, reduced mineralization, and abnormal osteoblast behavior in developing bone. *J Bone Miner Res* **19**: 1441–51.

29 Zhao C, Irie N, Takada Y, *et al.* (2006) Bidirectional ephrinB2-EphB4 signaling controls bone homeostasis. *Cell Metab* **4**: 111–21.

30 Ryu J, Kim HJ, Chang EJ, *et al.* (2006) Sphingosine 1-phosphate as a regulator of osteoclast differentiation and osteoclast-osteoblast coupling. *EMBO J* **25**: 5840–51.

31 Hauge EM, Qvesel D, Eriksen EF, *et al.* (2001) Cancellous bone remodeling occurs in specialized compartments lined by cells expressing osteoblastic markers. *J Bone Miner Res* **16**: 1575–82.

32 Brandi ML, Collin-Osdoby P (2006) Vascular biology and the skeleton. *Journal of Bone & Mineral Research* **21**: 183–92.

33 Eghbali-Fatourechi GZ, Lamsam J, *et al.* (2005) Circulating osteoblast-lineage cells in humans.[see comment]. *New England Journal of Medicine* **352**: 1959–66.

34 Kassem M, Risteli L, Mosekilde L, *et al.* (1991) Formation of osteoblast-like cells from human mononuclear bone marrow cultures. *APMIS* **99**: 269–74.

35 Veillette CJ, von Schroeder HP (2004) Endothelin-1 down-regulates the expression of vascular endothelial growth factor-A associated with osteoprogenitor proliferation and differentiation. *Bone* **34**: 288–96.

36 Tombran-Tink J, Barnstable CJ (2004) Osteoblasts and osteoclasts express PEDF, VEGF-A isoforms, and VEGF receptors: possible mediators of angiogenesis and matrix remodeling in the bone. *Biochemical & Biophysical Research Communications* **316**: 573–9.

37 Xiong H, Rabie AB (2005) Neovascularization and mandibular condylar bone remodeling in adult rats under mechanical strain. *Frontiers of Bioscience* **10**: 74–82.

38 Li G, Cui Y, McIlmurray L, Allen WE (2005), *et al*. rhBMP-2, rhVEGF(165), rhPTN and thrombin-related peptide, TP508 induce chemotaxis of human osteoblasts and microvascular endothelial cells. *Journal of Orthopaedic Research* **23**: 680–5.

39 Marotti G, Ferretti M, Muglia MA, *et al*. (1992) A quantitative evaluation of osteoblast-osteocyte relationships on growing endosteal surface of rabbit tibiae. *Bone* **13**: 363–8.

40 Bonewald LF (2004) Osteocyte biology: its implications for osteoporosis. *Journal of Musculoskeletal Neuronal Interactions* **4**: 101–4.

41 Silvestrini G, Ballanti P, Patacchioli F, *et al*. (2005) Detection of osteoprotegerin (OPG) and its ligand (RANKL) mRNA and protein in femur and tibia of the rat. *Journal of Molecular Histology* **36**: 59–67.

42 Eriksen EF, Qvesel D, Hauge EM, *et al*. (2005) Further evidence that vascular remodeling spaces are lined by cells of osteogenic origin: Characterization of a possible coupling structure. *Journal of Bone & Mineral Research* **15**: S371.

43 Mundy GR (1997) Mechanisms of bone metastasis. [Review] [99 refs]. *Cancer* **80**: 1546–56.

44 Andersen TL, Soe K, Sondergaard TE, *et al*. (2010) Myeloma cell-induced disruption of bone remodelling compartments leads to osteolytic lesions and generation of osteoclast-myeloma hybrid cells. *Br J Haematol* **148**: 551–61.

45 Polascik TJ (2009) Bisphosphonates in oncology: evidence for the prevention of skeletal events in patients with bone metastases. *Drug Des Devel Ther* **3**: 27–40.

46 Lindsay R, Hart DM, Forrest C, *et al*. (1980) Prevention of spinal osteoporosis in oophorectomised women. *Lancet* **2**: 1151–4.

47 Steiniche T, Hasling C, Charles P, *et al*. (1989) A randomized study on the effects of estrogen/gestagen or high dose oral calcium on trabecular bone remodeling in postmenopausal osteoporosis. *Bone* **10**: 313–20.

48 Recker RR, Kimmel DB, Parfitt AM, *et al*. (1988) Static and tetracycline-based bone histomorphometric data from 34 normal postmenopausal females. *J Bone Miner Res* **3**: 133–44.

49 Eriksen EF, Langdahl B, Vesterby A, *et al*. (1999) Hormone replacement therapy prevents osteoclastic hyperactivity: A histomorphometric study in early postmenopausal women. *J Bone Miner Res* **14**: 1217–21.

50 Pacifici R, Rifas L, Teitelbaum S, *et al*. (1987) Spontaneous release of interleukin 1 from human blood monocytes reflects bone formation in idiopathic osteoporosis. *Proc Natl Acad Sci USA* **84**: 4616–20.

51 Kassem M, Ankersen L, Eriksen EF, *et al*. (1997) Demonstration of cellular aging and senescence in serially passaged long-term cultures of human trabecular osteoblasts. *Osteoporos Int* **7**: 514–24.

52 Eriksen EF, Hodgson SF, Eastell R, *et al*. (1990) Cancellous bone remodeling in type I (postmenopausal) osteoporosis: quantitative assessment of rates of formation, resorption, and bone loss at tissue and cellular levels. *J Bone Miner Res* **5**: 311–19.

53 Dempster DW (1989) Bone histomorphometry in glucocorticoid-induced osteoporosis. *J Bone Miner Res* **4**: 137–41.

54 Eriksen EF (2010) Cellular mechanisms of bone remodeling. *Rev Endocr Metab Disord* **11**: 219–227.

CHAPTER 4

Fracture Risk Assessment

Ronald C. Hamdy

East Tennessee State University, Johnson City, TN, USA

Fracture risk assessment

The main goal of treating osteoporosis is to reduce the risk of fractures which are associated with profound psycho-socioeconomic implications. This is now a realistic and achievable goal given the availability of effective and relatively safe medications. Unfortunately, no medication is free of adverse effects and most available medications are expensive. At the time of preparing this manuscript only alendronate is available as a generic preparation. It is therefore important to target patients at risk of sustaining fractures to maximize potential benefits and cost-effectiveness and minimize potential adverse effects of prescribed medications.

The World Health Organization (WHO) diagnostic guidelines for osteoporosis are based entirely on bone mineral density (BMD) and subjects are classified into three categories: osteoporosis, low bone mass, and normal. A T-score cut-point of −2.5 has been chosen because it identifies the population most likely to sustain a fracture. Although the WHO classification originally was not meant to be used as a treatment guide, it is, and patients with osteoporosis are usually offered treatment because of their high fracture risk. The majority of patients who sustain fractures, however, do not have densitometric evidence of osteoporosis [1, 2]. Furthermore, in the low bone mass (osteopenia) category are a group of quite diverse patients: those who have a T-score as low as −2.4 and as high as −1.1. The fracture risk of a patient with a T-score of −2.4 is much higher than one with a T-score of −1.1, and yet both are in the same diagnostic category. There is therefore a need to better identify those at risk of fractures.

Two sets of factors interact to increase the risk of fractures: those reducing bone strength and those increasing the risk of falls. Although some osteoporotic fractures occur spontaneously and may be followed by a fall, most are the result of falls. Some of these factors are listed in the accompanying chart.

Osteoporosis: Diagnosis and Management, First Edition. Edited by Dale W. Stovall.
© 2013 John Wiley & Sons, Ltd. Published 2013 by John Wiley & Sons, Ltd.

Estimating the fracture risk based on BMD

BMD is probably the single most important factor affecting fracture risk: roughly for each standard deviation below the reference population, the risk of fracture is doubled [3, 4]. Marshall and coworkers examined data from 11 prospective studies which included over 90 000 person-years of observation and more than 2000 fractures, and derived a formula to estimate fracture risk entirely based on BMD. The fracture risk is estimated by raising 2.6, 2.3, or 1.8 to the power of the T-score of the hip, lumbar vertebrae, or distal radius, respectively, to calculate the relative risk of fracture at these sites [5]. In the process of estimating the relative risk of fracture, it is certainly debatable as to whether the patient's BMD should be compared to a young healthy reference population and therefore use the T-score, or whether the patient should be compared to an age- and sex-matched population, in which case the Z-score would be used. Although both positions can be defended, it seems more appropriate when estimating an individual patient's relative risk of sustaining a fracture that she be compared to a young healthy adult population with a low fracture risk, that is, use the T-score. The impact of aging on fracture risk is discussed later.

One of the main advantages of using T-scores to estimate fracture risk is that it takes into account only the BMD and therefore may be used to monitor the patient's response to treatment: as BMD increases, fracture risk decreases. Changes in BMD are indeed used as endpoints in most studies assessing the efficacy of medication for osteoporosis or low bone mass. Even though this is an over-simplistic view because it ignores medication induced changes in bone micro-architecture and that changes in BMD account for less than half of the treatment induced reduction in fracture risk [6], it may be used to encourage patients to adhere to the prescribed medication. Feedback is important to maintain the patient's motivation to continue taking a medication for an essentially asymptomatic condition.

On the other hand, basing the fracture risk assessment and subsequent management strategy entirely on BMD has important limitations because several factors apart from BMD modulate the fracture risk. The relationship between BMD and fracture risk is curvilinear with the risk for fracture increasing exponentially as BMD decreases. There is no BMD or T-score cut-off-point below which the fracture risk is not increased and above which it is increased [5]. For instance, the fracture risk of a patient with a T-score of −2.4 is not that different from a patient with a T-score of −2.5, although both are in different diagnostic categories: the former has low bone mass, the latter has osteoporosis. In fact, a patient with a T-score of −2.5 or −2.4 may be switched from one diagnostic category to the other

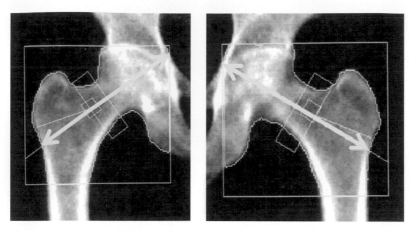

Figure 4.1 The hip axis length affects bone fragility.

based on the precision of the dual energy x-ray absorptiometry (DXA) center where the scan is done [7].

Bone geometry and fracture risk

Bone geometry affects bone strength and therefore fracture risk. The longer the hip axis length (HAL), that is, the distance between the inner pelvic brim to the outer edge of the greater trochanter along the femoral neck axis, the higher the fracture risk. For each standard deviation increase in HAL above the mean of a control population, the femoral neck fracture risk is increased by 1.9-fold and that of trochanteric fractures by 1.6-fold [8]. A number of other geometrical characteristics may affect the hip fracture risk, including femoral neck-shaft angle, femoral neck width, and upper femoral neck area (see Figures 4.1 and 4.2) [9].

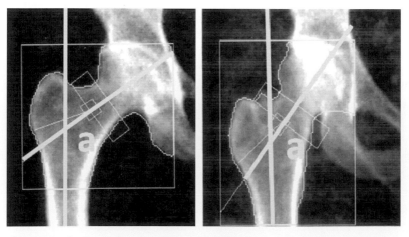

Figure 4.2 The femoral neck angle (a) may affect bone strength.

Age and fracture risk

Age directly affects the fracture risk independently of the BMD: at any given BMD level the fracture risk is higher in older than younger subjects. For instance, the probability of sustaining a hip fracture in women with a T-score of -2.5 is about five times greater among those individuals who are 80 years of age as compared to those who are 50 years old [10].

Bone turnover and fracture risk

Bone turnover also affects the fracture risk independently of BMD [11, 12]. A high rate of bone turnover may lead to abnormal bone micro-architecture and a low rate of bone turnover may lead to micro-damage accumulation. Both increase the risk of fractures. Postmenopausal women with bone resorption markers in the highest quartile are about twice as likely to sustain fractures compared to those in the three lower quartiles [13] and patients with high rates of bone turnover respond best to antiresorptive therapy [14]. Markers of bone turnover can be assayed commercially in the blood or urine. The most frequently used ones are the C-telopeptides (C-Tx) and N-telopeptides (N-Tx). A number of factors affect the serum and urine levels of these markers [15] and clinicians need to be aware of these while interpreting the results.

Other factors and fracture risk

Many other factors also modulate the relationship between BMD and fracture risk and should be taken into consideration when identifying patients at risk of sustaining fractures. Some are listed in the accompanying chart. Several attempts have been made to integrate clinical risk factors to better estimate the fracture risk and identify those patients who would benefit most from therapy.

The FRAX® tool

In February 2008 the WHO released its first version of the fracture risk assessment (FRAX®) tool [16]. FRAX is continually being updated and since its inception it has undergone several revisions. It is freely available on the web <http://www.shef.ac.uk/FRAX/> and has been included by densitometer manufacturers in their reporting software to automatically calculate the FRAX® score in the computer-generated report. FRAX® estimates the patient's ten-year probability of sustaining a hip or major (i.e., hip, clinical vertebral, proximal humerus or forearm) osteoporotic fracture. The probability is expressed as a percentage to help health care professionals and patients better understand and appreciate its potential impact and significance. The permutation is country-specific and takes into account the patient's life expectancy and, in the USA, the patient's ethnicity. It can also be used in men.

The FRAX® tool takes into account the patient's age, weight, height, and seven risk factors: a history of hip fractures in one of the biologic parents, a personal history of fragility fractures, cigarette smoking, alcohol abuse, rheumatoid arthritis, corticosteroid therapy, and secondary osteoporosis. The database from which FRAX® was initially developed included about 250 000 person-years and 5000 fractures and has been validated in 11 cohorts of patients [17]. FRAX® represents a major step forward in assessing the fracture risk of individual patients and developing management strategies geared towards specific patients.

FRAX can be used to make management decisions

Results of FRAX are used for treatment decisions [18–20]. In the USA, the National Osteoporosis Foundation (NOF) recommends treatment in patients with osteopenia if the risk of hip or major osteoporotic fractures is or exceeds 3% and 20%, respectively [18]. FRAX® results are also used for reimbursement purposes [21].

FRAX cannot be used for following up patients

A major limitation of FRAX® is that it can only be used in patients who have not been treated for low bone mass and therefore cannot be used for follow-up. Furthermore, as each FRAX® revision may change the fracture probability, using it repeatedly over a period of time in the same patient, even untreated, may be problematic as different probabilities may be obtained thus undermining its potential impact.

Response to risk factors is dichotomized

A major drawback of FRAX® is that all risk factors are dichotomized and have to be answered in a yes/no manner: there is no allowance for varying degrees of a given risk factor. For instance, a patient with a clinically silent morphometric vertebral compression fracture discovered during vertebral fracture assessment (VFA) while having a DXA scan done and a patient who has sustained a fragility hip fracture just prior to applying the FRAX® are rated equally, even though clustering of fractures tends to occur during the first year following an initial fracture. Although the 10-year probability is about the same in both patients, there should be some urgency treating the patient who has recently sustained a fragility fracture [22–25]. FRAX® also does not take into account the number of vertebral compression fractures or other fractures, although the risk of fractures is higher in patients who have sustained multiple vertebral compression fractures or multiple fractures than in those who have a single fracture [26].

The answer to the question about cigarette smoking is also yes/no, with no room to include the number of cigarettes and how long the patient has been smoking. Smoking three cigarettes a day for six months cannot have the same impact on bone mass and fracture risk as smoking 40 cigarettes a day for the past 30 years, and yet both are treated the same in the algorithm.

Similarly, although it is well known that the dosage of corticosteroids affects fracture risk, it is not possible to quantify the response to this question which has to be answered in binary fashion: yes/no. The FRAX® tool therefore underestimates the fracture risk in patients who are taking 7.5 mg of prednisone a day or more and overestimates the risk in those taking 2.5 mg orally a day or less or those who are on inhaled or topical corticosteroids. In this respect the nomogram developed by the American College of Rheumatology is quite useful (Figure 4.3) [27]. This nomogram is based on the patient's gender, ethnic group, and T-score and classifies patients on corticosteroids into three groups: high risk, medium risk, and low risk. See Chapter 6 for an in-depth discussion of glucocorticoid-induced osteprorosis.

FRAX® uses BMD of the femoral neck

Another disadvantage of the FRAX® model is that it uses the BMD of the femoral neck and not the lumbar vertebrae. The vertebrae are made up predominantly of trabecular bone which, given its vascularity and higher rate of turnover than cortical bone, tends to be affected earlier and to a larger extent than cortical bone. By only including the femoral neck BMD, which is predominantly made up of cortical bone and therefore affected later in the disease process, the fracture risk will be underestimated in many early postmenopausal women who therefore may not be offered treatment if the therapeutic strategy is based on the FRAX® score.

Several risk factors increasing the risk of fractures are not included in FRAX®

Another major weakness of the FRAX® tool is that it does not take into consideration the patient's propensity to fall, a major contributor to fractures [28–30]. FRAX® also does not take into account the serum vitamin D level, even though vitamin D deficiency is associated with an increased risk of fractures [26]. Several other risk factors for fractures also have not been taken into account by the FRAX® model, including diabetes mellitus, depression, malabsorption, and a number of medications (see Chapter 7) that can increase the risk of fractures either by leading to a reduced bone mass or impaired sense of balance, postural stability and increased risk of falls. Sedatives, hypnotics, and psychotropics may increase the risk of falls by impairing balance, postural control, and cognitive functions;

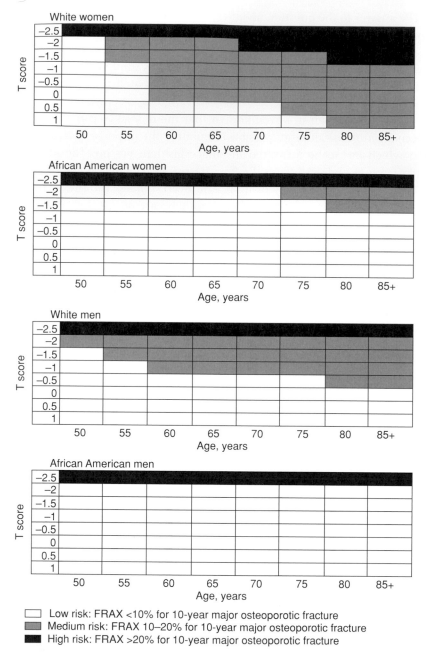

Figure 4.3 American College of Rheumatology fracture risk stratification. (*Source*: Grossman JM, Gordon R, Ranganath VK, *et al*. (2010) [27]).

medications that induce hypotension and diuretics may induce orthostatic hypotension and increase the risk of falls. Impaired vision also increases the risk of falls. Bifocal glasses may distort visual perception around the feet while using the lower lens which is meant for near vision.

It may be argued that including these risk factors in the FRAX® permutation will not be useful while treating low bone mass because no osteoporosis medication can improve balance, cognitive functions, or vision. Yet the main purpose of the tool is to quantify the fracture risk, besides, the patient's age and sex are included in the permutation and they too cannot be affected by the prescribed medication. It is hoped that future versions of FRAX® will take into consideration more risk factors to provide a more accurate reflection of the patient's true fracture risk.

FRAX® can be calculated without BMD

One of the advantages of FRAX® is that it can be calculated without BMD and therefore can be used to identify patients who would need a DXA scan [10, 31]. This could be very useful in countries or geographic locations with limited access to DXA scanners, where it may help identify patients at risk of fracture who would subsequently benefit from a DXA scan, thus improving the efficiency of DXA usage by detecting patients susceptible to fracture. It can, however, be a drawback if applied where access to DXA centers is not an issue, as it may deny DXA access to patients who have osteopenia or osteoporosis but fall below the threshold to have a DXA scan. These patients will not be identified, will not be treated, and may sustain fractures that could have been prevented had they been identified and treated before the fracture is sustained.

Prescribing a medication for low bone mass entirely based of a permutation of risk factors without measuring bone mass raises important issues. The results of the HIP risedronate study [32] provide eloquent evidence that when treatment is initiated based on clinical risk factors for fractures (the cohort of patients aged 80 years and older included in the study), the fracture risk reduction is not as pronounced as when patients were included based on a low T-score (the cohort aged 70–79 years). In the older cohort, compared to placebo, those receiving risedronate had a 20% reduction in the risk of hip fractures, whereas in the younger cohort, compared to placebo, risedronate reduced the risk of hip fractures by 60% in patients who had previously sustained a vertebral fracture and 40% in those who had not sustained such a fracture before inclusion in the study. Selecting patients for treatment based on DXA scans yields better results than when patients are selected based on clinical risk factors.

Patient follow-up is also problematic in patients selected for therapy without a DXA scan. In the absence of a baseline scan, it is not possible to

assess the patient's response to treatment especially if the assessment tool
(FRAX®) is not to be used in patients treated for osteoporosis/osteopenia.
Without having a baseline against which the patient's progress can be
monitored it will not be possible to determine whether the medication
has been effective at increasing the BMD. It also will be difficult to decide
when to stop the medication. Continuing the medication indefinitely raises
important concerns about safety and cost. Discontinuing the medication
after an arbitrary period is problematic. For instance, the discontinuation
of alendronate after a five-year treatment period is associated with an
increased fracture risk if the patient's T-score is −2.5 or lower, but not
if the patient's T-score is higher than −2.5 [33]. But how is one to know
what is the T-score unless a DXA scan is done?

Therefore although the use of FRAX® without BMD may be an expe-
dient way to triage patients, in the long term it may be a costly exercise,
may increase the risk of adverse effects, may deny treatment to patients
who need it, and may unnecessarily expose patients to medications they
do not need. The use of FRAX® without BMD to develop a management
strategy therefore cannot be encouraged in areas where access to DXA is
not an issue.

FRAX® is a work in evolution

Even with all these limitations, FRAX® remains a very useful tool to assess
fracture risk and identify patients at high risk of fractures. It has undergone
several revisions since its original release and is a work in evolution, con-
stantly updated and refined as more data become available. But like all
tools, it needs to be used skillfully.

The Garvan Fracture Risk Calculator (FRC)

The Garvan Fracture Risk Calculator predicts the five- and ten-year probability of sustaining fragility fractures [34, 35]. It takes into account the
patient's age and weight or BMD (lumbar spine or femoral neck), a history of falls in the previous 12 months quantified as 1, 2, or >2, and a
history of fragility fractures, also quantified as 1, 2, or >2. FRC does not
include other risk factors included in the FRAX® model and only applies
to subjects aged 60 years [36]. In a population study, conformity between
FRAX® and FRC for hip fractures was 79.5% [29]. In another study, 74%
of women in the highest-risk quartile of FRAX® were also in the highest
quartile FRC [37]. In men, however, FRC appears to discriminate better
than FRAX® [38].

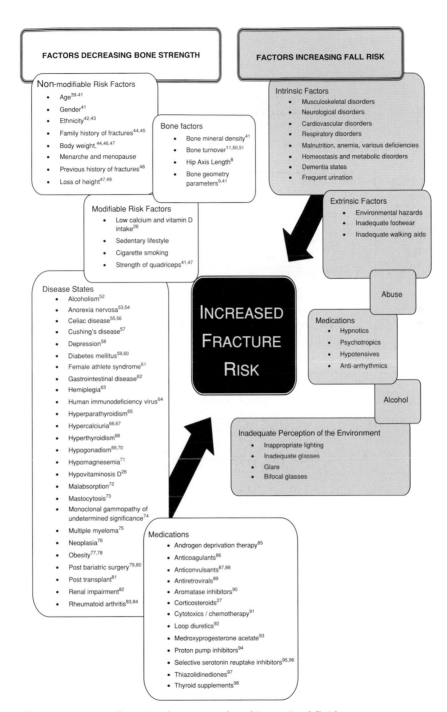

Figure 4.4 Factors decreasing bone strength and increasing fall risk.

Conclusion

The main goal of treating osteoporosis is to reduce the risk of fractures. Several tools are available to assess fracture risk, but none is comprehensive and none encompasses all possible risk factors (Figure 4.4).

The FRAX® tool developed by the World Health Organization is a major step forward: it estimates the patient's probability of sustaining a fracture in the next 10 years, can be used in men and women, is freely available on the web, and has been incorporated by densitometer manufacturers in their software. It is, however, still a work in evolution and at present has several limitations. The selection and management of patients with low bone mass; therefore, is at present anchored in the clinical rather than statistical arena, and clinicians need to integrate the evidence-based science with the art of practicing medicine.

Disclosures

Dr. Hamdy has no conflict of interest to declare for this chapter. His work has been performed outside the scope of his employment as a US government employee and represents his personal professional views and not those of the US government.

Acknowledgements

I would like to thank Ms. Jennifer Culp, BFA, and Ms. Lindy Russell, BA with East Tennessee State University for their assistance in preparing this manuscript for publication.

References

1 Siris ES, Chen YT, Abbott TA, *et al.* (2004) Bone mineral density thresholds for pharmacological intervention to prevent fractures. *Arch Intern Med* **164**(10): 1108–12.

2 Schuit SC, van der Klift M, Weel AE, *et al.* (2004) Fracture incidence and association with bone mineral density in elderly men and women: the Rotterdam Study. *Bone* **34**(1): 195–202.

3 Melton LJ 3rd, Atkinson EJ, O'Fallon WM, *et al.* (1993) Long-term fracture prediction by bone mineral assessed at different skeletal sites. *J Bone Miner Res* **8**(10): 1227–33.

4 Cummings SR, Bates D, Black DM (2002) Clinical use of bone densitometry: scientific review. *JAMA* **288**(15): 1889–97.

5 Marshall D, Johnell O, Wedel H (1996) Meta-analysis of how well measures of bone mineral density predict occurrence of osteoporotic fractures. *BMJ* **312**(7041): 1254–9.

6 Wasnich RD, Miller PD (2000) Antifracture efficacy of antiresorptive agents are related to changes in bone density. *J Clin Endocrinol Metab* **85**(1): 231–6.

7 Kiebzak GM, Faulkner KG, Wacker W, *et al.* (2007) Effect of precision error on T-scores and the diagnostic classification of bones status. *J Clin Densitom* **10**(3): 239–43.

8 Faulkner KG, Cummings SR, Black D, *et al.* (1993) Simple measurement of femoral geometry predicts hip fracture: the study of osteoporotic fractures. *J Bone Miner Res* **8**(10): 1211–17.

9 Bonnick SL (2004) *Bone Densitometry in Clinical Practice*. 2nd ed. Totowa, NJ: Humana Press Inc., pp. 257–63.

10 Kanis JA, McCloskey EV, Johansson H, *et al.* (2008) Case finding for the management of osteoporosis with FRAX – assessment and intervention thresholds for the UK. *Osteoporos Int* **19**(10): 1395–1408.

11 Chapurlat RD, Garnero P, Bréart G, *et al.* (2000) Serum type I collagen breakdown product (serum CTX) predicts hip fracture risk in elderly women: the EPIDOS study. *Bone* **27**(2): 283–6.

12 Gerdhem P, Ivaska KK, Alatalo SL, *et al.* (2004) Biochemical markers of bone metabolism and prediction of fracture in elderly women. *J Bone Miner Res* **19**(3): 386–93.

13 Garnero P, Sornay-Rendu E, Claustrat B, *et al.* (2000) Biochemical markers of bone turnover, endogenous hormones and the risk of fractures in postmenopausal women: the OFELY study. *J Bone Miner Res* **15**(8): 1526–36.

14 Bjarnason NH, Sarkar S, Duong T, *et al.* (2001) Six and twelve month changes in bone turnover are related to reduction in vertebral fracture risk during 3 years of raloxifene treatment in postmenopausal osteoporosis. *Osteoporos Int* **12**(11): 922–30.

15 Hannon R, Eastell R (2000) Preanalytical variability of biochemical markers of bone turnover. *Osteoporos Int* **11** (Suppl 6): S30–44.

16 Kanis JA, on behalf of the World Health Organisation Scientific Group (2007) *Assessment of Osteoporosis at the Primary Health Care Level*. WHO Collaborating Centre for Metabolic Bone Diseases, University of Sheffield.

17 Silverman SL, Calderon AD (2010) The utility and limitations of FRAX: A US perspective. *Curr Osteoporos Rep* **8**(4): 192–7.

18 National Osteoporosis Foundation (2008) *Clinician's Guide to Prevention and Treatment of Osteoporosis*. Washington, DC: National Osteoporosis Foundation.

19 Compston J, Cooper A, Cooper C, *et al.* (2009) Guidelines for the diagnosis and management of osteoporosis in postmenopausal women and men from the age of 50 years in the UK. *Maturitas* **62**(2): 105–8.

20 National Osteoporosis Guideline Group (2010) *Osteoporosis Clinical Guideline for Prevention and Treatment*. Executive summary, updated July 2010. Available at: <http://www.shef.ac.uk/NOGG/NOGG_Executive_Summary.pdf> Accessibility verified April 23, 2012.

21 Lippuner K, Johansson H, Kanis JA, *et al.* (2010) FRAX assessment of osteoporotic fracture probability in Switzerland. *Osteoporos Int* **21**(3): 381–9.

22 Lindsay R, Silverman SL, Cooper C, *et al.* (2001) Risk of new vertebral fracture in the year following a fracture. *JAMA* **285**(3): 320–3.

23 Center JR, Bliuc D, Nguyen TV, *et al.* (2007) Risk of subsequent fracture after low-trauma fracture in men and women. *JAMA* **297**(4): 387–94.

24 Ryg J, Rejnmark L, Overgaard S, *et al.* (2009) Hip fracture patients at risk of second hip fracture: a nationwide population-based cohort study of 169,145 cases during 1977–2001. *J Bone Miner Res* **24**(7): 1299–1307.

25 van Geel TA, van Helden S, Geusens PP, *et al.* (2009) Clinical subsequent fractures cluster in time after first fractures. *Ann Rheum Dis* **68**(1): 99–102.

26 Roux C, Briot K, Horlait S, *et al.* (2007) Assessment of non-vertebral fracture risk in postmenopausal women. *Ann Rheum Dis* **66**(7): 931–5.

27 Grossman JM, Gordon R, Ranganath VK, *et al.* (2010) American College of Rheumatology 2010 recommendations for the prevention and treatment of glucocorticoid-induced osteoporosis. *Arthritis Care Res* **62**(11): 1515–26.

28 Geusens P (2009) Strategies for treatment to prevent fragility fractures in postmenopausal women. *Best Pract Res Clin Rheumatol* **23**(6): 727–40.

29 Pluskiewicz W, Adamczyk P, Franek E, *et al.* (2010) Ten-year probability of osteoporotic fracture in 2012 Polish women assessed by FRAX and nomogram by Nguyen *et al.* – Conformity between methods and their clinical utility. *Bone* **46**(6): 1661–7.

30 Siris ES, Baim S, Nattiv A (2010) Primary care use of FRAX: absolute fracture risk assessment in postmenopausal women and older men. *Postgrad Med* **122**(1): 82–90.

31 Leslie WD, Morin S, Lix LM, *et al.* (2012) Fracture risk assessment without bone density measurement in routine clinical practice. *Osteoporos Int* **23**(1): 75–85.

32 McClung MR, Geusens P, Miller PD, *et al.* (2001) Effect of risedronate on the risk of hip fracture in elderly women. *Hip Intervention Program Study Group. N Engl J Med* **344**(5): 333–40.

33 Schwartz AV, Bauer DC, Cummings SR, *et al.* (2010) Efficacy of continued alendronate for fractures in women with and without prevalent vertebral fracture: the FLEX trial. *J Bone Miner Res* **25**(5): 976–82.

34 Nguyen ND, Frost SA, Center JR, *et al.* (2007) Development of a nomogram for individualizing hip fracture risk in men and women. *Osteoporos Int* **18**(8): 1109–17.

35 Nguyen ND, Frost SA, Center JR, *et al.* (2008) Development of prognostic nomograms for individualizing 5-year and 10-year fracture risks. *Osteoporos Int* **19**(10): 1431–44.

36 van den Bergh JP, van Geel TA, Lems WF, *et al.* (2010) Assessment of individual fracture risk: FRAX and beyond. *Curr Osteoporos Rep* **8**(3): 131–7.

37 Sambrook PN, Flahive J, Hooven FH, *et al.* (2011) Predicting fractures in an international cohort using risk factor algorithms without BMD. *J Bone Miner Res* **26**(11): 2770–7.

38 Sandhu SK, Nguyen ND, Center JR, *et al.* (2010) Prognosis of fracture: evaluation of predictive accuracy of the FRAX algorithm and Garvan nomogram. *Osteoporos Int* **21**(5): 863–71.

39 Siris ES, Brenneman SK, Barrett-Connor E, *et al.* (2006) The effect of age and bone mineral density on the absolute, excess, and relative risk of fracture in postmenopausal women aged 50–99: results from the National Osteoporosis Risk Assessment (NORA). *Osteoporos Int* **17**(4): 565–74.

40 Hui SL, Slemenda CW, Johnston CC Jr. (1988) Age and bone mass as predictors of fracture in a prospective study. *J Clin Invest* **81**(6): 1804–9.

41 Nguyen ND, Eisman JA, Center JR, *et al.* (2007) Risk factors for fracture in nonosteoporotic men and women. *J Clin Endocrinol Metab* **92**(3): 955–62.

42 Cummings SR, Cauley JA, Palermo L, *et al.* (1994) Racial differences in hip axis lengths might explain racial differences in rates of hip fracture. Study of Osteoporotic Fractures Research Group. *Osteoporos Int* **4**(4): 226–9.

43 Kim KM, Brown JK, Kim KJ, *et al.* (2011) Differences in femoral neck geometry associated with age and ethnicity. *Osteoporos Int* **22**(7): 2165–74.

44 Cummings SR, Nevitt MC, Browner WS, *et al.* (1995) Risk factors for hip fracture in white women. Study of Osteoporotic Fractures Research Group. *N Engl J Med* **332**(12): 767–73.

45 Kanis JA, Borgstrom F, De Laet C, *et al.* (2005) Assessment of fracture risk. *Osteoporos Int* **16**(6): 581–9.

46 Chapurlat RD, Bauer DC, Nevitt M, *et al.* (2003) Incidence and risk factors for a second hip fracture in elderly women. The Study of Osteoporotic Fractures. *Osteoporos Int* **14**(2): 130–6.

47 Nguyen TV, Eisman JA, Kelly PJ, *et al.* (1996) Risk factors for osteoporotic fractures in elderly men. *Am J Epidemiol* **144**(3): 255–63.

48 Kanis JA, Johnell O, De Laet C, *et al.* (2004) A meta-analysis of previous fracture and subsequent fracture risk. *Bone* **35**(2): 375–82.

49 Bennani L, Allali F, Rostom S, *et al.* (2009) Relationship between historical height loss and vertebral fractures in postmenopausal women. *Clin Rheumatol* **28**(11) 1283–9.

50 Garnero P, Hausherr E, Chapuy MC, *et al.* (1996) Markers of bone resorption predict hip fracture in elderly women: the EPIDOS Prospective Study. *J Bone Miner Res* **11**(10): 1531–8.

51 Unnanuntana A, Gladnick BP, Donnelly E, *et al.* (2010) The assessment of fracture risk. *J Bone Joint Surg Am* **92**(3): 743–53.

52 Maurel DB, Boisseau N, Benhamou CL, *et al.* (2012) Alcohol and bone: review of dose effects and mechanisms. *Osteoporos Int* **23**(1): 1–16.

53 Warren MP (2011) Endocrine manifestations of eating disorders. *J Clin Endocrinol Metab* **96**(2): 333–43.

54 Misra M, Klibanski A (2011) Bone health in anorexia nervosa. *Curr Opin Endocrinol Diabetes Obes* **18**(6): 376–82.

55 Stenson WF, Newberry R, Lorenz R, *et al.* (2005) Increased prevalence of celiac disease and need for routine screening among patients with osteoporosis. *Arch Intern Med* **165**(4): 393–9.

56 Bianchi ML, Bardella MT (2008) Bone in celiac disease. *Osteoporos Int* **19**(12): 1705–16.

57 Hadjidakis D, Tsagarakis S, Roboti C, *et al.* (2003) Does subclinical hypercortisolism adversely affect the bone mineral density of patients with adrenal incidentalomas? *Clin Endocrinol (Oxf)* **58**(1): 72–7.

58 Cizza G (2011) Major depressive disorder is a risk factor for low bone mass, central obesity, and other medical conditions. *Dialogues Clin Neurosci* **13**(1): 73–87.

59 Räkel A, Sheehy O, Rahme E, *et al.* (2008) Osteoporosis among patients with type 1 and type 2 diabetes. *Diabetes Metab* **34**(3): 193–205.

60 Hofbauer LC, Brueck CC, Singh SK, *et al.* (2007) Osteoporosis in patients with diabetes mellitus. *J Bone Miner Res* **22**(9): 1317–28.

61 Feingold D, Hame SL (2006) Female athlete triad and stress fractures. *Orthop Clin North Am* **37**(4): 575–83.

62 Bernstein CN, Leslie WD, Leboff MS (2003) AGA technical review on osteoporosis in gastrointestinal diseases. *Gastroenterology* **124**(3): 795–841.

63 Hamdy RC, Moore SW, Cancellaro VA, *et al.* (1995) Long-term effects of strokes on bone mass. *Am J Phys Med Rehabil* **74**(5): 351–6.

64 Triant VA, Brown TT, Lee H, *et al.* (2008) Fracture prevalence among human immunodeficiency virus (HIV)-infected versus non-HIV-infected patients in a large U.S. healthcare system. *J Clin Endocrinol Metab* **93**(9): 3499–3504.

65 Bilezikian JP, Khan AA, Potts JT Jr (2009) Third International Workshop on the Management of Asymptomatic Primary Hyperthyroidism. Guidelines for the management of asymptomatic primary hyperparathyroidism: summary statement from the Third International Workshop. *J Clin Endocrinol Metab* **94**(2): 335–9.

66 Sakhaee K, Maalouf NM, Kumar R, *et al.* (2011) Nephrolithiasis-associated bone disease: pathogenesis and treatment options. *Kidney Int* **79**(4): 393–403.

67 García-Nieto V, Navarro JF, Monge M, *et al.* (2003) Bone mineral density in girls and their mothers with idiopathic hypercalciuria. *Nephron Clin Pract* **94**(4): c89–93.

68 Bassett JH, O'Shea PJ, Sriskantharajah S, *et al.* (2007) Thyroid hormone excess rather than thyrotropin deficiency induces osteoporosis in hyperthyroidism. *Mol Endocrinol* **21**(5): 1095–1107.

69 Ebeling PR (2008) Clinical practice. Osteoporosis in men. *N Engl J Med* **358**(14): 1474–82.

70 Khosla S, Amin S, Orwoll E (2008) Osteoporosis in men. *Endocr Rev* **29**(4): 441–64.

71 Fatemi S, Ryzen E, Flores J, *et al.* (1991) Effect of experimental human magnesium depletion on parathyroid hormone secretion and 1,25-dihydroxyvitamin D metabolism. *J Clin Endocrinol Metab* **73**(5): 1067–72.

72 Harpavat M, Keljo DJ, Regueiro MD (2004) Metabolic bone disease in inflammatory bowel disease. *J Clin Gastroenterol* **38**(3): 218–24.

73 Chiappetta N, Gruber B (2006) The role of mast cells in osteoporosis. *Semin Arthritis Rheum* **36**(1): 32–6.

74 Abrahamsen B, Andersen I, Christensen SS, *et al.* (2005) Utility of testing for monoclonal bands in serum of patients with suspected osteoporosis: retrospective, cross sectional study. *BMJ* **330**(7495): 818.

75 Melton LJ 3rd, Kyle RA, Achenbach SJ, *et al.* (2005) Fracture risk with multiple myeloma: a population-based study. *J Bone Miner Res* **20**(3): 487–93.

76 Barton BE (2005) Interleukin-6 and new strategies for the treatment of cancer, hyperproliferative diseases and paraneoplastic syndromes. *Expert Opin Ther Targets* **9**(4): 737–52.

77 Compston JE, Watts NB, Chapurlat R, *et al.* (2011) Obesity is not protective against fracture in postmenopausal women: GLOW. *Am J Med* **124**(11): 1043–50.

78 Premaor MO, Pilbrow L, Tonkin C, *et al.* (2010) Obesity and fractures in postmenopausal women. *J Bone Miner Res* **25**(2): 292–7.

79 Fleischer J, Stein EM, Bessler M, *et al.* (2008) The decline in hip bone density after gastric bypass surgery is associated with extent of weight loss. *J Clin Endocrinol Metab* **93**(10): 3735–40.

80 Wang A, Powell A (2009) The effects of obesity surgery on bone metabolism: what orthopedic surgeons need to know. *Am J Orthop (Belle Mead NJ)* **38**(2): 77–9.

81 Ebeling PR (2009) Approach to the patient with transplantation-related bone loss. *J Clin Endocrinol Metab* **94**(5): 1483–90.

82 Jamal SA, Swan VJ, Brown JP, *et al.* (2010) Kidney function and rate of bone loss at the hip and spine: the Canadian Multicentre Osteoporosis Study. *Am J Kidney Dis* **55**(2): 291–9.

83 Ghazi M, Kolta S, Briot K, *et al.* (2012) Prevalence of vertebral fractures in patients with rheumatoid arthritis: revisiting the role of glucocorticoids. *Osteoporos Int* **23**(2): 581–7.

84 Hofbauer LC, Hamann C, Ebeling PR (2010) Approach to the patient with secondary osteoporosis. *Eur J Endocrinol* **162**(6): 1009–20.

85 Smith MR, Lee WC, Brandman J, *et al.* (2005) Gonadotropin-releasing hormone agonists and fracture risk: a claims-based cohort study of men with nonmetastatic prostate cancer. *J Clin Oncol* **23**(31): 7897–7903.

86 Carlin AJ, Farquharson RG, Quenby SM, *et al.* (2004) Prospective observational study of bone mineral density during pregnancy: low molecular weight heparin versus control. *Hum Reprod* **19**(5): 1211–14.

87 Ensrud KE, Walczak TS, Blackwell TL, *et al.* (2008) Antiepileptic drug use and rates of hip bone loss in older men: a prospective study. *Neurology* **71**(10): 723–30.

88 Pack AM, Morrell MJ, Randall A, *et al.* (2008) Bone health in young women with epilepsy after one year of antiepileptic drug monotherapy. *Neurology* **70**(18): 1586–93.

89 Brown TT, Qaqish RB (2006) Antiretroviral therapy and the prevalence of osteopenia and osteoporosis: a meta-analytic review. *AIDS* **20**(17): 2165–74.

90 Coleman RE, Banks LM, Girgis SI, *et al.* (2007) Skeletal effects of exemestane on bone-mineral density, bone biomarkers, and fracture incidence in postmenopausal women with early breast cancer participating in the Intergroup Exemestane Study (IES): a randomised controlled study. *Lancet Oncol* **8**(2): 119–27.

91 Molina JR, Barton DL, Loprinzi CL (2005) Chemotherapy-induced ovarian failure: manifestations and management. *Drug Saf* **28**(5): 401–16.

92 Lim LS, Fink HA, Kuskowski MA, *et al.* (2008) Loop diuretic use and increased rates of hip bone loss in older men: the Osteoporotic Fractures in Men Study. *Arch Intern Med* **168**(7): 735–40.

93 Guilbert ER, Brown JP, Kaunitz AM, *et al.* (2009) The use of depot-medroxyprogesterone acetate in contraception and its potential impact on skeletal health. *Contraception* **79**(3): 167–77.

94 Roux C, Briot K, Gossec L, *et al.* (2009) Increase in vertebral fracture risk in postmenopausal women using omeprazole. *Calcif Tissue Int* **84**(1): 13–19.

95 Wu Q, Bencaz AF, Hentz JG, *et al.* (2012) Selective serotonin reuptake inhibitor treatment and risk of fractures: a meta-analysis of cohort and case-control studies. *Osteoporos Int* **23**(1): 365–75.

96 Pitts CJ, Kearns AE (2011) Update on medications with adverse skeletal effects. *Mayo Clin Proc* **86**(4): 338–43.

97 Meier C, Kraenzlin ME, Bodmer M, *et al.* (2008) Use of thiazolidinediones and fracture risk. *Arch Intern Med* **168**(8): 820–5.

98 Stein E, Shane E (2003) Secondary osteoporosis. *Endocrinol Metab Clin North Am* **32**(1): 115–34, vii.

CHAPTER 5

Secondary Causes of Osteoporosis: Bone Diseases

Peter R. Ebeling
The University of Melbourne, Melbourne, VIC, Australia

Introduction

Secondary osteoporosis is defined as bone loss, microarchitecural deterioration, and fragility fractures caused by either an underlying disease or concurrent medication [1] (Table 5.1; see also Chapter 16 on medications). Secondary osteoporosis is a diagnostic and therapeutic challenge, as it frequently affects patient populations (premenopausal women or younger men) usually not affected by osteoporosis. The underlying conditions are diverse, often rare (Table 5.2), and require specialized tests for diagnosis [1].

Apart from well-known endocrine disorders, including Cushing's syndrome, male or female hypogonadism, hyperthyroidism and hyperparathyroidism, diabetes mellitus can also result in osteoporosis [2]. Patients with type 1 diabetes mellitus (T1DM) have a 12-fold higher risk of osteoporotic fractures, compared with nondiabetic controls [3]. Although patients with type 2 diabetes mellitus (T2DM) usually have preserved bone mass, they also have an increased risk of fractures implying there may be a reduction in the quality of bone and its material properties. In addition, chronic inflammation present in inflammatory bowel disease and rheumatoid arthritis cause osteoporosis [4], in part because of the proinflammatory cytokine milieu. Bariatric surgery [5] has also emerged as an important cause of secondary osteoporosis.

Pathophysiology

Endocrine diseases
Hyperthyroidism
A history of overt hyperthyroidism is an established risk factor for osteoporotic fractures [6]. A large study of 686 postmenopausal women

Osteoporosis: Diagnosis and Management, First Edition. Edited by Dale W. Stovall.
© 2013 John Wiley & Sons, Ltd. Published 2013 by John Wiley & Sons, Ltd.

Table 5.1 More common causes of secondary osteoporosis.

- Cushing's syndrome or exogenous corticosteroids (e.g. > 5 mg/day for > 3 mths)
- Excessive alcohol use (> 2 units or 18 g/d)
- Primary or secondary hypogonadism
  - e.g. associated with medications (corticosteroids, opioids, androgen deprivation therapy for prostate cancer, aromatase therapy for breast cancer)
- Low calcium intake and vitamin D deficiency or insufficiency (serum 25(OH)D < 60 nmol/L)
- Smoking
- Family history of minimal trauma fracture (possible genetic cause)

demonstrated that a serum TSH level of <0.1 mU/l was associated with a 4- and 5-fold risk of hip and vertebral fractures, respectively [7]. Based on animal models, thyroid hormone excess [8] as well as suppressed thyrotropin levels [9] have been implicated. Activation of thyroid hormone receptor (TR)-α on osteoblasts and osteoclasts results in both enhanced bone resorption and bone loss [8].

Primary hyperparathyroidism

Women are three times more often affected by primary hyperparathyroidism (PHPT) than men [10]. Chronic PTH excess is catabolic to the skeleton, and preferentially affects cortical rather than cancellous bone. Thus, bone loss is most prominent at skeletal sites that comprise cortical bone (middle third of the forearm and femoral neck), while the spine, mainly composed of cancellous bone, is less severely affected by bone loss. However, the risk of spinal fractures is also increased in PHPT. In patients

Table 5.2 Less common causes of secondary osteoporosis.

- Low BMI (< 20) and associated eating disorders
- Lack of or excessive exercise
- Anti-epileptic drugs (phenytoin, phenobarbitone, primidone, carbamazepine)
- Thyrotoxicosis or thyroxine over-replacement
- Primary hyperparathyroidism
- Chronic liver or kidney disease
- Malabsorption, including coeliac disease
- Hypercalciuria
- Rheumatoid arthritis or ankylosing spondylosis
- Type 1 and type 2 diabetes mellitus
- Multiple myeloma and other monoclonal gammopathies
- HIV or its treatment with protease inhibitors
- Mastocytosis
- Organ transplant or immunosuppressives (cyclo & tacrolimus)
- Osteogenesis imperfecta
- Gaucher and Fabre disease

with PHPT, the presence of either fragility fractures or a T-score < -2.5 is an indication for parathyroid surgery in an otherwise asymptomatic patients [10]. A recent observational study over the course of 15 years showed that parathyroidectomy normalized biochemical indices of bone turnover and preserved BMD, whereas cortical bone density decreased in the majority of subjects without surgery during long-term follow-up [11]. Furthermore, bone density at both the spine and at numerous cortical bone sites has been shown to increase following parathyroidectomy.

Idiopathic hypercalciuria

Idiopathic hypercalciuria occurs in the setting of normocalcemia when the 24-hour urinary calcium excretion exceeds 4 mg/kg/day, regardless of gender and when no other cause of increased urine calcium excretion is present (e.g., Cushing's syndrome or PHPT) [12]. In patients with idiopathic hypercalciuria, there is a propensity to form calcium-containing renal calculi and BMD is often reduced, while bone turnover is increased. The pathogenesis of this condition is unclear.

Male hypogonadism

Androgens are crucial for the accrual of peak bone mass in men and the maintenance of their bone strength thereafter [4, 13, 14]. The effects of androgens on bone in men are mediated through the conversion of androgens to estradiol via the aromatase enzyme [15]. Hypogonadism is a major risk factor for low BMD and fragility fractures in men and results in increased bone remodeling with rapid bone loss [14].

Pregnancy-associated osteoporosis

Bone loss occurs in normal pregnancies and during lactation, but is reversible. This bone loss is exaggerated in pregnancy-associated osteoporosis, but the mechanisms underlying its pathogenesis are not known. Implicated factors include preexisting vitamin D deficiency, low dietary intake of calcium and protein, low BMD, increased parathyroid hormone-related protein (PTHrP) and high bone turnover rates [16, 17]. Multiple pregnancies with prolonged periods of lactation [18] and the use of heparins for thromboembolic disorders [19] are other risk factors.

Diabetes mellitus type 1

The risk of osteoporotic fractures is increased by 12-fold in patients with T1DM [3]. Lack of the bone-anabolic actions of insulin and other beta cell-derived proteins such as amylin may contribute to low BMD and increased fracture risk in patients with T1DM [2]. In long-standing disease, diabetic complications, such as retinopathy, polyneuropathy, and nephropathy are the major determinants of low bone mass and increased fracture risk, in part due to an increased risk of falls [2]. Data from the Women's Health Initiative (WHI) Study indicated a 20% higher risk for fractures in women with T2DM even after adjustment for frequent falls and increased BMD (4-5% higher at the hip [20]). This may be due to deteriorations in bone quality secondary to effects of glycosylation products on bone collagen. An important additional risk factor for fractures in postmenopausal women with T2DM is the use of thiazolidinedione drugs, which has been associated with fractures of the hip, proximal humerus and small bones of the hands and feet [21].

Growth hormone deficiency

Insulin-like growth factor (IGF)-1 and IGF binding proteins (IGFBPs), which are produced upon stimulation of its hepatic receptor by human growth hormone (hGH), represent a potent stimulator of osteoblastic functions and bone formation [22, 23]. Patients with untreated adult-onset growth hormone (GH) deficiency have a 2- to 3-fold higher risk of osteoporotic fractures [23], with the degree of osteopenia being related to the severity of GH deficiency [24]. Accurate measurement of areal BMD using DXA in patients with pediatric-onset GH deficiency is complicated because of short stature and small bone size and it is recommended that one measure volumetric BMD using peripheral QCT in these patients.

Gastrointestinal diseases
Celiac disease

Chronic diarrhea and malabsorption due to villous atrophy are the traditional hallmarks of celiac disease, but may be absent clinically. In patients with celiac disease, intestinal absorption of calcium is impaired and vitamin D deficiency is common, resulting in osteomalacia and secondary hyperparathyroidism [25]. Associated autoimmune disorders such as type A gastritis with achlorhydria, Graves' disease with hyperthyroidism, and T1DM may further impair skeletal health. A recent study demonstrated a 17-fold higher prevalence of celiac disease among patients with osteoporosis compared with normal individuals, supporting a recommendation for serologic screening with anti-tissue transglutaminase antibodies in all patients with osteoporosis to exclude celiac disease [26].

Inflammatory bowel disease

The pathogenesis of osteoporosis in inflammatory bowel disease is complex, and patients with Crohn's disease have lower BMD compared with those with ulcerative colitis [27]. Chronic inflammation, diarrhea, malabsorption, low body mass index, and intermittent or chronic use of systemic glucocorticoid therapy for flares are major causes of osteoporosis in patients with inflammatory bowel disease. In addition, vitamin D deficiency in those with short bowel syndrome or functional loss of terminal ileum integrity, repeated hospitalizations, and prolonged immobility may contribute to low bone mass in these patients [27].

Gastrectomy and chronic proton pump inhibitor therapy

Osteoporosis after gastrectomy may affect up to one third of patients postoperatively, and is due to decreased calcium absorption secondary to higher gastrointestinal pH values [28]. These findings are consistent with a report indicating a 3.5-fold increase risk of vertebral fractures in postmenopausal women using omeprazole, a widely used proton pump inhibitor [29]. However, decreased calcium absorption may not be the cause of the bone loss and fractures associated with proton pump inhibitor therapy [30]. For more information on this subject, see Chapter 12 on calcium and vitamin D.

Bariatric surgery

Bone loss after bariatric surgery has become a clinical challenge [31]. The various procedures, including biliopancreatic diversion with duodenal switch, laparascopic gastric banding, and Roux-en-Y gastric bypass, are associated with variable degrees of reduced fractional calcium absorption and vitamin D malabsorption [5, 31]. Bone loss may be moderately severe after one of these procedures and appears to be closely related to the degree of weight loss [5]. A preliminary study indicated a doubling of fracture risk after bariatric surgery. In addition, the associated calcium and vitamin D deficiency following bariatric surgery may be both difficult to treat and long-lasting.

Hematological and immunological diseases

Myeloma bone disease and monoclonal gammopathy of undetermined significance

Various cytokines secreted by myeloma cells have a significant impact on bone cells and contribute to both osteoporosis and fractures, primarily affecting the axial skeleton. Expression of receptor activator of NF-κB ligand (RANKL) and other pro-osteoclastogenic factors (IL-6, Il-11, TGF β) by myeloma cells results in enhanced osteoclastogenesis and increased bone resorption [32]. In addition, myeloma cells secrete dickkopf-1, a soluble Wnt signaling inhibitor, which suppresses osteoblastic differentiation and reduces bone formation [33]. A population-based retrospective cohort study that followed 165 patients with myeloma for 537 person-years reported that in the year before myeloma was diagnosed, 16-times more fractures were observed than expected, particularly spinal or rib fractures [34]. Up to 5% of patients with newly diagnosed osteoporosis have either multiple myeloma or monoclonal gammopathy of undetermined significance (MGUS) [35]. Patients with MGUS, a disease that can progress to multiple myeloma, also have a 2.7-fold increased risk of axial fractures [36].

Systemic mastocytosis

Bone loss due to mastocytosis may be rapid and severe and affects both the long bones and the spine. Osteoporosis results from excessive degranulation of mast cell products, including IL-1, IL-3, IL-6, and histamine, which promote osteoclast differentiation from precursor cells [37]. An activating mutation of the tyrosine kinase c-kit (D816V mutation), present in over 90% of adult patients with mastocytosis, also contributes to elevated bone resorption. Patchy osteosclerosis may also occur as bone formation can be increased by histamine and other mediators released by mast cells.

HIV disease and Highly Active Antiretroviral Therapy (HAART)

Both women and men with HIV disease are at increased risk of spinal, hip, distal radius and other fractures due to osteoporosis. In older individuals with HIV disease, fracture risk is increased 3 to 4-fold compared with non-HIV infected controls [38]. In a large Danish study, although HIV-infected patients had increased risk of fracture compared with population controls, in the HIV-infected patients the increased fracture risk was observed for low-energy but not for high-energy fractures, and the increased risk of low-energy fracture was only observed in highly active antiretroviral therapy (HAART)-exposed patients [39]. Up to 27% of HIV-infected males have vertebral fractures, compared with 13% in controls. Multiple vertebral fractures were also more common in cases than in controls [40]. The risk of having osteoporotic bone density is also increased 3.7-fold for HIV-infected individuals compared with controls [41]. In addition to HAART use, the increase in osteoporosis risk is related to low body mass index, hypogonadism, infection, inflammation, vitamin D deficiency, growth hormone deficiency, smoking and alcohol abuse. An assessment of bone health, including measurement of BMD and vitamin D status, is therefore important in all individuals with HIV disease.

Prospective studies, mostly small and/or nonrandomized, have generally found that HAART initiation reduces BMD by 1% to 5% over 1 to 2 years [42], although this initial short-term bone loss may not be ongoing [43]. Therapy with tenofovir (TDF) has been associated with greater reductions in BMD than with stavudine or abacavir (ABC) [44–46]. In a trial of HAART-naive patients, individuals randomized to TDF-emtricitabine

(FTC) had greater bone loss and greater increases in markers of bone turnover over 24 weeks of therapy compared to patients who were randomized to ABC-lamivudine (3TC) [45]. In a randomized trial of TDF-emtricitabine (FTC) treatment, lower baseline bone formation marker levels and lower fat mass predicted subsequent bone loss [47]. The largest prospective study of HIV infected+ participants (n = 4640) assessed fractures over 5 years. In this study, fracture rates among HAART-naïve participants were higher within the first 2 years after HAART initiation (0.53/100 person-years) than in subsequent years (0.30/100 person-years) and fracture risk was independently associated with current smoking and glucocorticoid use, but not with exposure to specific HAART [48].

Gaucher disease

Gaucher disease (GD) is an autosomal recessive inherited lysosomal storage disorder affecting multiple organs. Nonneuronopathic GD (GD1), the most common form, can present with hepatosplenomegaly, anemia, bleeding tendencies, thrombocytopenia, skeletal pathology, growth retardation and, in severe cases, pulmonary disease [49]. Bone involvement is present in up to 90% of patients when assessed by MRI and is the major cause of morbidity in patients with GD1. Osteopenia and/or osteoporosis is present in up to 76% of patients with GD1 and increases in BMD occur following initiation of enzyme replacement therapy [50]. Bone infarcts, avascular necrosis, lytic lesions, osteosclerosis, and, rarely, acute osteomyelitis, also occur in these patients. The diagnosis should be considered in patients presenting with bone infarcts when no other cause can be identified.

Diagnosis

The initial evaluation of patients with suspected secondary osteoporosis should include a detailed history of clinical risk factors for osteoporosis, symptoms of common underlying medical conditions and medications that result in bone loss, a complete physical examination and appropriate laboratory tests.

A comprehensive review of medications is essential, as is an assessment of past and current smoking and alcohol use, and a family history of osteoporosis or fractures. Particular attention should be given to diabetes mellitus, anorexia nervosa, and prolonged sex hormone deficiency, as well as potentially reversible endocrine disorders, such as Cushing's syndrome or acromegaly. Based on initial findings and the clinical index of suspicion, further laboratory and imaging studies, as well as more invasive tests may be required.

Bone mineral densitometry using DXA is the method of choice for the diagnosis of secondary osteoporosis and should be measured at the lumbar spine and hip [51]. Aortic calcification and osteophytes, particularly common in older men, may artificially increase spinal BMD measurement making hip DXA measurements more reliable in this population. A Z-score (age- and sex-matched BMD) of < -2 is indicative of a higher likelihood of a secondary cause for osteoporosis, and helps to identify individuals who should be more thoroughly evaluated. In the presence of a secondary cause, fracture risk may be increased independently of BMD [51]. For example, patients with chronic kidney disease (CKD) or Cushing's syndrome may have increased skeletal fragility despite normal BMD. Spinal X-rays should be performed in those with localized back pain, recent spinal deformities or height loss of more than 3 cm to detect prevalent vertebral fractures, osteolytic lesions or tumors. An alternative to spinal x-rays is the use of vertebral fracture assessment (VFA) using DXA, which provides lateral vertebral morphometry.

Routine renal and liver function tests, a full blood count, serum calcium and phosphate levels, C-reactive protein, bone-specific alkaline phosphatase, serum 25-hydroxyvitamin D_3, serum levels of thyrotropin and serum testosterone levels in men should be performed initially. Serum levels of parathyroid hormone, serum protein electrophoresis, serum free light chains and a 24-hour urinary calcium excretion are also useful screening tests.

Anti-tissue transglutaminase antibodies should be measured to test for celiac disease, especially if iron-deficiency anemia and low 25-hydroxyvitamin D_3 levels are present, and if positive, a duodenal biopsy is required to confirm the diagnosis. To exclude Cushing's syndrome, a fasting morning serum cortisol level after administration of 1 mg dexamethasone at midnight the previous day should be performed. If systemic mastocytosis is suspected, serum tryptase or a 24-hour urinary excretion of histamine, should be measured. If available, urinary excretion of N-methylhistamine or 11-β prostaglandin $F_{2\alpha}$ may be more robust and reliable than urinary histamine excretion. *COL1A* genetic testing is required to confirm the diagnosis of osteogenesis imperfecta.

Performance of iliac crest bone biopsy and bone histomorphometry, using double tetracycline labeling to measure bone formation rate, is reserved for young individuals with severe osteoporosis, including multiple fractures or fractures occurring after antiresorptive treatment. In these situations, bone histomorphometry may distinguish osteomalacia from osteoporosis; and establish the presence of either systemic mastocytosis or infiltrating malignant diseases such as multiple myeloma, lymphoma, leukemia, and disseminated carcinoma. Bone histomorphometry may also detect an osteoblast defect in premenopausal women or men with idiopathic osteoporosis, where all secondary causes have been excluded.

Biochemical markers of bone turnover may reveal high rates of bone remodeling despite antiresorptive therapy, which may indicate reduced therapeutic efficacy or poor patient adherence with treatment.

Management of secondary osteoporosis

Management of secondary osteoporosis aims to: (1) treat the underlying disease, and (2) increasing bone mass to prevent future fractures. A practical approach with patient-centered, individualized therapy is warranted.

Treatment of the underlying disease
Endocrine diseases
Cushing's syndrome and primary hyperparathyroidism should be surgically treated if osteoporosis is present. Endogenous hyperthyroidism should be treated with antithyroid drugs, radioiodine therapy, or surgery, while exogenous hyperthyroidism requires adjustment of the L-thyroxine dosage with a target serum thyrotropin level between 0.4 and 2.0 mU/l, except if TSH-suppressive therapy for differentiated thyroid carcinoma is required.

Sex hormone deficiency in premenopausal women and men with osteoporosis should be replaced. Although fracture risk reduction has not been studied for testosterone replacement therapy, increases in BMD are seen in hypogonadal men treated with testosterone [4]. A balance of the benefits and risks of sex hormone therapy, such as breast cancer and thromboembolic diseases in women, and sleep apnea, benign prostatic hypertrophy and prostate cancer in men, should be carefully considered before initiating therapy.

While growth hormone replacement therapy in adult growth hormone deficiency increases BMD in men [52, 53], no data on fracture reduction are available and the benefit-risk ratio of this expensive therapy remains unclear. Patients with T1DM and low bone mass benefit from intensive insulin therapy [54] and aggressive prevention of diabetic vascular complications, including retinopathy, nephropathy and polyneuropathy to help prevent falls [2]. Patients with both T1DM and T2DM require falls risk assessment.

Gastrointestinal diseases
Patients with celiac disease need to adhere to a gluten-free diet, and if supplemented with adequate vitamin D and calcium, large and significant increases in BMD may be seen. Exocrine pancreatic enzymes should be

replaced in states of malabsorption due to pancreatic insufficiency. For patients with inflammatory bowel disease, in particular those with Crohn's disease, attempts should be made to modify the immunosuppressive regimen to control inflammation and to reduce glucocorticoid doses, as in other inflammatory disorders or following transplantation. Small bowel surgery in Crohn's disease should be as conservative as possible to preserve the terminal ileum and vitamin D deficiency should be treated. The bone health of patients undergoing bariatric surgery should be monitored lifelong, and vitamin D and calcium deficiency should be treated.

General measures

All patients with secondary osteoporosis should also limit alcohol consumption to no more than two standard drinks per day and stop smoking. Patients with hypercalciuria may benefit from a thiazide (12.5–25 mg hydrochlorothiazide per day) to reduce urinary calcium excretion and increase BMD.

Specific osteoporosis treatment
Vitamin D and calcium

An adequate intake of calcium (800–1200 mg/day) via dietary intake or supplements when this is not achievable is recommended. Vitamin D supplementation (≥ 800 IU/day) is recommended as vitamin D deficiency may contribute both to low bone mass and an increased propensity to fall [55]. In addition, the efficacy of anti-osteoporotic drugs has largely been demonstrated in the presence of vitamin D and calcium supplementation. Therapy should be titrated with doses that result in normocalcemia and serum 25-hydroxyvitamin D_3 concentrations of at least 30 ng/ml (75 nmol/L).

Intestinal calcium and vitamin D absorption may be severely impaired in widespread Crohn's disease, after gastrectomy or with chronic use of proton-pump inhibitors, and after bariatric surgery. In these circumstances, higher doses of vitamin D may be required. An alternative is oral vitamin D administered at 50 000–100 000 IU once a week, if required to 25-hydroxyvitamin D_3 concentrations of at least 30 ng/ml (75 nmol/L).

Bisphosphonates

Either oral or intravenous bisphosphonates are effective in the treatment of secondary osteoporosis. In patients with osteoporosis secondary to gastrointestinal diseases or in those not tolerating, or adhering to, oral bisphosphonates and those, in whom oral bisphosphonates are contraindicated, intravenous bisphosphonates are preferred. Intravenous bisphosphonates are also preferred to oral bisphosphonates in patients with malabsorption. Zoledronic acid (4 or 5 mg/year) has recently been evaluated in various forms of secondary osteoporosis in which it has prevented bone loss, and in some conditions, has increased BMD more than with oral bisphosphonates.

Osteoporosis in men

Studies of treatment in men with osteoporosis have been smaller and fewer in number than those in women. Treatment efficacy in men is mostly based on positive effects on BMD and bone turnover. In both hypogonadal and eugonadal men, alendronate (10 mg/day) increased spinal and femoral neck BMD and reduced the incidence of vertebral fractures by 80% over 2 years [56]. Risedronate (5 mg/day) increased spinal and femoral neck BMD and reduced spinal fractures by 60% over 1 year in an uncontrolled study [57]. Both studies had insufficient statistical power to measure differences in fracture rates at nonvertebral sites. Zoledronic acid (5 mg annually) given to elderly men after hip fractures increased femoral neck BMD, reduced risk of all clinical fractures by 35%, and lowered all-cause mortality by 28% over 3 years [58]. In another study, the administration of zoledronic acid increased BMD to a similar extent to alendronate over 2 years in both hypogonadal and eugonadal men with osteoporosis [59]. For more information see the chapter devoted to male osteoporosis.

Miscellaneous

Oral alendronate (70 mg/week or 10 mg/day) has been shown to increase BMD in patients with primary hyperparathyroidism [60, 61], T2DM [62], in those who are pregnant, and in lactation-associated osteoporosis [63]. However, none of these studies was powered to assess fractures. Furthermore, semi-annual therapy with 4 mg of zoledronic acid prevented bone loss in patients with monoclonal gammopathy of undetermined significance [64]. Treatment with zoledronic acid (4 mg given 5 times per year) has also been shown to prevent bone loss after liver transplantation [65] and after allogeneic bone marrow transplantation [66, 67]. Similarly, treatment with IV ibandronate (2 mg given 4 times per year) has been shown to prevent bone loss and reduced fractures in men after cardiac transplantation [68].

Teriparatide

Bone formation is impaired in many men and premenopausal women with idiopathic osteoporosis, thus providing a rationale to use the bone-anabolic drug, teriparatide. See also the chapter on PTH.

Osteoporosis in men

In hypogonadal and eugonadal men with osteoporosis, teriparatide (20 µg/day subcutaneously) increased spinal and proximal femur BMD

[69], and in follow-up studies reduced the risk of spinal fractures. The concurrent use of alendronate and teriparatide blunted the bone-anabolic effect of teriparatide in men [70]. Thus, oral bisphosphonates should be used only after teriparatide has been completed. This strategy may preserve the BMD gain and increase BMD further. Due to the high cost and need for daily injection, teriparatide is generally recommended for severe osteoporosis or individuals not responding adequately to bisphosphonates. Recent studies conducted in postmenopausal women indicated that the combination therapy with either teriparatide and zoledronic acid or teriparatide and denosumab [71] caused a greater increase in hip BMD than monotherapy with either agent alone.

Denosumab

Denosumab is a human monoclonal antibody directed against receptor activator of NF-κB ligand (RANKL), an essential cytokine for osteoclast differentiation and activation and has potent antiresorptive properties [72].

Osteoporosis in men

In hypogonadal and eugonadal men with osteoporosis, denosumab (60 mg every six months subcutaneously) increased spinal and proximal femur BMD [73]. For more information, see the chapter devoted to denosumab.

Conclusion

Fragility fractures in men or premenopausal women, very low BMD, and fractures that occur after 12 months of antiresorptive therapy should all prompt a work-up for secondary osteoporosis. Bone mineral density should be measured at the hip and spine using DXA, and the presence of prevalent vertebral fractures with lateral X-rays of the thoracic and lumbar spine or VFA, using DXA, should be sought. A detailed clinical history and physical examination combined with laboratory testing may reveal an underlying disease that needs to be confirmed by more definitive diagnostic tests. Treatment of the underlying disease is critical to reverse adverse effects on bone. All patients with secondary osteoporosis should receive adequate calcium and vitamin D supplementation, ensuring normal serum 25-hydroxyvitamin D_3 concentrations of at least 30 ng/ml (75 nmol/L). Oral bisphosphonates (e.g., alendronate and risedronate) given once per week are proven antiresorptive agents and prevent bone loss. Poor compliance, malabsorption, or gastrointestinal intolerance of oral bisphosphonates may favor the use of parenteral bisphosphonates (e.g., ibandronate and zoledronic acid). In this regard, zoledronic acid infused intravenously once per year increases BMD and has also been shown to reduce mortality in the elderly after hip fractures. However, an acute phase reaction is a frequent side effect, particularly after the first infusion. Teriparatide may be used in patients with severe GIO or men with vertebral fractures and very low BMD when antiresorptive therapy has failed. Denosumab is effective in hypogonadal and eugonadal men with osteoporosis. New therapies for osteoporosis, including odanacatib, a specific cathepsin K inhibitor, and third-generation selective estrogen receptor modulating drugs, are currently under investigation and may have a role in management of secondary osteoporosis in the future. For more information on these agents, see Chapter 14 on emerging therapies.

Disclosure

PRE has received research funding from Amgen, Merck, Eli-Lilly and Novartis.

Acknowledgements

The author thanks Drs. Lorenz Hofbauer and Christine Hamman for their prior assistance.

References

1 Painter SE, Kleerekoper M, Camacho PM (2006) Secondary osteoporosis: a review of the recent evidence. *Endocr Pract* **12**: 436–45.

2 Hofbauer LC, Brueck CC, Singh SK, Dobnig H (2007) Osteoporosis in patients with diabetes mellitus. *J Bone Miner Res* **22**: 1317–28.

3 Nicodemus KK, Folsom AR; Iowa Women's Health Study (2001) Type 1 and type 2 diabetes and incident hip fractures in postmenopausal women. *Diabetes Care* **24**: 1192–7.

4 Ebeling PR (2008) Clinical practice. Osteoporosis in men. *N Engl J Med* **358**: 1474–82.

5 Coates PS, Fernstrom JD, Fernstrom MH, Schauer PR, Greenspan SL (2004) Gastric bypass surgery for morbid obesity leads to an increase in bone turnover and a decrease in bone mass. *J Clin Endocrinol Metab* **89**: 1061–5.

6 Cummings SR, Nevitt MC, Browner WS, Stone K, Fox KM, Ensrud KE, Cauley J, Black D, Vogt TM (1995) Risk factors for hip fracture in white women. Study of Osteoporotic Fractures Research Group. *N Engl J Med* **332**: 767–73.

7 Bauer DC, Ettinger B, Nevitt MC, Stone KL; Study of Osteoporotic Fractures Research Group (2001) Risk for fracture in women with low serum levels of thyroid-stimulating hormone. *Ann Intern Med* **134**: 561–8.

8 Bassett JH, O'Shea PJ, Sriskantharajah S, Rabier B, Boyde A, Howell PG, Weiss RE, Roux JP, Malaval L, Clement-Lacroix P, Samarut J, Chassande O, Williams GR (2007) Thyroid hormone excess rather than thyrotropin deficiency induces osteoporosis in hyperthyroidism. *Mol Endocrinol* **21**: 1095–1107.

9 Abe E, Marians RC, Yu W, Wu XB, Ando T, Li Y, Iqbal J, Eldeiry L, Rajendren G, Blair HC, Davies TF, Zaidi M (2003) TSH is a negative regulator of skeletal remodelling. *Cell* **115**: 151–62.

10 Bilezikian JP, Khan A, Arnold A, Brandi ML, Brown E, Bouillon R, Camacho P, Clark O, D'Amour P, Eastell R, Goltzman D, Hanley DA, Lewiecki EM, Marx S, Mosekilde L, Pasieka JL, Peacock M, Rao D, Reid IR, Rubin M, Shoback D, Silverberg S, Sturgeon C, Udelsman R, Young JE, Potts JT (2009) Guidelines for the management of asymptomatic primary hyperparathyroidism: summary statement from the Third International Workshop. *J Clin Endocrinol Metab* **94**: 335–9.

11 Rubin MR, Bilezikian JP, McMahon DJ, Jacobs T, Shane E, Siris E, Udesky J, Silverberg SJ (2008) The natural history of primary hyperparathyroidism with or without parathyroid surgery after 15 years. *J Clin Endocrinol Metab* **93**: 3462–70.

12 Worcester EM, Coe FL (2008) New insights into the pathogenesis of idiopathic hypercalciuria. *Semin Nephrol* **28**: 120–32.

13 Riggs BL, Khosla S, Melton LJ 3rd (2002) Sex steroids and the construction and conservation of the adult skeleton. *Endocr Rev* **23**: 279–302.

14 Khosla S, Amin S, Orwoll E (2008) Osteoporosis in men. *Endocr Rev* **29**:441–64.

15 Khosla S, Melton LJ 3rd, Riggs BL (2002) Clinical review 144: Estrogen and the male skeleton. *J Clin Endocrinol Metab* **87**: 1443–5.

16 Kovacs CS (2001) Calcium and bone metabolism in pregnancy and lactation. *J Clin Endocrinol Metab* **86**: 2344–8.

17 Kovacs CS, Fuleihan G-H (2006) Calcium and bone disorders during pregnancy and lactation. *Endocrinol Metab Clin North Am* **35**: 21–51.

18 Barbour LA, Kick SD, Steiner JF, LoVerde ME, Heddleston LN, Lear JL, Barón AE, Barton PL (1994) A prospective study of heparin-induced osteoporosis in pregnancy using bone density. *Am J Obstet Gynecol* **170**: 862–9.

19 Dahlman TC (1993) Osteoporotic fractures and the recurrence of thromboembolism during pregnancy and the puerperium in 184 women undergoing thromboprophylaxis with heparin. *Am J Obstet Gynecol* **168**: 1265–70.

20 Bonds DE, Larson JC, Schwartz AV, Strotmeyer ES, Robbins J, Rodriguez BL, Johnson KC, Margolis KL (2006) Risk of fracture in women with type 2 diabetes: the Women's Health Initiative Observational Study. *J Clin Endocrinol Metab* **91**: 3404–10.

21 Schwartz AV, Sellmeyer DE, Vittinghoff E, Palermo L, Lecka-Czernik B, Feingold KR, Strotmeyer ES, Resnick HE, Carbone L, Beamer BA, Park SW, Lane NE, Harris TB, Cummings SR (2006) Thiazolidinedione use and bone loss in older diabetic adults. *J Clin Endocrinol Metab* **91**: 3349–54.

22 Ebeling PR, Jones JD, O'Fallon WM, Janes CH, Riggs BL (1993) Short-term effects of recombinant human insulin-like growth factor I on bone turnover in normal women. *J Clin Endocrinol Metab* **77**: 1384–7.

23 Giustina A, Mazziotti G, Canalis E (2008) Growth hormone, insulin-like growth factors, and the skeleton. *Endocr Rev* **29**: 535–59.

24 Colao A, Di Somma C, Pivonello R, Loche S, Aimaretti G, Cerbone G, Faggiano A, Corneli G, Ghigo E, Lombardi G (1999) Bone loss is correlated to the severity of growth hormone deficiency in adult patients with hypopituitarism. *J Clin Endocrinol Metab* **84**: 1919–24.

25 Bianchi ML, Bardella MT (2008) Bone in celiac disease. *Osteoporos Int* **19**: 1705–16.

26 Stenson WF, Newberry R, Lorenz R, Baldus C, Civitelli R (2005) Increased prevalence of celiac disease and need for routine screening among patients with osteoporosis. *Arch Intern Med* **165**: 393–9.

27 Bernstein CN, Leslie WD, Leboff MS (2003) AGA technical review on osteoporosis in gastrointestinal diseases. *Gastroenterology* **124**: 795–841.

28 Lim JS, Kim SB, Bang HY, Cheon GJ, Lee JI (2007) High prevalence of osteoporosis in patients with gastric adenocarcinoma following gastrectomy. *World J Gastroenterol* **13**: 6492–7.

29 Roux C, Briot K, Gossec L, Kolta S, Blenk T, Felsenberg D, Reid DM, Eastell R, Glüer CC (2008) Increase in vertebral fracture risk in postmenopausal women using omeprazole. *Calcif Tissue Int* **84**: 13–19.

30 Hansen KE, Jones AN, Lindstrom MJ, Davis LA, Ziegler TE, Penniston KL, Alvig AL, Shafer MM (2010) Do proton pump inhibitors decrease calcium absorption? *J Bone Miner Res* **25**: 2786–95.

31 Wang A, Powell A (2009) The effects of obesity surgery on bone metabolism: what orthopedic surgeons need to know. *Am J Orthop* **38**: 77–9.

32 Sezer O, Heider U, Zavrski I, Kuehne CA, Hofbauer LC (2003) RANK ligand and osteoprotegerin in myeloma bone disease. *Blood* **101**: 2094–8.

33 Tian E, Zhan F, Walker R, Rasmussen E, Ma Y, Barlogie B, Shaughnessy JD Jr. (2003) The role of the Wnt-signaling antagonist DKK1 in the development of osteolytic lesions in multiple myeloma. *N Engl J Med* **349**: 2483–94.

34 Melton LJ 3rd, Kyle RA, Achenbach SJ, Oberg AL, Rajkumar SV (2005) Fracture risk with multiple myeloma: a population-based study. *J Bone Miner Res* **20**: 487–93.

35 Abrahamsen B, Andersen I, Christensen SS, Skov Madsen J, Brixen K (2005) Utility of testing for monoclonal bands in serum of patients with suspected osteoporosis: retrospective, cross sectional study. *BMJ* **330**: 818.

36 Melton LJ 3rd, Rajkumar SV, Khosla S, Achenbach SJ, Oberg AL, Kyle RA (2004) Fracture risk in monoclonal gammopathy of undetermined significance. *J Bone Miner Res* **19**: 25–30.

37 Chiappetta N, Gruber B (2006) The role of mast cells in osteoporosis. *Semin Arthritis Rheum* **36**: 32–6.

38 Triant VA Brown TT, Lee H, Grinspoon SK (2008) Fracture prevalence among human immunodeficiency virus (HIV)-infected versus non-infected patients in a large U.S. healthcare system. *J Clin Endocrinol Metab* **93**: 3499–3504.

39 Hansen AB, Gerstoft J, Kronborg G, Larsen CS, Pedersen C, Pedersen G, Obel N (2012) Incidence of low and high-energy fractures in persons with and without HIV infection: a Danish population-based cohort study. *AIDS* **26**: 285–93.

40 Torti C, Mazziotti G, Soldini PA, Focà E, Maroldi R, Gotti D, Carosi G, Giustina A (2012) High prevalence of radiological vertebral fractures in HIV-infected males. *Endocrine* **41**: 512–17.

41 Brown TT, Qaqish RB (2006) Antiretroviral therapy and the prevalence of osteopenia and osteoporosis: a meta-analytic review. *AIDS* **20**: 2165–74.

42 Mallon PWG (2010) HIV and bone mineral density. *Current Opinion in Infectious Diseases* **23**: 1–8.

43 Bolland MJ, Wang TK, Grey A, Gamble GD, Reid IR (2011) Stable bone density in HAART-treated individuals with HIV: a meta-analysis. *J Clin Endocrinol Metab* **96**: 2721–31.

44 Gallant JE, Staszewski S, Pozniak AL, DeJesus E, Suleiman JM, Miller MD, Coakley DF, Lu B, Toole JJ, Cheng AK; 903 Study Group (2004) Efficacy and safety of tenofovir DF vs stavudine in combination therapy in antiretroviral-naive patients: a 3-year randomized trial. *JAMA* **292**: 191–201.

45 Stellbrink H-J, Orkin C, Arribas JR, Compston J, Gerstoft J, Van Wijngaerden E, Lazzarin A, Rizzardini G, Sprenger HG, Lambert J, Sture G, Leather D, Hughes S, Zucchi P, Pearce H; ASSERT Study Group (2010) Comparison of changes in bone density and turnover with abacavir-lamivudine versus tenofovir-emtricitabine in HIV-infected adults: 48-week results from the ASSERT study. *Clinical Infectious Diseases* **51**: 963–72.

46 McComsey GA, Kitch D, Daar ES, Tierney C, Jahed NC, Tebas P, Myers L, Melbourne K, Ha B, Sax PE (2011) Bone mineral density and fractures in antiretroviral-naive persons randomized to receive abacavir-lamivudine or tenofovir disoproxil fumarate-emtricitabine along with efavirenz or atazanavir-ritonavir: aids clinical trials group A5224s, a substudy of ACTG A5202. *J Infect Dis* **203**: 1791–1801.

47 Haskelberg H, Hoy JF, Amin J, Ebeling PR, Emery S, Carr A, STEAL Study Group (2012) Changes in bone turnover and bone loss in HIV-infected patients changing treatment to tenofovir-emtricitabine or abacavir-lamivudine. *PLoS One* **7**: e38377. Epub 2012 Jun 15.

48 Yin MT, Kendall MA, Wu X, Tassiopoulos K, Hochberg M, Huang JS, Glesby MJ, Bolivar H, McComsey GA (2012) Fractures afterantiretroviral initiation: An analysis of the ACTG longitudinal linked randomized trial (ALLRT) study. *AIDS*. Aug 28 [Epub ahead of print].

49 Mikosch P (2011) Gaucher disease and bone. *Best Pract Res Clin Rheumatol* **25**: 665–81.

50 Mistry PK, Weinreb NJ, Kaplan P, Cole JA, Gwosdow AR, Hangartner T (2011) Osteopenia in Gaucher disease develops early in life: response to imiglucerase enzyme therapy in children, adolescents and adults. *Blood Cells Mol Dis* **46**: 66–72.

51 Khan AA, Hanley DA, Bilezikian JP, Binkley N, Brown JP, Hodsman AB, Josse RG, Kendler DL, Lewiecki EM, Miller PD, Olszynski WP, Petak SM, Syed ZA, Theriault D, Watts NB; Canadian Panel of the International Society for Clinical Densitometry (2006) Standards for performing DXA in individuals with secondary causes of osteoporosis. *J Clin Densitom* **9**: 47–57.

52 Baum HB, Biller BM, Finkelstein JS, Cannistraro KB, Oppenhein DS, Schoenfeld DA, Michel TH, Wittink H, Klibanski A (1996) Effects of physiologic growth hormone therapy on bone density and body composition in patients with adult-onset growth hormone deficiency. A randomized, placebo-controlled trial. *Ann Intern Med* **125**: 883–90.

53 Snyder PJ, Biller BM, Zagar A, Jackson I, Arafah BM, Nippoldt TB, Cook DM, Mooradian AD, Kwan A, Scism-Bacon J, Chipman JJ, Hartman ML (2007) Effect of growth hormone replacement on BMD in adult-onset growth hormone deficiency. *J Bone Miner Res* **22**: 762–70.

54 Campos Pastor MM, Lopez-Ibarra PJ, Escobar-Jimenez F, Serrano Pardo MD, Garcia-Cervigon AG (2000) Intensive insulin therapy and bone mineral density in type 1 diabetes mellitus: a prospective study. *Osteoporos Int* **11**: 455–9.

55 Holick MF (2007) Vitamin D deficiency. *N Engl J Med* **357**: 266–81.

56 Orwoll E, Ettinger M, Weiss S, Miller P, Kendler D, Graham J, Adami S, Weber K, Lorenc R, Pietschmann P, Vandormael K, Lombardi A (2000) Alendronate for the treatment of osteoporis in men. *N Eng J Med* **343**: 604–10.

57 Ringe JD, Faber H, Farahmand P, Dorst A (2006) Efficacy of risedronate in men with primary and secondary osteoporosis: results of a 1-year study. *Rheumatol Int* **355**: 427–31.

58 Lyles KW, Colón-Emeric CS, Magaziner JS, Adachi JD, Pieper CF, Mautalen C, Hyldstrup L, Recknor C, Nordsletten L, Moore KA, Lavecchia C, Zhang J, Mesenbrink P, Hodgson PK, Abrams K, Orloff JJ, Horowitz Z, Eriksen EF, Boonen S; HORIZON Recurrent Fracture Trial (2007) Zoledronic acid and clinical fractures and mortality after hip fracture. *N Engl J Med* **357**: 1799–1809.

59 Orwoll ES, Miller PD, Adachi JD, Brown J, Adler RA, Kendler D, Bucci-Rechtweg C, Readie A, Mesenbrink P, Weinstein RS (2010) Efficacy and safety of a once-yearly i.v. Infusion of zoledronic acid 5-mg versus a once-weekly 70-mg oral alendronate in

the treatment of male osteoporosis: a randomized, multicenter, double-blind, active-controlled study. *J Bone Miner Res* **25**: 2239–50.

60 Rossini M, Gatti D, Isaia G, Sartori L, Braga V, Adami S (2001) Effects of oral alendronate in elderly patients with osteoporosis and mild primary hyperparathyroidism. *J Bone Miner Res* **16**: 113–19.

61 Chow CC, Chan WB, Li JK, Chan NN, Chan MH, Ko GT, Lo KW, Cockram CS (2003) Oral alendronate increases bone mineral density in postmenopausal women with primary hyperparathyroidism. *J Clin Endocrinol Metab* **88**: 581–7.

62 Keegan TH, Schwartz AV, Bauer DC, Sellmeyer DE, Kelsey JL; fracture intervention trial (2004) Effect of alendronate on bone mineral density and biochemical markers of bone turnover in type 2 diabetic women: the fracture intervention trial. *Diabetes Care* **27**: 1547–53.

63 O'Sullivan SM, Grey AB, Singh R, Reid IR (2006) Bisphosphonates in pregnancy and lactation-associated osteoporosis. *Osteoporos Int* **17**: 1008–12.

64 Berenson JR, Yellin O, Boccia RV, Flam M, Wong SF, Batuman O, Moezi MM, Woytowitz D, Duvivier H, Nassir Y, Swift RA (2008) Zoledronic acid markedly improves bone mineral density for patients with monoclonal gammopathy of undetermined significance and bone loss. *Clin Cancer* **14**: 6289–95.

65 Crawford BA, Kam C, Pavlovic J, Byth K, Handelsman DJ, Angus PW, McCaughan GW (2006) Zoledronic acid prevents bone loss after liver transplantation: a randomized, double-blind, placebo-controlled trial. *Ann Intern Med* **144**: 239–48.

66 D'Souza AB, Grigg AP, Szer J, Ebeling PR (2006) Zoledronic acid prevents bone loss after allogeneic haemopoietic stem cell transplantation. *Intern Med J* **36**: 600–3.

67 Chae YS, Kim JG, Moon JH, Kim SN, Lee SJ, Kim YJ, Sohn SK (2009) Pilot study on the use of zoledronic acid to prevent bone loss in allo-SCT recipients. *Bone Marrow Transplant* **44**: 35–41.

68 Fahrleitner-Pammer A, Piswanger-Soelkner JC, Pieber TR, Obermayer-Pietsch BM, Pilz S, Dimai HP, Prenner G, Tscheliessnigg KH, Hauge E, Portugaller RH, Dobnig H (2009) Ibandronate prevents bone loss and reduces vertebral fracture risk in male cardiac transplant patients: a randomized double-blind, placebo-controlled trial. *J Bone Miner Res* **24**: 1335–44.

69 Orwoll ES, Scheele WH, Paul S, Adami S, Syversen U, Diez-Perez A, Kaufmann JM, Clancy AD, Gaich GA (2003) The effect of teriparatide [human parathyroid hormone (1-34)] therapy on bone density in men with osteoporosis. *J Bone Miner Res* **18**: 9–17.

70 Finkelstein JS, Hayes A, Hunzelman JL, Wyland JJ, Lee H, Neer RM (2003) The effects of parathyroid hormone, alendronate, or both in men with osteoporosis. *N Engl J Med* **349**: 1216–26.

71 Tsai JN, Uihlein AV, Lee H, Kumbhani R, Siwila-Sackman E, McKay EA, Burnett-Bowie S-A M, Neer RM, Leder BZ (2013) Teriparatide and denosumab, alone or combined, in women with postmenopausal osteoporosis: The DATA study randomised trial. *Lancet.* May 15 [Epub ahead of print].

72 Hofbauer LC, Schoppet M (2004) Clinical implications of the osteoprotegerin/RANKL/RANK system for bone and vascular diseases. *JAMA* **292**: 490–5.

73 Orwoll E, Teglbjærg CS, Langdahl BL, Chapurlat R, Czerwinski E, Kendler DL, Register JY, Kivitz A, Lewiecki EM, Miller PD, Bolognese MA, McClung MR, Bone HG, Ljunggren O, Abrahamsen B, Gruntmanis U, Yang YC, Wagman RB, Siddhanti S, Grauer A, Hall JW, Boonen S (2012) A randomized, placebo-controlled study of the effects of denosumab for the treatment of men with low bone mineral density. *J Clin Endocrinol Metab* **97**: 3161–9.

CHAPTER 6

Glucocorticoid-induced Osteoporosis

Stuart Silverman & Swamy Venuturupalli
Cedars-Sinai Medical Center, Los Angeles, CA, USA

Introduction

Glucocorticoids are widely used in medical treatment. The prevalence of glucocorticoid use in postmenopausal women was estimated to be between 2.7% and 4.6% in an observational cohort of postmenopausal women [1]. Furthermore, glucocorticoid use is known to be associated with a reduction in bone mineral density (BMD) and an increase in one's relative risk for fracture. This chapter will discuss the effects of glucocorticoids on BMD and fractures including the prevalence, pathophysiology, evaluation, and treatment of this problem.

Epidemiology

Oral glucocorticoids are associated with bone loss which is most rapid in the first 3–6 months of therapy [2]. The risk for fracture is directly related to one's daily dose [3]. The greatest increase in fracture risk is for vertebral fractures, although an increase in the risk for hip fractures has also been reported. Data from the General Practitioners Research Database in the UK have shown increased fracture risk with daily doses of 2.5 mg to 7.5 mg of prednisone or its equivalent with a dose-dependent effect. The association between daily dose and fracture risk has been shown to be stronger than the association between fracture risk and cumulative dose. In patients taking doses of >= 7.5 mg daily, a relative risk of 5.18 (4.25–6.31) has been reported for vertebral fractures, compared to a relative risk in nonvertebral fractures of 2.27 (2.16–3.10) [2]. There is evidence of a possible reduction in BMD and a small increase in fracture risk in individuals who have taken

Osteoporosis: Diagnosis and Management, First Edition. Edited by Dale W. Stovall.
© 2013 John Wiley & Sons, Ltd. Published 2013 by John Wiley & Sons, Ltd.

either high doses of inhaled glucocorticoids [4] or intermittent oral gluco-corticoid [5]. Premenopausal women and younger men have been shown to be at decreased risk of glucocorticoid induced bone changes based on data from randomized controlled trials [6]. Cessation of glucocorticoid use is associated with decreased fracture risk and partial reversal of bone loss [2]. Nevertheless, some increased risk for fracture remains, possibly related to the disorder for which the glucocorticoids were initially prescribed.

FRAX

Glucocorticoid exposure has a negative effect on one's risk for fracture that is independent of its effects on BMD. Based on this fact, ever use of oral glucocorticoids for three months or more is one of the clinical risk factors in the WHO Fracture Risk Assessment Tool (FRAX). However, the current FRAX algorithm uses data from the UK General Practitioners Database which is largely based on doses of 2.5–7.5 mg of daily prednisone use or its equivalent [7]. Therefore, a correction factor based on dose has been proposed. Using the UK data base, the average adjustment for hip fracture for daily doses under 2.5 mg/day is 0.65, and the adjustment for doses over 7.5 mg is 1.2. The average adjustment for major osteoporotic fracture is 0.8 for daily doses of glucocorticoids under 2.5 mg and 1.15 for doses over 7.5 mg/day [8].

Workup

It is important to assess the risk for fracture in any individual who is either initially prescribed glucocorticoid therapy or who is currently tak-ing glucocorticoids. Individuals who are newly prescribed glucocorticoid therapy who have an anticipated duration of glucocorticoid use that is greater than three months should have a baseline BMD measurement in both their spine and hip. In addition, a lateral spine DXA should be con-sidered to rule out vertebral fracture. Furthermore, these patients should have their serum 25-hydroxy vitamin D levels drawn and a 24-hour urine for hypercalciuria should be considered. Finally, the clinician should con-sider a further work-up for secondary causes of osteoporosis in these patients including a sensitive TSH, celiac panel, gonadal hormones, liver function, renal function, blood count and sedimentation rate. Both BMD and height should be measured over time. If other causes of osteoporo-sis, including secondary osteoporosis are identified in these patients, they should be treated [9].

Pathophysiology

Although glucocorticoid induced osteoporosis (GIO) and postmenopausal osteoporosis share some common pathophysiology, significant differences exist between the two. Increased bone turnover occurs in both GIO and postmenopausal osteoporosis, but they differ in their time course [6]. Glucocorticoids upregulate production of RANKL resulting in increased bone resorption and osteoclastogenesis [10]. Glucocorticoid therapy also results in a prolonged reduction in bone formation due to a decrease in osteoblast function and an increase in apoptosis of osteoblasts and osteocytes, resulting in decreased bone turnover. In postmenopausal women, this increased bone turnover state may persist [11]. Effects on trabecular microarchitecture have been reported in the two conditions, with greater trabecular thinning in GIO and greater trabecular perforation in menopause [12]. Glucocorticoids also alter both the intestinal and renal metabolism of calcium [6]. Furthermore, glucocorticoid use is associated with hypogonadism [12].

The effects of glucocorticoids have been studied in a murine model. These data reveal that glucocorticoid therapy results in significant reduction in both trabecular bone volume and whole bone strength. Furthermore, these studies have demonstrated that glucocorticoids have independent effects on trabecular and cortical bone. Initially, glucocorticoids impact trabecular bone the most due to its higher metabolic activity [11]. However, with prolonged glucocorticoid use, cortical bone metabolism is also affected [11].

Glucocorticoids have an impact on osteoblasts via several mechanisms. They inhibit the differentiation of mesenchymal precursor cells into osteoblasts by directing the precursors toward adipocyte development, which results in a decreased osteoblast pool [13]. Furthermore, glucocorticoids increase the expression of Wnt signaling antagonists, such as Dickkopf-1 and sclerostin, which inhibit osteoblast maturation [14, 15].

Treatment studies in an animal model have demonstrated a direct effect of glucocorticoids on osteocytes, resulting in a modification of their microenvironment [16]. Lane *et al.* [17] showed an enlargement of lacunar space and the generation of a surrounding area of hypomineralized bone and reduced elastic modulus around the lacunae with a reduced mineral-to-matrix ratio determined by Raman microspectroscopy, suggesting that glucocorticoids may alter bone material properties. Other potential effects of glucocorticoids on bone include an increase in osteoclastic maturation; however, despite the high numbers of osteoclasts on the bone surface, it is not clear that a significant increase occurs in bone resorption. Finally, glucocorticoids induce significant effects on the endocrine system.

Glucocorticoid therapy reduces the production of both adrenal and gonadal hormones, including estrogen and testosterone, with possible deleterious effects on bone cells [18].

Treatment

In regards to the treatment of patients with GIO, there are several general measures that should be considered in all patients. Included are the following: (1) Minimize glucocorticoid dose, for example consider steroid sparing agents and alternate day dosing. (2) Consider alternate formulations or routes of administration, for example intraarticular or topical may be preferred over oral systemic administration. (3) Provide adequate calcium and vitamin D. (4) Instruct the patient regarding adequate exercise and physical activity. (5) Avoid alcohol and tobacco. (6) Assess fall risk and balance, for example consider balance training and environmental measures to reduce the risk of falling [6].

In general, patients who are at increased risk of fracture should be treated. Important risk factors are glucocorticoid dose and duration, age, FRAX score, and BMD T score <= −1.5. Based on available data in 2012, available therapies for both men and women include bisphosphonates such as alendronate, risedronate, etidronate, and intravenous zoledronate; and anabolic agents such as teriparatide. The evidence for medication efficacy for these agents was primarily based on BMD effects since fractures were not a primary endpoint. Unfortunately, there is little data on the long-term safety of these medications in GIO, although there is long-term safety data in postmenopausal osteoporosis. One should consider bone protective therapy at the onset of glucocorticoid exposure in patients at risk [9]. If glucocorticoids are stopped, the clinician should reevaluate the fracture risk and consider withdrawing therapy. If glucocorticoids are continued long-term therapies should be continued. Although one can consider a drug holiday in postmenopausal women after five years of oral bisphosphonate therapy or three years of IV bisphosphonate therapy, there is no data regarding the use of therapeutic holidays in GIO. Patients with a history of fracture on therapy should be considered for long-term therapy with the same or an alternate agent.

Treatment studies in GIO are complicated by several factors, for example, studies often combine patients with multiple rheumatic disorders (e.g., polymyalgia rheumatica, rheumatoid arthritis with different comorbidities) as well as pulmonary and gastrointestinal disorders. In addition, studies often combine patients of different ages and both genders. Finally, most studies have been short-term (i.e., 1-year studies with BMD as the primary endpoint) [6].

Regulatory agencies have allowed BMD to be the primary endpoint for agents that have demonstrated fracture efficacy in postmenopausal osteoporosis [6]. Most of the patients studied include postmenopausal women, with smaller numbers of premenopausal women and men. Trials traditionally have been separated into two types: prevention and treatment. Prevention trials refer to patients at the start of glucocorticoid therapy, and treatment refers to patients with at least 3 months of glucocorticoid therapy. Recent guidelines, such as Group for the Respect of Ethics and Excellence in Science, suggest that this differentiation may not be necessary. All patients should be given calcium and vitamin D [19].

Treatment with oral bisphosphonates

Risedronate and alendronate have been shown to increase bone density compared with placebo in patients treated with glucocorticoids, with a reduction in the risk of new vertebral fractures. Alendronate was compared with a placebo in a trial of patients who had received glucocorticoids for greater than 3 months [20, 21] and a group that had received glucocorticoids for less than 3 months. In these studies, there was a BMD increase of the lumbar spine of 2% to 3% in patients receiving 5–10 mg of alendronate daily versus a loss of 0.5% in the placebo group after 1 year, with a 1% increase in femoral neck on treatment versus –1% with placebo therapy. These data revealed a 40% relative risk reduction [20, 21]. Fewer new vertebral fractures occurred in the alendronate groups; however, the number of events was very small. There were only two in the alendronate group and three in the placebo group. Risedronate was studied in two trials, a prevention trial and a treatment trial [22, 23]. Combining data, the relative risk of vertebral fracture was reduced by 70%. Risedronate has been approved to prevent and treat GIO, whereas alendronate has only received approval to treat GIO. In the risedronate treatment trial, lumbar spine BMD increased 2.7% and femoral neck BMD increased 1.8% in patients taking risedronate, whereas no change occurred in the placebo group.

Treatment with other agents

Calcitonin has been shown to prevent glucocorticoid-induced bone loss by injection or intranasally; no data has shown that it reduces fracture risk [24, 25]. Raloxifene has been shown to prevent glucocorticoid induced bone loss [26].

Treatment with intravenous bisphosphonates

The safety and efficacy of intravenous zoledronic acid was recently compared to oral risedronate in the prevention and treatment of GIO [27]. A single 5-mg infusion of zoledronate and daily oral risedronate, 5 mg, were compared in a 1-year randomized, double-blind, double-dummy study of patients with less than 3 months' exposure to glucocorticoids and those in treatment for longer than 3 months. There were about 150 patients in each group in the prevention population and 270 in the treatment population. After 12 months, lumbar spine BMD increased significantly more with zoledronate than risedronate in the two subpopulations. For example, in the treatment population zoledronate increased lumbar spine BMD 4.1% versus 2.7% with risedronate ($P = 0.0001$); in the prevention population, zoledronate increased lumbar BMD 2.6% versus risedronate 0.6% ($P < 0.0001$). Zoledronate was also more effective than risedronate in terms of increasing BMD at the femoral neck, trochanter, and total hip. This superior effect was apparent at 6 months. Zoledronate reduced a resorption marker, serum C-terminal collagen crosslinked telopeptide of type 1 collagen(serum CTX) significantly more than risedronate in the treatment and prevention population [27]. Researchers found a significant correlation between the lumbar spine BMD change and serum biomarkers at 12 months. The results indicate that a single infusion of zoledronate suppresses bone turnover significantly more than daily oral risedronate for up to 1 year in different subgroups of patients with GIO. Bone markers were suppressed as early as days 9–11 and throughout the 12 months of study onward. Sambrook [28] reported similar positive results in 265 men randomized to risedronate or zoledronic acid, concluding that once yearly zoledronic acid increased BMD within one year to a greater extent than risedronate.

Treatment with bone formation agents

Saag *et al.* [29] reported results of a 36-month clinical trial in patients who had taken glucocorticoids for at least 3 months and were randomized to recombinant human parathyroid hormone (rhPTH (1-34)) daily by subcutaneous injections or alendronate, 70-mg tablets by mouth, once a week. The two treatment groups had gains in lumbar spine BMD, 5.3% in the alendronate comparative group versus 11.0% in the teriparatide group. Femoral neck BMD gains compared to baseline were 2.6% with alendronate and 5.1% with teriparatide. Fewer patients had new radiographic vertebral fractures in the teriparatide group, 1.7% (3/173), versus the alendronate group of 7.7% (13/169, $P = 0.007$). The number of patients with new vertebral fractures was not significantly different between the two groups. The two treatments were generally well tolerated. These data suggest that in patients at high risk for fracture, an anabolic agent may be preferred.

Guidelines for managing GIO

Several groups have published guidelines for the management of GIO [9, 30, 31]. The publication of guidelines by numerous groups reflects the variations in the availability of screening tools, DEXA scanning, as well as racial, and ethnic differences in fracture risk and the availability of pharmaceutical interventions.

In 2001, the American College of Rheumatology (ACR) published guidelines for the management of GIO. These guidelines were updated in 2010 using the RAND/UCLA method of guideline development [30]. The hallmark of these guidelines is the recommendation for treatment based on the risk of fracture. The guidelines discuss two methods of assessing risk of fracture: they provide descriptive case examples to assign risk of fracture and also use the FRAX tool to assess fracture risk. Based on the risk of fracture calculated by either of these methods, patients are classified as being at low, medium or high risk for fracture. Treatment recommendations are then made based on the dose and duration of steroid exposure (summarized in Figure 6.1).

The treatment recommendations for postmenopausal women and men over 50 who are at high risk, follows guidelines from the National Osteoporosis Foundation (NOF) to treat anyone with a FRAX determined risk for fracture >20% over 10 years. Hence, duration of exposure <1 month warrants treatment in this group. In the low- and medium-risk patients, treatment recommendations are based on an anticipated duration of glucocorticoid treatment of over 3 months, and the dose is calculated as the average intended dose over that period of time.

Premenopausal women and men <50 years of age are also addressed with a separate set of guidelines, given that the FRAX tool is not validated in these groups of patients. Additionally, the long-term safety of pharmacologic agents in this group are not clear, and hence recommendations for treatment are made only for those at clearly the highest risk of fracture in this group of patients. Additionally, for women of childbearing potential, those drugs with shorter half life have been recommended (see Figure 6.2).

These criteria are particularly relevant to the United States where bone density testing is freely available. The major limitations of the 2010 ACR guidelines are also the limitations of the FRAX tool, which are summarized in an earlier part of this chapter. These include the possible underestimation of spinal fracture risk using the FRAX, as well as underestimation

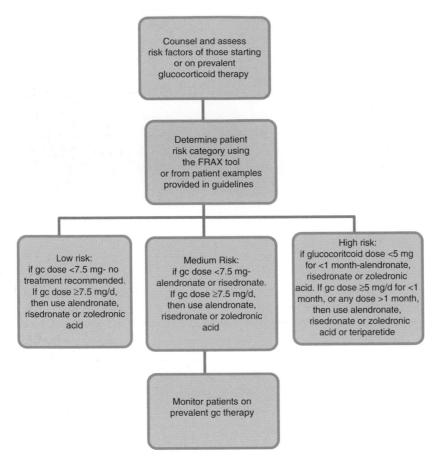

Figure 6.1 The ACR guidelines for the treatment of GIO in post-menopausal women and in men ≥50 years of age. For low and medium risk patients, the duration of glucocorticoid (gc) exposure is assumed to be >3 months.

of fracture risk when higher than the average dose of steroid is used. A correction factor for the FRAX tool based on the dose of steroid used has been suggested and will likely need to be added when these guidelines are updated [8]. Additionally, these guidelines do not address the incremental risk that specific diseases such as rheumatoid arthritis add to the absolute fracture risk of fracture in GIO.

IOF guidelines

The ACR guidelines assume that DEXA screening is freely available. However, in several countries in Europe and the rest of the world, DEXA

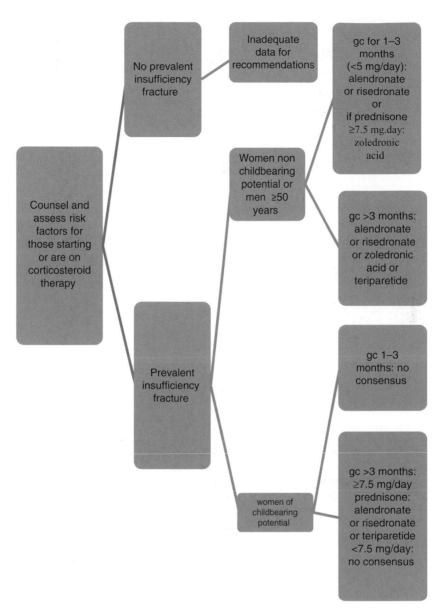

Figure 6.2 The ACR guidelines for the treatment of GIO in premenopausal women and in men <50 years of age. Gc, glucocorticoids; pred, prednisone.

screening is either limited in availability or not available at all. Recognizing these discrepancies, in 2012, the International Osteoporosis Foundation published a framework for the development of guidelines for GIO for individual countries and regions. Guidance for the management of GIO will vary between countries because of differences in resources, availability, and cost of treatment as well as health care policies. Hence, a unified

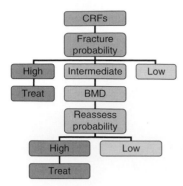

Figure 6.3 Management algorithm for the assessment of individuals at risk of fracture. (*Source*: Lekamwasam S. (2012) [9]).

set of guidelines is not recommended; rather the document encourages the development of local guidelines in each country or region based on their recommendations.

A general approach to risk assessment as advocated by the National Osteoporosis guideline Group is recommended as shown in Figure 6.3 [9]. Fracture probability and risk categorization based on age, sex, BMI and clinical risk factors is shown. Those patients at high risk are offered treatment without BMD testing. Those patients at low risk do not need to be offered treatment and BMD testing is not required. The size of the intermediate group will vary in different countries, and DEXA testing is helpful in risk assessment of this group.

In this document, while FRAX remains an important method of fracture risk assessment, several limitations of FRAX and adjustments are discussed and adjustments are suggested. Adjustments for higher or lower than average daily doses of prednisone have been advocated for postmenopausal women and men aged ≥50 years. For hip fracture, these are 0.65 for <2.5 mg/d and 1.20 for ≥7.5 mg/d and for major osteoporotic fracture, 0.8 and 1.15, respectively. For high doses of glucocorticoids, greater upward adjustment of fracture probability may be required [32]. Additionally the guidelines emphasize the limitations of FRAX in the assessment of GIO (whether with or without adjustment) in underestimating the risk of vertebral fractures. Other adjustments to FRAX estimated probabilities based on ancillary clinical information such as high falls risk, multiple prior fractures, immobility or severe rheumatoid arthritis are suggested [33]. FRAX does not specifically assess the risk of vertebral fractures, a risk that is prominent in patients treated with glucocorticoids. While an algorithm has been suggested to adjust the fracture risk estimates based on differences between hip and spine BMD, it is unclear if this correction captures the total increased risk of vertebral fractures seen in patients treated with glucocorticoids.

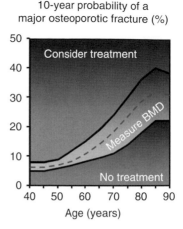

10-year probability of a
major osteoporotic fracture (%)

Figure 6.4 Assessment guidelines of the UK
National Osteoporosis Guideline Group based
on the ten-year probability of a major fracture
(%). The dotted line denotes the intervention
threshold where assessment is made in the
absence of BMD, a BMD test is recommended
for individuals where the probability
assessment lies in the mid region. Adapted
from [9]. Note that virtually all patients on
corticosteroids fall into the "measure BMD" or
"consider treatment" groups.

National guidelines for the treatment of GIO have been published in several countries including Canada, France, Italy, Spain and the UK. The IOF
document does not prescribe a set intervention threshold for treatment of
GIO. In the UK, the intervention threshold in women without a prior fracture is set at the age-specific fracture probability equivalent (using FRAX)
to a woman with a prior fracture and thus rises with age [34]. Using these
criteria as an example, the intervention threshold will vary from country
to country because the risks of fracture and death vary.

An example of a strategy that has been adopted in the UK is used to
highlight the approach that can be applied based on the resources available (see Figure 6.4). If no access to BMD is available, assessment of fracture probability is determined using FRAX and treatment considered in
those in whom the fracture probability lies above the intervention threshold. If access to DXA is available, the use of FRAX is used to determine not
only the fracture probability at which one needs to intervene (intervention threshold) but also the fracture probability for BMD testing (assessment thresholds) [34, 35]. Assessment thresholds for the UK are shown in
Figure 6.4.

If limited access to DXA is available, those with fracture probabilities
above the lower assessment threshold but below the upper assessment
threshold can be considered for BMD testing and their fracture probability reassessed. Treatment can then be considered in those with a fracture probability above the intervention threshold. If unlimited access to
DXA is available, all those with fracture probabilities above the lower
assessment threshold can be considered for BMD testing and their fracture
probability reassessed. Treatment can then be considered in those with a
fracture probability above the intervention threshold.

Based on the example from the UK, all patients over 70 years, those on doses of steroids >7.5 mg and those with prior fragility fractures should be considered for treatment. FRAX is then used to determine the fracture risk and in those who are above the intervention threshold treatment is initiated and in those above the assessment threshold, DEXA scanning is performed and those above the intervention threshold are treated. After treatment is initiated, continued monitoring is recommended.

The intervention threshold in the ACR guidelines for treatment of GIO in those with a fracture risk of 10–20% is lower than that suggested in the IOF framework. However, the IOF framework provides tool for the development of guidelines that are more suitable to the local conditions. As with all guidelines, these sets of guidelines are limited by the quality of clinical evidence that is available and will likely need to updated in the near future.

References

1 Diez-Perez A, Hooven FH, Adachi JD, *et al.* (2001) Regional differences in treatment for osteoporosis. *The Global Longitudinal Study of Osteoporosis in Women* [GLOW] *Bone* [in press].

2 Van Staa TP, Leufkens HG, Abenhaim L, Zhang B, Cooper C (2000) Use of oral corticosteroids and risk of fractures. *J Bone Miner Res* **15**: 933–1000.

3 Van Staa TP, Leufkens HG, Cooper C (2002) The epidemiology of corticosteroid-induced osteoporosis: a meta-analysis. *Osteoporos Int* **13**: 777–87.

4 Van Staa TP, Leufkens HG, Cooper C (2001) Use of inhaled corticosteroids and risk of fractures. *J Bone Miner Res* **16**: 581–8.

5 de Vries F, Bracke M, Leufkens HG, Lammers JW, Cooper C, van Staa TP (2007) Fracture risk with intermittent high-dose oral glucocorticoid therapy. *Arthritis Rheum* **56**: 208–14.

6 Silverman S, Lane NE (2009) Glucocorticoid induced osteoporosis. *Current Osteoporosis Reports* **7**: 23–6.

7 Kanis JA on behalf of the World Health Organization Scientific Group (2009) *Assessment of Osteoporosis at the Primary-care Level. Technical Report.* http://www.shefacuk /FRAX/indexhtm(accessed 15 August 2011).

8 Kanis JA, Johansson H, Oden A, McCloskey E (2011) Guidance for the adjustment of FRAX according to the dose of glucocorticoids. *Osteoporos Int* **22**: 809–16.

9 Lekawasam S, Adachi JD, Agnusdii D, *et al.* (2012) A Framework for the development of guidelines for management of glucocorticoid induced osteoporosis. IOF/ECTS GIO Guidelines working group. *Osteoporos Int,* epub.

10 Weinstein RS, O'Brien CA, Almeida M, *et al.* (2011) Osteoprogerin prevents glucocorticoid induced osteoporosis in mice. *Endocronology* **152**: 3323–31.

11 Yao W, Cheng Z, Busse C, *et al.* (2008) Glucocorticoid excess in mice results in early activation of osteoclastogenesis and adipogenesis and prolonged suppression of osteogenesis: a longitudinal study of gene expression in bone tissue from glucocorticoid-treated mice. *Arthritis Rheum* **58**: 1674–86.

12 Dalle Carbonare L, Arlot ME, Chavassieux PM, *et al.* (2001) Comparison of tra-
    becular bone microarchitecture and remodeling in glucocorticoid-induced and post-
    menopausal osteoporosis. *J Bone Miner Res* **16**: 87–103.

13 Baron R, Rawadi G (2007) Targeting the Wnt/beta-catenin pathway to regulate bone
    formation in the adult skeleton. *Endocrinology* **148**: 2635–2643.

14 Ohnaka K, Tanabe M, Kawate H, *et al.* (2005) Glucocorticoid suppresses the canon-
    ical Wnt signal in cultured human osteoblasts. *Biochem Biophys Res Commun* **329**:
    177–81.

15 Wang FS, Ko JY, Yeh DW, Ke HC, wu HL (2008) Modulation of Dickkopf-1 attenu-
    ates glucocorticoid induction of osteoblast apoptosis, adipocytic differentiation, and
    bone mass loss. *Endocrinology* **149**: 1793–1801.

16 Weinstein RS, Jilka RL, Parfitt AM, Manolagas SC (1998) Inhibition of osteoblasto-
    gensis and promotion of apoptosis of osteoblasts and osteocytes by glucocorticoids.
    Potential mechanisms of their deleterious effects on bone. *J Clin Invest* **102**: 274–82.

17 Lane NE, Luckert B (1998) The science and therapy of glucocorticoid induced bone
    loss. *Endocrinol Metab Clinic North Amer* **27**(2): 465–83.

18 Lane NE, Yao W, Balooch M, *et al.* (2006) Glucocorticoid-treated mice have localized
    changes in trabecular bone material properties and osteocyte lacunar size that are not
    observed in placebo-treated or estrogen-deficient mice. *J Bone Miner Res* **21**: 466–76.

19 Compston J, Reid DM, Boisdron J, *et al.* (2008) Recommendations for the registration
    of agents and prevention and treatment of glucocorticoid-induced osteoporosis: an
    update from the Group for the Respect of Ethics and Excellence in Science. *Osteoporos
    Int* **19**: 1247–50.

20 Saag KG, Emkey R, Schnitzer TJ, *et al.* (1998) Alendronate for the prevention and
    treatment of glucocorticoids-induced osteoporosis. Glucocorticoids-Induced Osteo-
    porosis Intervention Study Group. *N Engl J Med* **339**: 292–9.

21 Adachi JD, Saag KG, Delmas PD, *et al.* (2001) Two-year effects of alendronate on
    bone mineral density and vertebral fracture in patients receiving glucocorticoids:
    a randomized, double-blind, placebo-controlled extension trial. *Arthritis Rheum* **44**:
    202–11.

22 Reid DM, Hughes RA, Laan RF, *et al.* (2000) Efficacy and safety of daily risedronate in
    the treatment of corticosteroid-induced osteoporosis in men and women: a random-
    ized trial. European Corticosteroid-Induced Osteoporosis Treatment Study. *J Bone
    Mine Res* **15**: 1006–13.

23 Cohen S, Levy RM, Keller M, *et al.* (1999) Risedronate therapy prevents
    corticosteroid-induced bone loss: a twelve-month, multicenter, randomized, double-
    blind, placebo-controlled, parallel-group study. *Arthritis Rheum* **42**: 2309–18.

24 Luengo M, Pons F, Marrtinez de Osaba MJ, Picado C (1994) Prevention of further
    bone mass loss by nasal calcitonin in patients on long term glucocortipoids therapy
    for asthma: a two-year follow up study. *Thorax* **49**: 1099–1102.

25 Montemurro L, Schiraldi G, Fraioli P, *et al.* (1991) Prevention of corticosteroid-
    induced osteoporosis with salmon calcitonin in sarcoid patients. *Calcif Tissue Int* **49**:
    71–6.

26 Mok CC, Ying KY, To CH, *et al.* (2011) Raloxifene for prevention of glucocorticoid
    induced bone loss: a 12 month randomized double blinded placebo controlled trial.
    Ann Rheum Dis **70**: 778–84.

27 Sambrook PN, Roux C, Devogelaer JP, Saag K, Lau CS, Reginster JY, Bucci-Rechtweg
    C, Su G, Reid DM (2012) Bisphosphonates and glucocorticoid osteoporosis in men:
    results of a randomized controlled trial comparing zoledronic acid with risedronate.
    Bone **50**(1): 289–95. Epub 2011 Oct 29. Erratum in: Bone. 2012 Mar; 50(3): 811.

28 P Roux C, Reid DM, Devogelaer JP, Saag K, Lau CS, Reginster JY, Papanastasiou P, Bucci-Rechtweg C, Su G, Sambrook PN (2012) Post hoc analysis of a single IV infusion of zoledronic acid versus daily oral risedronate on lumbar spine bone mineral density in different subgroups with glucocorticoid-induced osteoporosis.*Osteoporos Int* **23**(3): 1083–90.

29 Saag K, Shane E, Boonen S, *et al.* (2007) Teriparatide or alendronate in glucocorticoid induced osteoporosis. *N Engl J Med* **357**: 2028–39.

30 American College of Rheumatology ad hoc Committee on Glucocorticoid-induced Osteoporosis (2011). Recommendations for the prevention and treatment of glucocorticoid-induced osteoporosis: 2001 update. *Arthritis Rheum* **44**: 1496–1503.

31 Devogelaer JP *et al.* (2006) Evidence-based guidelines for the prevention and treatment of glucocorticoid-induced osteoporosis: a consensus document of the Belgian Bone Club. *Osteoporos Int* **17**: 8–19, doi:10.1007/s00198-005-2032-z.

32 Leib ES *et al.* (2011) Official Positions for FRAX((R)) clinical regarding glucocorticoids: the impact of the use of glucocorticoids on the estimate by FRAX((R)) of the 10 year risk of fracture from Joint Official Positions Development Conference of the International Society for Clinical Densitometry and International Osteoporosis Foundation on FRAX((R)). *J Clin Densitom* **14**: 212–19, doi:S1094-6950(11)00126-0 [pii]10.1016/j.jocd.2011.05.014.

33 Kanis JA *et al.* (2011) Interpretation and use of FRAX in clinical practice. *Osteoporos Int* **22**: 2395–2411, doi:10.1007/s00198-011-1713-z.

34 Kanis JA *et al.* (2008) Case finding for the management of osteoporosis with FRAX® – Assessment and intervention thresholds for the UK. *Osteoporos Int* **19**: 1395–1408; Erratum 2009 *Osteoporos Int* **20**: 499–502.

35 Compston JE *et al.* (2009) Guidelines for the diagnosis and management of osteoporosis in postmenopausal women and men from the age of 50 years in the UK. *Maturitas* **62**: 105–8.

CHAPTER 7

Secondary Causes of Osteoporosis: Other Medications

Diane M. Biskobing
Virginia Commonwealth University School of Medicine, Richmond, VA, USA

Introduction

Osteoporosis is a skeletal disorder characterized by a decrease in bone mass and quality leading to increased fracture risk. Osteoporosis is diagnosed using bone densitometry which compares the bone mineral density (BMD) of the patient to that of a young, healthy adult matched for gender and race (T-score). Low bone mass is defined as a T-score between –1.0 and –2.5 and osteoporosis is a T-score less than–2.5 [1]. Low BMD is recognized as a strong risk factor for fracture. When a patient is identified with low bone mass or osteoporosis, secondary causes must be considered. One such cause is medical therapies that are used for a variety of other indications. Osteoporosis and fractures can be attributed to a multitude of pharmacologic agents. The medications most commonly associated with bone loss and fracture are glucocorticoids which were discussed in Chapter 6. However, bone loss and fractures are also seen with a number of other commonly prescribed medications which are discussed in this chapter. The most common medications that can lead to bone loss are shown in Table 7.1.

Aromatase inhibitors

Aromatase is the enzyme that converts androgens to estrogens. Aromatase inhibitors (AI) are commonly used as adjunct therapy or to prevent recurrence in postmenopausal women with estrogen receptor positive breast cancer [2]. Included in this category of agents are anastrazole, letrozole, and exemestrane. Because these agents significantly decrease estrogen levels in postmenopausal women, bone turnover is accelerated [3]. In a study comparing anastrazole and tamoxifene alone or in combination, both bone

Osteoporosis: Diagnosis and Management, First Edition. Edited by Dale W. Stovall.
© 2013 John Wiley & Sons, Ltd. Published 2013 by John Wiley & Sons, Ltd.

Table 7.1 Medications
that cause osteoporosis.

Aromatase inhibitors
Anti-depressants
Anti-epileptics
Calcineurin inhibitors
Depot medroxyprogesterone
GnRH agonists
Proton pump inhibitors
Thiazolidinediones

resorption and formation markers were significantly increased in the anastrazole alone group compared to tamoxifene alone [4]. The enhanced bone turnover resulted in decreased bone density as well: spine BMD decreased 4% and hip 3.2% after 2 years of anastrazole compared to a gain of 1.9% at the spine and 1.2% at the hip with tamoxifen, a selective estrogen receptor modulator (SERM) [4]. The nonrandomized controls showed minimal change in BMD. Bone loss was greatest in women within 4 years of menopause. The BMD loss in these patients leads to increased fracture risk as seen in multiple studies [5]. A large 5-year clinical trial comparing letrozole to tamoxifene reported a 40% increase in fracture rate in the letrozole group [6]. In a ten-year follow up study that included women who had received either 5 years of anastrazole or tamoxifene, increased fractures in the anastrazole arm were reported during treatment, but no difference in fractures were reported during the follow up period off active drug [7]. These findings led to the recommendation by the European Society for Clinical and Economical aspects of Osteoporosis that all women receiving AI should be evaluated for fracture risk. In addition, they recommended that all women on AI aged 75 years or older as well as women with osteoporosis or a FRAX 10 year risk of hip fracture of 3% or greater be placed on osteoporosis treatment [2]. Both oral and intravenous bisphosphonates have been shown to prevent bone loss when used concurrently with AI [3]. Recently, denosumab has also been shown to be effective in preventing AI-associated bone loss [8].

Antidepressants

In 2010 antidepressants were the second most commonly prescribed therapeutic drug class in the US [9]. In this class, selective serotonin reuptake inhibitors (SSRI) are more commonly prescribed because of perceived fewer side effects. Antidepressants have been reported to be associated with decreases in BMD as well as an increased rate of fractures [10]. SSRI users exhibited higher rates of bone loss compared to tricyclic antidepressants (TCA) users or controls in the Study of Osteoporotic Fractures [11]. Despite this, Liu *et al.* reported increased hip fracture risk with current use of both TCA as well as SSRI [12]. Some studies suggested that higher fracture risk is associated with antidepressants that have a higher affinity for the serotonin reuptake transporter [13,14] whereas other studies have not demonstrated a difference in risk based on affinity for the transporter [15]. A recent meta-analysis reported a relative risk for fracture of 1.72 (1.51–1.95, 95% CI) with use of SSRI [10]. Depression itself has been associated with increased fracture risk but even after adjustment for depression, use of SSRI still confer increased fracture risk [10].

The mechanism for increased fracture risk associated with antidepressants is not entirely clear. One hypothesis is that antidepressants use results in less physical activity leading to unloading induced bone loss. However, Warden *et al.* was unable to confirm this theory in a mouse model [16]. They demonstrated that while neither SSRI nor TCA treatment impacted activity levels in mice, both treatments negatively impact bone mass. Serotonin receptors are found on osteoblasts, osteocytes, and osteoclasts [17]. Mice deficient in $5HT_{2B}$ receptor exhibit bone loss due to decreased osteoblast number [17]. In vivo animal studies show decreased bone formation with SSRI use [16, 18, 19]. Effects on bone resorption are mixed; two studies showed no effect of SSRI on osteoclast number or activity [16,19] whereas another study showed increased osteoclast number with high dose fluoxetine treatment [18]. Taken together, these data suggest SSRI negatively impact osteoblast formation and function leading to diminished bone formation with minimal impact on bone resorption.

Anti-epileptic drugs

Patients with seizure disorders are known to have an increased rate of fractures. Furthermore, anti-epileptic drugs (AED) are associated with bone loss and increased fracture risk. In one study, over 10% of both men and women of less than 50 years of age who were treated with long-term AED therapy were found to have osteoporosis as compared to an expected rate of 0.6% [20]. Multiple studies have shown a 2–6 fold increase in fracture risk associated with AED use [21]. In addition, the risk of fracture increases progressively with increasing duration and cumulative dose of AED [22] and the number of AEDs prescribed [23]. More specifically, greater than 12 years of AED use has been shown to result in a relative risk for fracture of 4.15 (95% CI 2.71–6.34) [22]. Some studies have shown that the increased risk for fractures associated with AEDs only occurs with enzyme inducing AEDs while other studies have not shown a difference between enzyme inducers and noninducers [22, 24]. In a large case-control study, increased fractures were seen with carbamazepine, valproate, phenobarbital, and phenytoin monotherapy but not with lamotrigine [22]. Fracture rates were 60% higher with the use of more than one AED as compared to monotherapy [22].

The mechanism for bone loss due to AED use is not clear. Animal studies and in vitro studies show increased bone turnover with phenytoin treatment [25, 26]. Markers of bone metabolism in subjects on long-term AED therapy display elevated bone formation and resorption makers consistent with increased bone turnover [27]. Early reports in patients on long-term AED therapy reported decreased 25-hydroxyvitamin D with development of secondary hyperparathyroidism. Some recent studies have confirmed these findings [28]; however, other studies have not shown vitamin D deficiency in this population of patients [29]. Furthermore, treatment with calcium and vitamin D has not been shown to decrease fracture rate in patients taking AEDs [30]. Other proposed mechanisms include alteration of vitamin K metabolism, decreased calcitonin and IGF-1 levels and increased homocysteine [21]. However, the clinical impact of these alterations has not been well studied.

Calcineurin inhibitors

Calcineurin inhibitors such as cyclosporine and tacrolimus are immune modulators commonly used in transplant patients [31]. The impact of calcineurin inhibitors on bone stems from the role of calcineurin in normal bone metabolism. Calcineurin Aα knock-out mice exhibit significantly decreased BMD characterized by reduced bone formation attributed to a reduction in osteoblast differentiation [32]. In addition, calcineurin is also necessary for normal osteoclast differentiation [33]. In vivo animal studies have shown increased bone resorption and bone loss with both cyclosporine and tacrolimus [34, 35]. However, understanding the effects of these agents posttransplant is complex since most patients are initially treated with combination immunosuppression including glucocorticoids making it difficult to determine the effect of a single agent. Thiebaldl et al. demonstrated high bone turner exhibited by elevated osteocalcin levels up to 18 months after heart transplant [36]. They attributed the elevated levels of osteocalcin to cyclosprorin therapy since glucocorticoids are known to suppress bone formation. One retrospective study in renal transplant patients showed a similar degree of bone loss in patients treated with cyclosporine monotherapy versus prednisolone and azathioprine therapy [37]. The degree of bone loss associated with tacrolimus appears to be comparable to cyclosporine [31]. In addition to significant bone loss associated with these agents there is an increased risk of fracture. In a retrospective study, 59% of patients experienced a fracture after solid organ transplant [38]. The fractures occurred between 5 and 80 months after transplant. All patients in this study were treated with glucocorticoids for the first 6 months posttransplant but were transitioned to a glucocorticoid sparing immunosuppressive regimen thereafter. The fracture risk was increased 10–15 fold in men and 20–30 fold in women despite the use of the glucocorticoid sparing regimen [38]. These results imply that immunosuppressive agents incur increased fracture risk independent of glucocorticoids.

Depot medroxyprogesterone acetate

Depot medroxyprogesterone acetate (DMPA) is a long-acting contraceptive used frequently in teens and young adults to improve compliance with contraception. It is administered as a once every 90-day intramuscular injection. DMPA decreases serum gonadotropin levels through negative feedback resulting in decreased ovarian estradiol production [39]. As a result bone turnover is increased leading to a decreased BMD. Because DMPA is often used during a time when many woman are still accruing bone mass, there is concern that prolonged use of DMPA negatively impacts peak BMD accrual. Harel *et al.* prospectively studied BMD in 12–18 year old girls for up to 60 months after initiating DMPA therapy [40]. They found that 47% of the subjects lost less than 5% of their BMD, 16% lost between 5% and 8%, and 37% lost more than 8% of their BMD. Subjects who received a greater number of DMPA injections displayed higher rates of bone loss [40]. Clark confirmed these findings in an older group of women aged 18–35 who were followed prospectively over 2 years after initiation of therapy [41]. At two years, BMD at the spine and hip were decreased by 5.7% compared to a stable BMD seen in nonusers [41]. However, multiple studies have demonstrated recovery of BMD after discontinuation of DMPA. More specifically, teenage girls who stopped DMPA after 5 years of use showed recovery of bone mass at all sites over the following 5 years [40]. Calcium intake did not significantly impact the recovery of bone mass (Figure 7.1). Other studies in older woman also demonstrated recovery of BMD to near baseline after discontinuation [42]. Finally, two studies have demonstrated no difference in BMD in postmenopausal women who used DMPA compared to nonusers [39, 43]. Ultimately however, the long-term effect of DMPA on fracture risk was the primary concern which led to an FDA black box warning for DMPA. Unfortunately, data on fracture risk after DMPA use is sparse. Meier *et al.* reported on a case-control study of fracture risk related

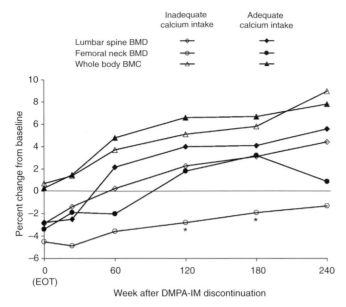

Figure 7.1 Recovery of BMD and BMC shown as mean percent change in BMD and BMC from the end of treatment (EOT) with DMP. Also shown is the effect of calcium intake on BMD and BMC recovery. Calcium intake did not significantly impact BMD recovery after adjusting for end of treatment BMD and risk factors. (*Source:* Harel Z, Cole Johnson C, Gold, MA *et al.* (2010) [40]).

to current or previous use of DMPA [44]. Current use of three or more DMPA prescriptions significantly increased the odds ratio (OR) of sustaining a fracture in all age groups. Past use of DMPA also resulted in a significantly increased OR of fracture but appeared to be dependent on age. Increased fracture risk was only seen in women greater than 30 years of age with past use of 10 or more DMPA prescriptions (ibid). The difference in risk between age groups is likely a reflection of recovery of bone mass in the younger women. To summarize, significant bone loss is seen across all age groups with the use of DPMA use and increasing length of therapy is associated with increased bone loss. However, recovery of BMD is seen after discontinuation of therapy and postmenopausal women with past use of DPMA do not on average have lower BMD than nonusers. Concerning though is the small increase in fractures seen in current users as well as past users over the age of 30.

GnRH agonists

Long acting gonadotropin releasing hormone (GnRH) agonists are used for sex hormone responsive conditions such as prostate cancer in men and endometriosis in women. These agents result in markedly reduced gonadotropin levels leading to hypogonadism and enhanced bone turnover. GnRH agonists are typically given as an intramuscular depot injection over several months of treatment. In prostate cancer, treatment leads to significant bone loss within 12 months of initiating therapy with an average bone loss at the total hip of 3.3% [45]. Long-term, the degree of bone loss correlates with the number of years on therapy for prostate cancer [46]. In addition, fracture rate is significantly increased in prostate cancer patients treated with GnRH agonists [47, 48]. A large retrospective study of men with prostate cancer demonstrated that fracture risk rises progressively with an increasing number of doses of GnRH agonists [47]. More than nine doses resulted in a fracture risk similar to orchiectomy. A similar study in Sweden showed a 60% increase in fracture risk with GnRH agonist therapy [48]. The effects of GnRH agonists may be reversible with short-term treatment. Surrey *et al.* reported on a study in premenopausal women with endometriosis who were randomized to leuprolide acetate alone or in combination with estrogen and/or progesterone [49]. At the end of treatment, women treated with leuprolide alone lost 5.4% BMD at the spine compared to a 1.2% decrease with addition of norethinedrone and no loss with the addition of estrogen plus norethinedrone [49]. After completion of therapy, follow-up BMD showed recovery, although BMD remained significantly lower than baseline in the leuprolide alone group. A six-year study in the United Kingdom, though, showed no difference in BMD between women who had previously received goserelin alone compared to goserelin with estrogen and progesterone [50]. Therefore, it appears that the combination of estrogen and progestin therapy, commonly referred to as ad-back therapy, can prevent bone loss associated with the use of GNRH agonists.

Proton pump inhibitors

Proton pump inhibitors (PPI) were introduced in 1989 and are commonly prescribed for suppression of gastric acid production in the management of gastroesophageal reflux, dyspepsia, and peptic ulcer disease [51]. In 2010, 53 million prescriptions were written for omeprozole, making it the 6th most frequently prescribed medication in the United States [9]. In 2011, the FDA raised concerns about potential increased risk of fractures with long term use of PPI [52]. The FDA advisory board noted evidence of increased fracture rate in long-term users of PPI. The advisory was based on results from seven epidemiologic studies; six reported an increased fracture risk associated with PPI use [53–58]. A recent meta-analysis, using the seven studies cited by the FDA as well as 4 others, reported a relative risk for any fracture of 1.16 (95% CI 1.02–1.32), hip fracture of 1.3 (95% CI 1.19–1.43), and vertebral fracture of 1.56 (95% CI 1.31–1.85) [51]. In addition several of these studies demonstrated increasing risk for fracture with increasing duration of PPI use [57, 58, 59] and/or increasing dose of PPI [55, 57, 61].

The purported primary mechanism for the PPI-associated increase fracture risk is related to the effects of acid suppression on calcium absorption. In vitro calcium carbonate dissolution is dependent on an acidic environment. To study the effect of proton pump inhibition on calcium absorption, O'Connell performed a randomized, crossover trial [60]. Subjects were given either placebo or omeprozole and 400 units of vitamin D daily for 7 days. Radiolabeled calcium absorption was then measured after an overnight fast. Fractional calcium absorption fell from 9.1% with placebo to 3.5% after omeprozole demonstrating a significant decrease in calcium absorption after just one week of PPI therapy (Figure 7.2) [60]. Mizinushi *et al.* demonstrated decreased calcium absorption in men who were switched from a H2 blocker to PPI with a subsequent increase in PTH and markers of bone resorption and formation [61]. Despite these findings seen with PPI use, studies have been mixed regarding effects on

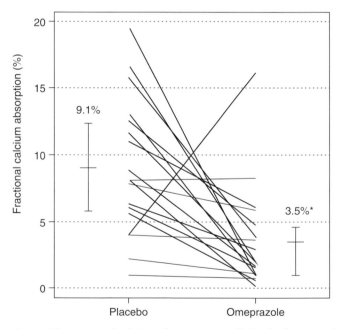

Figure 7.2 Fractional calcium absorption in individual subjects. Each subject was given 1 week of placebo followed by 1 week of omeprozole. P = 0.003 for difference between placebo and omeprozole. (*Source:* O'Connell M. *et al.* (2005) [60]).

BMD. One study reported that men taking PPIs had slightly lower total hip BMD compared to nonusers [54]. However, other studies have demonstrated that subjects taking PPIs do not have significantly lower BMD [58, 62]. Longitudinal studies evaluating rates of bone loss in users of PPIs also are mixed with two studies showing no difference in rates of bone loss between PPI users and nonusers [58, 62] and one study showing a diminished improvement in BMD with calcium and vitamin D treatment in PPI users compared to nonusers [54]. Many patients with osteoporosis treated with bisphosphonates are also taking PPIs. In a post-hoc analysis of three prospective clinical trials of the antifracture efficacy of risedronate (Vertebral Efficacy with Risedronate Trial – Multinational; Vertebral Efficacy with Risedronate Trial – North America; risedronate Hip Intervention Program), risedronate significantly decreased fractures in both PPI users and nonusers implying that bisphosphonate efficacy is not impaired by PPI use [63].

Thiazolidinediones

Thiazolidinediones (TZD) are frequently used in the management of type 2 DM. In 2007 the FDA reported increased fractures in women treated with TZD [64, 65]. These fractures were reported as adverse events in two large clinical trials of glucose control with TZD versus comparator diabetic therapy. In A Diabetes Outcome and Prevention Trial, women treated with rosiglitazone had a fracture rate of 2.74 per 100 person-years compared to 1.54 with metformin and 1.29 with glyburide [66]. Men did not exhibit a higher rate of fracture with either drug. In a study to investigate the effects of TZDs on bone metabolism, nondiabetic postmenopausal women were randomized to placebo or rosiglitazone for 14 weeks. Woman receiving rosiglitazone showed lower levels of bone formation markers with no effect on bone resorption markers. BMD at the spine and hip significantly declined compared to placebo [67]. A separate study in postmenopausal women with type 2 DM randomized to rosiglitazone or placebo confirmed these findings showing decreased levels of markers of bone formation [68]. After two years the women on rosiglitazone exhibited significantly greater bone loss at the spine and trochanter than women on placebo [68]. These results imply a direct effect of TZDs on osteoblast function resulting in decreased bone formation. There are few studies evaluating fracture risk with use of TZDs. A retrospective analysis of the clinical trials for rosiglitazone and pioglitazone did demonstrate increased number of fractures reported as adverse events [69]. A case control study showed a 57% increased fracture risk with greater than one year of TZD use in postmenopausal women greater than 65 years of age [70]. Men and women less than 65 years of age did not exhibit an accelerated risk of fracture.

The mechanism for the negative effects of TZD on bone derives from its impact on osteoblast differentiation. TZDs activate PPARγ (peroxisome proliferator-activated receptor gamma), a member of the nuclear receptor superfamily of transcription factors [71]. In this role, PPARγ appears to be a significant regulator of bone cell differentiation. Osteoblasts evolve from pluripotent mesenchymal stem cells that have the potential to enter the osteoblast or adipocyte differentiation pathway. Activation of PPARγ inhibits osteoblast differentiation and promotes adipocyte formation. In addition, PPARγ has been shown to affect both osteocytes and osteoclasts. In vitro, treatment of osteocytes with TZDs leads to increased apoptosis and increased production of sclerostin, a potent inhibitor of bone formation [72]. Interestingly, the effect of TZDs on osteocytes can be prevented by the addition of estradiol to the cell culture [72]. An in vivo animal study showed decreased bone density in mice treated with rosiglitazone [73]. Further analysis showed decreased osteoblast numbers and markers of bone formation due to accelerated apoptosis of both osteocytes and osteoblasts. There was no impact on osteoclast numbers or function [73]. In summary, these studies demonstrate that TZDs have a direct effect on osteoblast formation and survival as well as osteocyte survival resulting in decreased bone formation.

Summary

Many commonly prescribed medications impact bone health and ultimately fracture risk. The mechanism for their effect on bone metabolism is summarized in Table 7.2. Most of the agents discussed accelerate bone turnover leading to bone loss and increased fracture risk. In these cases,

Table 7.2 Effect of medications on bone turnover.

Drug	Bone formation	Bone resorption
Aromatase inhibitors	↑	↑
Anti-depressants	↓	↔↑
Anti-epileptics	↑	↑
Calcineurin inhibitors	↑	↑
Depot medroxyprogesterone	↑	↑
GnRH agonists	↑	↑
Proton pump inhibitors	↑	↑
Thiazolidinediones	↓	↔

prevention or treatment of bone loss with antiresorptive agents such as bisphosphonates is an effective strategy. SSRIs and TZDs, though, appear to have a unique effect on bone formation by inhibiting osteoblast differentiation. In patients with underlying bone disease or at high risk for osteoporosis, these agents should be used with caution and awareness of their potential long-term adverse effects.

References

1 Watts N, Bilezekian J, Camacho P, *et al.* (2010) American Association of Clinical Endocrinologists medical guidelines for clinical practice for the diagnosis and treatment of postmenopausal osteoporosis. *Endocrin Prac* **16**(supp 3): 1–37.

2 Rizzoli R, Body J, DeCensi A, *et al.* (2012) Guidance for the prevention of bone loss and fractures in postmenopausal women treated with aromatase inhibitors for breast cancer: an ESCEO position paper. *Osteoporos Int* Jan 20 epub.

3 Geisler J, Lonning P (2010) Impact of aromatase inhibitors on bone health in breast cancer patients. *J Steroid Biochem Mol Biol* **118**: 294–9.

4 Eastell R, Hannon R, Cuzick J, *et al.* (2006) Effect of an aromatase inhibitor on BMD and bone turnover markers: 2-year results of the anastrozole, tamoxifen, alone or in combination (ATAC) trial. *J Bone Miner Res* **21**: 1215–23.

5 Lonning P, Geisler J (2008) Indications and limitations of third-generation aromatase inhibitors. *Expert Opin Investig Drugs* **17**: 723–39.

6 Rebaglio M, Sun Z, Price K, *et al.* (2009) Bone fractures among postmenopausal patients with endocrine-responsive early breast cancer treated with 5 years of letrozole or tamoxifen in the BIG 1-98 trial. *Annals of Oncology* **20**: 1489–98.

7 Cuzick J, Sestak I, Baum M, *et al.* (2010) Effect of anastrozole and tamoxifen as adjuvant treatment for early-stage breast cancer: 10-year analysis of the ATAC trial. *Lancet Oncol* **11**: 1135–41.

8 Ellis G, Bone H, Chlebowski R, *et al.* (2008) Randomized trial of denosumab in patients receiving adjuvant aromatase inhibitors for nonmetastatic breast cancer. *J Clin Oncol* **26**: 4875–82.

9 IMS Health Incorporated (2010) Top-line market data: 2010 top therapeutic class by US dispensed prescriptions. *IMS Health Incorporated.* http://www.imshealth. com/portal/site/ims/menuitem.5ad1c081663fdf9b41d84b903208c22a/?vgnextoid= fbc65890d33ee210VgnVCM10000071812ca2RCRD&vgnextfmt=default (accessed January 18, 2012).

10 Wu Q, Bencaz A, Hentz J, *et al.* (2012). Selective serotonin reuptake inhibitor treatment and risk of fractures: a meta-analysis of cohort and case-control studies. *Osteoporos Int* **23**: 365–75.

11 Diem S, Blackwell T, Stone K, *et al.* (2007) Use of antidepressants and rates of hip bone loss in older women. *Arch Intern Med* **167**: 1240–5.

12 Liu B, Anderson G, Mittmann N, *et al.* (1998) Use of selective serotonin-reuptake inhibitors or tricyclic antidepressants and risk of hip fractures in elderly people. *Lancet* **351**: 1303–7.

13 Bolton J, Metge C, Lix L, *et al.* (2008) Fracture risk from psychotropic medications: a population-based analysis. *J Clin Psychopharmacol* **38**: 384–91.

14 Verdel M, Souverein P, Egberts T, *et al.* (2010) Antidepressant drugs and risk of osteoporotic and non-osteoporotic fractures. *Bone* **47**: 604–9.

15 Gagne J, Patrick A, Mogun H, *et al.* (2011) Antidepressants and fracture risk in older adults: a comparative safety analysis. *Clinical Pharmacology Therapeutics* **89**: 880–7.

16 Warden S, Hassett S, Bond J, *et al.* (2010) Psycotropic drugs have contrasting skeletal effects that are independent of their effects on physical activity levels. *Bone* **46**: 985–92.

17 Bab I, Yirmiya R (2010) Depression, selective serotonin reuptake inhibitors, and osteoporosis. *Curr Osteoporos Rep* **8**: 185–91.

18 Warden S, Nelson I, Fuchs R, *et al.* (2008) Serotonin (5-hydroxytryptamine) transporter inhibition causes bone loss in adult mice independently of estrogen deficiency. *Menopause* **15**: 1176–83.

19 Bonnet N, Bernard P, Beaupied H, *et al.* (2007) Various effects of antidepressants on bone microarchitecture, mechanical properties and bone remodeling. *Toxicology and Applied Pharmacology* **221**: 111–18.

20 Pack A, Olarte L, Morrell M, *et al.* (2003) Bone mineral density in an outpatient population receiving enzyme-inducing antiepileptic drugs. *Epilepsy and Behavior* **4**: 169–74.

21 Nakken K, Tauboll E (2010) Bone loss associated with use of antiepileptic drugs. *Expert Opin Drug Saf* **9**: 561–71.

22 Souverein P, Webb D, Weil J, *et al.* (2006) Use of antiepileptic drugs and risk of fractures: case-control study among patients with epilepsy. *Neurology* **66**: 1318–24.

23 Beerhorst K, Schouwenaars F, Tan I, *et al.* (2012) Epilepsy: fractures and the role of cumulative antiepileptic drug load. *Acta Neurol Scand* **125**: 54–9.

24 Sato Y, Kondo I, Motooka H, *et al.* (2001) Decreased bone mass and increased bone turnover with valproate therapy in adults with epilepsy. *Neurology* **57**: 445–9.

25 Takahashi A, Onodera K, Shinoda H, *et al.* (2000) Phenytoin and its metabolite, 5-(4-hydroxyphenyl)-5-phenylhydantoin, show bone resorption in cultured neonatal mouse calvaria. *Jpn J Pharmacol* **82**: 82–4.

26 Lau K, Nakade O, Barr B, *et al.* (1995) Phenytoin increases markers of osteogenesis for the human species *in vitro* and *in vivo*. *J Clin Endocrinol Metab* **80**: 2347–53.

27 Lyngstad-Brechan M, Tauboll E, Nakken K, *et al.* (2008) Reduced bone mass and increased bone turnover in postmenopausal women with epilepsy using antiepileptic drug monothreapy. *Scand J Clin Lab Invest* **68**: 759–66.

28 Kim S, Lee J, Choi K, *et al.* (2007) A 6-month longitudinal study of bone mineral density with antiepileptic drug monotherapy. *Epilepsy and Behavior* **10**: 291–5.

29 Pack A, Morrell M, Marcus R, *et al.* (2005) Bone mass and turnover in women with epilepsy on antiepileptic drug monotherapy. *Ann Neurol* **57**: 252–7.

30 Espinosa P, Perez D, Abner E, *et al.* (2011) Association of antiepileptic drugs, vitamin D, and calcium supplementation with bone fracture occurrence in epilepsy patients. *Clin Neurol Neurosurg* **113**: 548–51.

31 Tamler R, Epstein S (2006) Nonsteroid immune modulators and bone disease. *Ann NY Acad Sci* **1068**: 284–96.

32 Sun L, Blair H, Peng Y, *et al.* (2005) Calcineurin regulates bone formation by the osteoblast. *PNAS* **102**: 17130–5.

33 Sun L, Peng Y, Zaidi N, *et al.* (2007) Evidence that calcineurin is required for the genesis of bone-resorbing osteoclasts. *Am J Physiol Renal Physiol* **292**: F285–F291.

34 Movsowitz C, Epstein S, Fallon M, *et al.* (1998) Cyclosporin-A *in vivo* produces severe osteopenia in the rat: effect of dose and duration of administration. *Endocrinology* **123**: 2571–7.

35 Romero D, Buchinsky F, Rucinski B, *et al.* (1995) Rapamycin: a bone sparing immunosuppressant? *J Bone Mineral Res* **10**: 760–8.

36 Thiebaud D, Krieg M, Gillard-Berguer D, *et al.* (1996) Cyclosporine induces high bone turnover and may contribute to bone loss after transplantation. *Eur J Clin Invest* **25**: 549–55.

37 Cueto-Manzano A, Konel S, Crowley V, *et al.* (2003) Bone histopathology and densitometry comparison between cyclosporine A monotherapy and prednisolone plus azathioprine dual immunosuppression in renal transplant patients. *Transplantation* **75**: 2053–8.

38 Edwards B, Desai A, Tsai J, *et al.* (2011) Elevated incidence of fractures in solid-organ transplant recipients on glucocorticoid-sparing immunosuppressive regimens. *J Osteoporosis*, epub article 591793.

39 Kaunitz A, Arias R, McClung M (2008) Bone density recovery after depot medroxyprogesterone acetate injectable contraception use. *Contraception* **77**: 67–76.

40 Harel Z, Johnson C, Gold M, *et al.* (2010) Recovery of bone mineral density in adolescents following the use of depot medroxyprogesterone acetate contraceptive injection. *Contraception* **81**: 281–91.

41 Clark M, Sowers M, Nichols S, *et al.* (2004) Bone mineral density changes over two years in first-time users of depot medroxyprogesterone acetate. *Fertil Steril* **82**: 1580–6.

42 Kaunitz A, Miller P, Rice V, *et al.* (2006) Bone mineral density in women aged 25–35 years receiving depot medroxyprogesterone acetate: recovery following discontinuation. *Contraception* **74**: 90–9.

43 Orr-Walker B, Evans M, Ames R, *et al.* (1998) The effect of past use of the injectable contraceptive deopt medroxyprogesterone acetate on bone mineral density in normal post-menopausal women. *Clin Endocrinol* **49**: 615–18.

44 Meier C, Brauchli Y, Jick S, *et al.* (2010) Use of depot medroxyprogesterone acetate and fracture risk. *J Clin Endocrinol Metab* **95**: 4909–16.

45 Mittan D, Lee S, Miller E, *et al.* (2001) Bone loss following hypogonadism in men with prostate cancer treated with GnRH analogs. *J Clin Endocriol Metab* **87**: 3656–61.

46 Kiratli B, Srinivas S, Perkash I, *et al.* (2001) Progressive decrease in bone density over 10 years of androgen deprivation therapy in patients with prostate cancer. *Urology* **57**: 127–32.

47 Shahinian V, Kuo Y, Freeman J, *et al.* (2005) Risk of fracture after androgen deprivation for prostate cancer. *N Engl J Med* **352**: 154–64.

48 Thorstenson A, Bratt O, Akre O, *et al.* (2012) Incidence of fractures causing hospitalisation in prostate cancer patients: results from the population-based PCBaSe Sweden. *Eur J Cancer* Feb 29 epub.

49 Surrey E, Hornstein M (2002) Prolonged GnRH agonist and add-back therapy for symptomatic endometriosis: long-term follow-up. *Obstet Gynecol* **99**: 709–19.

50 Pierce S, Gazvani R, Farquharson R (2000) Long-term use of gonadotropin-releasing hormone analogs and hormone replacement therapy in the management of endometriosis: a randomized trial with a 6-year follow-up. *Fertil Steril* **74**: 964–8.

51 Yu E, Bauer S, Bain P, *et al.* (2011) Proton pump inhibitors and risk of fractures: a meta-analysis of 11 international studies. *A J Med* **124**: 519–26.

52 FDA Drug Safety Communication (2011) Possible increased risk of fractures of the hip, wrist, and spine with the use of proton pump inhibitors. http://www.fda.gov/drugs/drugsafety/postmarketdrugsafetyinformationforpatientsandproviders/ucm213206.htm (accessed January 19, 2012).

53 Corley D, Kubo A, Zhao W, *et al.* (2010) Proton pump inhibitors and histamine-2 receptor antagonists are associated with hip fractures among at-risk patients. *Gastroenterology* **139**: 93–101.

54 Gray S, LaCroix A, Larson J, *et al.* (2010) Proton pump inhibitor use, hip fracture, and change in bone mineral density in postmenopausal women. *Arch Intern Med* **170**: 765–71.

55 Targownik L, Lix L, Metge C, *et al.* (2008) Use of proton pump inhibitors and risk of osteoporosis-related fractures. *CMAJ* **179**: 319–26.

56 Vestergaard P, Rejnmark L, Mosekilde L (2006) Proton pump inhibitors, histamine H2 receptor antagonists, and other antacid medications and the risk of fracture. *Calcif Tissue Int* **79**: 76–83.

57 Yang Y, Lewis J, Epstein S, *et al.* (2006) Long-term proton pump inhibitor therapy and risk of hip fracture. *JAMA* **296**: 2947–53.

58 Yu E, Blackwell, T, Ensrud K, *et al.* (2008) Acid-suppressive medications and risk of bone loss and fracture in older adults. *Calcif Tissue Int* **83**: 251–9.

59 deVries F, Cooper A, Cockle S, *et al.* (2009) Fracture risk in patients receiving acid-suppressant medication alone and in combination with bisphosphonates. *Osteoporos Int* **20**: 1989–98.

60 O'Connell M, Madden D, Murray A, *et al.* (2005) Effects of proton pump inhibitors on calcium carbonate absorption in women: a randomized crossover trial. *A J Med* **118**: 778–81.

61 Mizunashi K, Furukawa Y, Katano K, *et al.* (1993) Effect of emeprazole, an inhibitor of H^+, K^+-ATPase, on bone resorption in humans. *Calcif Tissue Int* **53**: 21–5.

62 Targownik L, Lix L, Leung S, *et al.* (2010) Proton-pump inhibitor use is not associated with osteoporosis or accelerated bone mineral density loss. *Gastroenterology* **138**: 896–904.

63 Roux C, Goldstein J, Zhou X, *et al.* (2012) Vertebral fracture efficacy during risedronate therapy in patients using proton pump inhibitors. *Osteoporos Int* **23**: 277–84.

64 FDA Safety (2007) *Actos* February. http://www.fda.gov/Safety/MedWatch/SafetyInformation/SafetyAlertsforHumanMedicalProducts/ucm150451.htm (accessed March 7, 2012).

65 FDA Safety (2007) *Avandia* February. http://www.fda.gov/Safety/MedWatch/SafetyInformation/SafetyAlertsforHumanMedicalProducts/ucm150833.htm (accessed March 7, 2012).

66 FDA Safety (2007) GlaxoSmithKline letter to health care providers February. http://www.fda.gov/downloads/Safety/MedWatch/SafetyInformation/SafetyAlertsforHumanMedicalProducts/UCM153903.pdf (accessed March 7, 2012).

67 Grey A, Bolland M, Gamble G, *et al.* (2007) The peroxisome proliferator-activated receptor agonist rosiglitazone decreases bone formation and bone mineral density in healthy postmenopausal women: a randomized, controlled trial. *J Clin Endocrinol Metab* **92**: 1305–10.

68 Berberoglu Z, Yazic A, Demirag N (2010) Effects of rosiglitazone on bone mineral density and remodeling parameters in postmenopausal diabetic women: a 2-year follow-up study. *Clinical Endocrinology* **73**: 305–12.

69 Grey A 2008. Skeletal consequences of thiazolidinedione therapy. *Osteoporos Int* **19**: 129–37.

70 Habib Z, Havstad S, Wells K, *et al.* (2010) Thiazolidinedione use and the longitudinal risk of fractures in patients with type 2 diabetes mellitus. *J Clin Endocrinol Metab* **95**: 592–600.

71 Wei W, Wan Y (2011) Thiazolidinediones on PPARγ: the roles in bone remodeling. *PPAR Res*; **2011**:867180. Epub 2011 Oct 29.

72 Mabilleau G, Mieczkowska A, Edmonds M (2010) Thiazolidinediones induce osteocyte apoptosis and increase sclerostin expression. *Diabet Med* **27**: 925–32.

73 Sorocéanu M, Miao D, Bai X, *et al.* (2004) Rosiglitazone impacts negatively on bone by promoting osteoblast/osteocyte apoptosis. *Journal of Endocrinology* **183**: 203–16.

CHAPTER 8

Hormone Therapy for Osteoporosis

Pilar Valenzuela Mazo[1] & James A. Simon[2]
[1]Pontificia Universidad Católica de Chile School of Medicine, Santiago, Chile
[2]The George Washington University *and* Women's Health & Research Consultants®, Washington, DC, USA

Inroduction

Reifenstein and Albright first established the association between the menopausal characteristic estrogen deficient state that defines menopause and osteoporosis in their original publications in the 1940s. They also demonstrated that the addition of estrogen reversed the negative calcium balance seen in this disease, suggesting that estrogen increased the rate of bone formation [1]. In the past 50 years many studies have subsequently shown that hormone therapy (HT) prevents bone loss and fracture [2], but only recently has our knowledge of HT and fractures been confirmed by a large randomized controlled clinical trial (RCT).

The Women's Health Initiative (WHI) hormone study included two HT treatment arms: estrogen alone with approximately 10 000 hysterectomized women who received conjugated equine estrogens (CEE; 0.625 mg/day) and estrogen plus a progestin with approximately 16 000 women with a uterus who received CEE (0.625 mg/day) plus medroxyprogesterone acetate (MPA; 2.5 mg/day). Study participants were between 50 and 79 years of age, and were not selected for a prevalent prior fracture or for osteoporosis. Results of the study showed that estrogen alone [3] and estrogen plus a progestin [4] reduced the risk of all fractures including fractures of the hip. These are extremely relevant data, as these WHI study participants represented a low-fracture risk population. Nevertheless, both estrogen alone and estrogen plus a progestin showed a statistically significant reduction in clinical fracture incidence including hip fracture in this unique population.

Osteoporosis: Diagnosis and Management, First Edition. Edited by Dale W. Stovall.
© 2013 John Wiley & Sons, Ltd. Published 2013 by John Wiley & Sons, Ltd.

Mechanism of action

Estrogen preserves bone and has an antiresorptive effect that is mediated by estrogen receptor alpha and/or estrogen receptor beta present in osteoblasts [5]. Estrogenic action on the osteoblast results in production of cytokines and other factors (see Chapter 3 on bone remodeling) that reduce osteoclast number, activity, and life span. Additionally, estrogen acts directly on the osteoclast progenitor cell decreasing its responsiveness to receptor activator of NFKB ligand (RANKL); a cytokine secreted by osteoblasts, and thereby prevents the maturation of osteoclasts. Estrogen also has anabolic effects which include increasing the proliferation, differentiation and function of osteoblasts [6]. The net effect of estrogen deficiency on the skeleton appears to be an increase in activation of bone remodeling and perhaps increased activity and efficiency of the osteoclast population of cells [2].

Estrogens are among the group of agents that reduce bone resorption in the skeleton. Other compounds in this group include bisphosphonates and selective estrogen receptor modulators (SERMs) which are also known as selective estrogen agonist/antagonists. It has been assumed that the reduction in fracture risk seen with these agents is secondary to the associated increase in BMD measured by dual x-ray absorptiometry (DEXA), but this association is not as clear as once imagined. In large prospective cohort studies, the reduction in fracture risk associated with estrogen therapy becomes evident too soon after initiation to be explained solely by increases in BMD [7, 8]. Therefore, the beneficial effects of HT on the prevention of vertebral and nonvertebral fractures in nonosteoporotic postmenopausal women must be attributed to other features besides increased bone mass. In several RCTs the positive effects of estrogen therapy on fracture risk have been shown to persist even after adjusting for changes in bone density [9–11] and this protection has been shown to rapidly decline following discontinuation of HT [8]. It has been suggested, based on observations from large clinical trials [12], that it is the decline in bone remodeling associated with bone-sparing therapy that leads to this initial rapid reduction in fracture risk. Estrogen's multiple actions on different systems may account for additional mechanisms resulting in fracture risk reduction. For example, HT is associated with a decreased risk of falls in general [13, 14] and falling tendency is one of the main determinants of fractures [15]. Estrogen's favorable effect on postural balance [16, 17], muscle strength [18, 19], overactive bladder symptoms [20] and conditions that impair vision such as cataracts [21] and age-related maculopathy [22] may also explain this reduction in one's risk of falling. Additionally, estrogen plays a crucial role in regulating the calcium-vitamin D-PTH axis. Estrogens increase intestinal calcium absorption [23] and renal reabsorption [24]. They facilitate vitamin D hydroxylation [25] to its metabolically active form, and estrogens decrease the age-related PTH increase [26]. Further, estrogens regulate PTH synthesis, secretion and homeostatic set point [27, 28].

The effect of estrogen therapy on bone

Estrogen either with or without a progestin, in different doses and administered via various routes, has been proven to be effective in protecting against bone loss at all skeletal sites and reducing the incidence of fracture in postmenopausal women. The strongest evidence comes from RCTs in which fracture incidence reduction is the primary outcome, but as these "fracture as an endpoint" trials are very expensive and take years to complete, many studies have used other measurements, such as change in BMD and bone turnover markers, as surrogate endpoints for fracture.

Changes in bone mineral density

A large meta-analysis published in 2002 [29] reviewed the efficacy of HT for prevention and treatment of osteoporosis in postmenopausal women. This meta-analysis included 57 studies that randomized postmenopausal women to either estrogen with or without a progestin, or to a placebo and were of at least one year in duration. In 55 of these studies BMD was measured at the lumbar spine, forearm, or femoral neck either by single-photon absorptiometry, DEXA, or quantitative computed tomography (QCT). The results showed that the pooled percent change in bone density was statistically significant in favor of HT at all measurement sites. After 1 year of treatment, the change in bone density with HT was 5.4% greater at the lumbar spine and 3.0% and 2.5% greater at the forearm and femoral neck, respectively (Figure 8.1). In the WHI trials, which were not included in the aforementioned meta-analysis, BMD of the lumbar spine, and total hip was measured by DEXA at baseline and at years 1, 3 and 6 in a subgroup consisting of 1024 and 938 women in the estrogen plus a progestin and estrogen alone groups, respectively. In the estrogen plus a progestin arm total hip BMD increased 3.7% at year 3 in the treatment group compared with 0.14% in the placebo group (P < 0.001) [10]; in the WHI's estrogen alone arm, total hip BMD increased 1.8% at year 6 in women receiving CEE compared with a loss of 1.9% in those receiving placebo (P < 0.0001) [30]. As for the lumbar spine, in the estrogen plus a progestin arm the mean percentage change in BMD was 3.3%, 4.5% and 7.5% greater at years 1, 3 and 6, respectively [10]. Similar results were observed in the estrogen alone arm with a statistically significant,

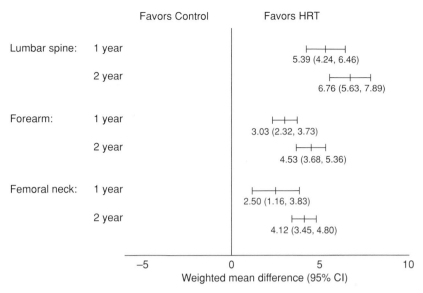

Figure 8.1 Meta-analysis of the efficacy of hormone replacement therapy in treating and preventing osteoporosis in postmenopausal women: weighted mean difference in percent change in bone density after treatment with HT.
(*Source*: Wells G *et al.* (2002) [29]).

5.1%, gain in BMD observed in the treatment group after 6 years of therapy [30].

Fractures

Fracture risk reduction is the ultimate measure of HT's bone protection. Before the results from the WHI trials were available, all evidence supporting estrogen's efficacy in preventing fracture came from observational studies. In two meta-analyses that included RCT's involving HT with available data on vertebral [31] and nonvertebral fractures [32], the authors concluded that HT was associated with a 33% (95% confidence interval (CI) 0.45 to 0.98; P = 0.04) and a 27% (95% [CI], 0.56–0.94; P = 0.02) reduction in vertebral and nonvertebral fractures, respectively.

In the WHI trials which evaluated estrogen alone and estrogen plus progestin therapy, women assigned to active treatment had fewer fractures. For estrogen alone the relative risks (RR) for hip, clinical vertebral and total fracture were 0.65 (95% CI, 0.45–0.94), 0.64 (95% CI, 0.44–0.93) and 0.71 (95% CI, 0.64–0.80), respectively [4]. In the estrogen plus progestin group in the WHI trial, the RR for hip, clinical vertebral and total fractures were 0.67 (95% CI, 0.47–0.96), 0.65 (95% CI, 0.46–0.92) and 0.76 (95% CI, 0.69–0.83), respectively [3].

Furthermore, the prospective Million Women's Study in the United Kingdom found that current users of hormone therapy had a significantly reduced incidence of fracture, with a RR of 0.62 (95% CI 0.58–0.66; P < 0.001). This RR of fracture did not vary significantly whether estrogen was used alone, in combination with a progestin, by estrogen dose, or with various estrogenic or progestogenic compounds [8].

Specific compounds

Conjugated equine estrogens (CEE) have been the most studied oral preparation of HT in postmenopausal women. In the WHI trial, both CEE 0.625 mg/day given alone and in combination with MPA 2.5 mg/day, proved effective in increasing BMD at the hip and spine and reducing fractures, in general, including fractures of the hip (Figure 8.2) [3, 4, 10, 30]. Where fracture is the assessed endpoint, there exist no equivalent RCT's that have evaluated the efficacy of other estrogen preparations for prevention or treatment of osteoporosis in postmenopausal women. But, there is evidence from meta-analyses and observational studies suggesting a similar effect on bone for estradiol.

In the meta-analysis by Wells *et al.* [29], when HT was grouped by estrogen preparation, the authors found no differences in the percent change in bone density between estradiol and CEE.

In the Million Women Study, compared to never-users of HT, users of different preparations of estradiol presented similar risk of incident fractures, RR 0.68 (95% CI 0.59–0.77) as users of equine estrogens, RR 0.62 (0.54–0.71). In the later study, the risk of fracture did not vary significantly if estrogen was used alone or in combination with a progestin nor according to the type of progestin [8].

Tibolone, a synthetic steroid that has mixed estrogenic, androgenic and progestogenic properties, is approved in many countries except for the U.S. for the management of menopausal symptoms and prevention of osteoporosis. In early postmenopausal and older osteoporotic women, treatment with tibolone reduces bone turnover markers and increases BMD at several different skeletal sites [33]. This medication has proven effective in significantly reducing vertebral and nonvertebral fractures in postmenopausal women of 60 years of age and older [34].

The effects of raloxifene, a selective estrogen receptor modulators (SERM) or estrogen agonist/antagonist, on bone are well established. In postmenopausal women with osteoporosis, treatment with raloxifene decreases bone turnover markers and increases BMD at different skeletal sites [35]. Raloxifene is effective in decreasing the incidence of vertebral

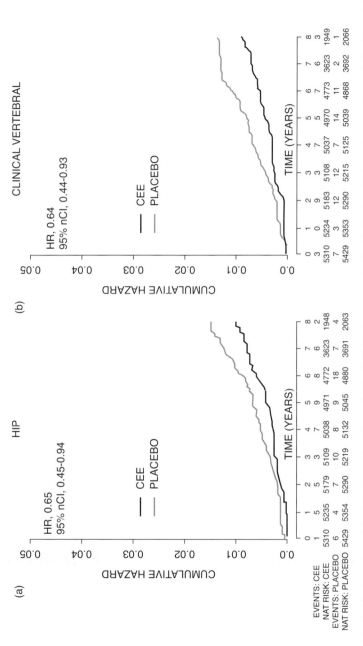

Figure 8.2 Effects of estrogen on risk of fracture. The Women's Health Initiative randomized trial. Kaplan-Meier estimates of cumulative hazards for hip (a) and vertebral (b) fracture. HR indicates hazard ratio; Nci, nominal confidence interval. (*Source*: Jackson RD, Wactawski-Wende J, LaCroix AZ (2006) [30]).

fractures, but has not been shown to decrease the rate of hip fractures [36]. Lasofoxifene and bazedoxifene, two other approved SERMs (neither available in the USA at present) reduce the risk of vertebral fracture in postmenopausal women with osteoporosis, and lasofoxifene may reduce nonvertebral fractures as well [37, 38]. See also the chapter on SERMs.

Lower doses of estrogen therapy

Due to the risks, both perceived and real, associated to estrogen therapy and the fact that many of these risks seem to be dose dependent (e.g., deep vein thrombosis), efforts have been made to determine the lowest effective dose for the management of menopause-related symptoms. Lower doses of estrogen are associated with a lower risk of endometrial hyperplasia than standard doses, and lower dose estrogen preparations also attenuate cardiovascular risks, as they increase C-reactive protein and coagulation factors to a lesser degree and appear to be associated with a lower risk of venous thromboembolism and stroke [39–41]. Compared with users of standard doses of estrogens, women using low-doses of estrogens are less likely to have unacceptable side effects, such as vaginal bleeding or breast tenderness [42], which are some of the main reasons for discontinuation of HT [43].

Data from the WHI demonstrated that HT in standard doses reduced the risk of hip and clinical spine fractures by about one-third [3, 4]. No similar trials using lower doses of estrogen to evaluate fracture risk have been performed; however, recent studies have shown no threshold level for estrogen activity on the skeleton. Rather a linear dose response in which an increment in BMD increase is observed with each increment in dose has been demonstrated [39].

Estrogen's favorable effect on bone mass has been evidenced at both low and ultra-low doses; 0.3 mg/day CEE [44, 45], 0.25 to 1 mg/day oral estradiol [46, 47], 0.014 to 0.25 mg/day transdermal estradiol [48, 49] and "local" estrogen delivered via vaginal ring (7.5 ug/24 hours) [50], all have been shown to significantly increase BMD at different skeletal sites in postmenopausal women. Remarkable is the fact that in one of these studies, which demonstrated significant increases in bone density, serum estradiol and estrone levels after treatment did not increase significantly compared to baseline [50].

In the Million Women Study, the reduction in fracture incidence associated with HT did not vary significantly according to the dose of estrogen used (equine estrogen <0.625 vs. ≥0.625 mg, P = 0.91; oral estradiol <1 vs ≥1 mg, P = 0.69; transdermal estradiol <50 vs. ≥50 μg, P = 0.53) [8]. Whether the absence of a dose response in this study was due to the methodology or simply the lack of sensitivity is unknown.

Route of administration

Due to the unfavorable cardiovascular effects associated with oral HT in the aforementioned data from the WHI, attention has turned to other modes of estrogen delivery, particularly the transdermal route. This route of administration may not be associated with the negative cardiovascular outcomes observed for oral HT. The particular feature of avoiding "first pass" hepatic metabolism is believed to explain the different effects of oral vs. transdermal HT on coagulation, fibrinolysis and lipid metabolism. To date, the available evidence suggests that, compared to oral estrogen therapy, transdermal estrogen therapy is associated to a lower risk of venous thromboembolism and stroke [51, 52]. The majority of clinical trials that have evaluated the effect of estrogen on BMD and fracture incidence have used CEE or estradiol delivered orally. Therefore, there is substantial evidence that oral estrogen in standard doses increases BMD and decreases the risk of fracture [2, 31, 32].

Estradiol in transdermal patches delivering between 14 to 100 ug of estradiol/day has been proven to prevent bone loss in postmenopausal women [53–57]. In postmenopausal women with established osteoporosis, a small study with a transdermal patch that delivered 100 ug of estradiol per day for 3 of 4 weeks was associated with a lower vertebral fracture rate [58].

Evidence from observational studies suggests that both oral and transdermal HT would have a similar protective effect on the risk of fracture. In a Swedish case-control study which included 1327 women aged 50–81 years with a hip fracture and 3262 controls, compared to never-use, oral estrogen ever-use was associated with an odds ratio (OR) of 0.63 (95% CI 0.45–0.88) and transdermal (patches) estrogen with an OR of 0.73 (95% CI 0.38–1.40); oral estrogen plus progestin was associated with an OR of 0.46 (95% CI 0.32–0.67) and transdermal estrogen plus progestin with an OR of 0.49 (95% CI 0.24–1.00). The authors concluded that transdermal estrogen treatment gave similar risk estimates for fracture risk reduction as compared to oral regimens [59]. In a Danish case-control study which including 64 548 women with a fracture and 193 641 controls, multivariable-adjusted ORs for risk reduction of any fracture were not different between oral and transdermal preparations [60].

In the Million Women's Study the relative risk reduction of incident fracture did not vary significantly according to whether estrogen was delivered orally, transdermally or by subcutaneous implant. Compared with never-users, multivariable-adjusted RRs of fracture were 0.60 (95% CI 0.53–0.68) for current use of oral estrogen and 0.75 (95% CI 0.65–0.86) for current use of transdermal estrogen [8].

Vaginal rings delivering systemic doses of estradiol represent an additional parenteral alternative. Vaginal rings delivering estradiol at a rate equivalent to 0.05 mg/day or 0.1 mg/day are approved for the treatment of both systemic (vasomotor) and local (vulvovaginal atrophy) menopausal symptoms for a period of 3 months, these have shown to increase BMD of the lumbar spine and total hip in healthy postmenopausal women [61]. Fracture reduction data of all types remains a significant deficiency in the non-oral estrogen therapy compendium of information.

Duration of therapy

The authors of the observational National Osteoporosis Risk Assessment (NORA) study, which included 170 852 postmenopausal women, evaluated the effects of duration of HT on BMD and fracture risk. Women who were currently using HT for any duration had higher T–scores than never users, and among women currently using estrogen, those who had used HT longest had the highest BMD levels at each bone site measured. In this study HT for 5 years or less was shown to preserve bone and reduce fracture risk while it was being used [62]; however, bone density and fracture benefits disappear shortly after discontinuation of HT (see below).

In the Postmenopausal Estrogen/Progestin Interventions (PEPI) randomized controlled trial there was a significant increase in both spine and hip BMD in women assigned to all active treatment groups from baseline to the 12-month visit. The trial lasted 3 years and between 70% and 90% of the increase in BMD seen in women assigned to active treatment occurred during the first 12 months of the study [63].

In the Million Women's Study, a significant reduction in the RR for fracture was found in women who had been taking HT for less than a year; RR 0.75 (0.60–0.93). The RR of fracture demonstrated in this study decreased further in a linear trend with increasing duration of HT, up to 5–9 years of use [8].

Cessation of therapy

Women who discontinue estrogen therapy are at increased risk for developing osteoporosis; the protective effect of HT on BMD and fracture risk declines after cessation of therapy at an unpredictable rate.

The pattern of accelerated bone loss observed after withdrawal of estrogen therapy is similar to that which occurs within the first years after the menopause [64, 65], and in women who stop HT the rates of BMD loss are not significantly different than those observed in women who do not receive HT [66].

Data from a large longitudinal observational study that evaluated the impact of HT cessation on hip fracture incidence showed a 55% increased risk for hip fracture in women who discontinued HT compared to those who remained on HT. The association between HT use and hip fracture prevention disappeared within two years of HT cessation [67]. Further, it has been shown that women who have used HT, regardless of duration, and stopped more than 5 years previously, have similar T-scores [62] and risk for hip fracture as women who have never used HT [68].

In general past use of HT confers no significant protection against fractures and incidence rates return to those of never-users within about a year or two after ceasing use [8]. Reviews of the impact of HT discontinuation on the skeleton are available [69].

Benefits and risks of estrogen therapy

It is necessary to interpret a complex body of existing data in order to understand the actual benefits and risks of HT. After extensive analysis of the available information, different specialized medical societies have produced elaborate position statements on the use of postmenopausal HT [70–72].

There is consensus that areas of benefit include relief of vasomotor and urogenital symptoms, prevention of early postmenopausal bone loss and osteoporotic fractures, and prevention of diabetes. Risks of HT include venous thromboembolism, stroke cholelithiasis, and cholecystitis. Some of these risks may be mitigated by a reduced dose and/or non-oral route of administration.

Recent data analyses from the WHI support initiation of HT for treatment of menopausal symptoms in younger women. In the subgroup of women starting HT who were either between 50 and 59 years of age or who were less than 10 years after menopause, the evidence suggests a reduction in "all cause" mortality and coronary artery disease. Furthermore, there is mounting evidence of an additional "window of opportunity" for long-term neuroprotection if HT is started near the onset of menopause. In this same subgroup of women, estrogen plus some progestins, but not estrogen alone, was associated with an increased risk of breast cancer. Available data on HT (with progestogen) has shown a beneficial effect on colon and endometrial cancer and a possible harmful effect on ovarian cancer, associations which would fall into the rare or very rare category.

Conclusions

Hormone therapy is part of a general strategy including recommendations for lifestyle modification including diet, exercise, smoking cessation and moderate alcohol consumption. HT should be individualized according to symptoms, personal and family history, results from relevant clinical trials and the woman's preferences; in addition to annual control and oversight by a healthcare professional.

The dose indicated should be the minimal effective dose in managing symptoms and there is no evidence-based argument to arbitrarily limit the duration of treatment.

In women with a uterus, a progestin should be added to their estrogen therapy for endometrial protection. In women who have undergone a hysterectomy, estrogen can be used alone.

HT is effective in preventing menopause-associated bone loss and decreases the risk of osteoporotic fractures, including vertebral and hip fractures. In postmenopausal women younger than 60 years of age who are at increased risk for fracture, HT can be considered as one of the first-line choices of therapy for the prevention and treatment of osteoporosis. In women older than 60 years, the initiation of HT solely for the purpose of preventing fractures is not recommended. The continuation of HT after the age of 60 years for prevention of fractures should balance the possible risks and other benefits associated with that specific HT, compared to other approved nonhormonal therapies for osteoporosis.

Hormone therapy is contraindicated in women with a personal history of breast cancer or a personal history of other estrogen-dependent malignancies such as endometrial cancer, genital bleeding of unknown cause, untreated endometrial hyperplasia, congenital or acquired thrombophilia or personal history of thromboembolism, coronary artery disease, uncontrolled hypertension and acute hepatic illness.

References

1 Reifenstein EC, Albright F (1947) The metabolic effects of steroid hormones in osteoporosis. *J Clin Invest* **26**: 24–56.
2 Lindsay R (2004) Hormones and bone health in postmenopausal women. *Endocrine* **24**(3): 223–30.
3 Rossouw JE *et al.* (2002) Risks and benefits of estrogen plus progestin in healthy postmenopausal women: principal results From the Women's Health Initiative randomized controlled trial. *JAMA* **288**(3): 321–33.
4 Anderson GL *et al.* (2004) Effects of conjugated equine estrogen in postmenopausal women with hysterectomy: The Women's Health Initiative randomized controlled trial. *JAMA* **291**: 1701–12.
5 Vidal O, KindblomLg, Ohlsson C (1999) Expression and localization of estrogen receptor-beta in murine and human bone. *J Bone Miner Res* **14**(6): 923–9.
6 Stepan JJ, Alenfeld F, Boivin G, Feyen JH, Lakatos P (2003) Mechanisms of action of antiresorptive therapies of postmenopausal osteoporosis. *Endocr Regul* **37**(4): 225–38.
7 Naessen T, Persson I, Adami HO, Bergström R, Bergkvist L (1990) Hormone replacement therapy and the risk for first hip fracture. A prospective, population-based cohort study. *Ann Intern Med* **113**(2): 95–103.

8 Banks E *et al.* (2004) Million women study collaborators. Fracture incidence in relation to the pattern of use of hormone therapy in postmenopausal women. *JAMA* **291**: 2212–20.

9 Cauley JA, Seeley DG, Ensrud K, Ettinger B, Black D, Cummings SR (1995) Estrogen Replacement Therapy and fractures in older women. *Ann Internal Med* **122**: 9–16.

10 Cauley JA, Robins J, Chen Z, *et al.* (2003) Effects of estrogen plus progestin on risk of fracture and bone mineral density. The Women's Health Initiative randomized trial. *JAMA* **290**: 1729–38.

11 Komulainen MH *et al.* (1998) HRT and Vitamin D in prevention of non-vertebral fractures in postmenopausal women; a 5 year randomized trial. *Maturitas* **31**(1): 45–54.

12 Eastell R, Barton I, Hannon RA, Chines A, Garnero P, Delmas PD (2003) Relationship of early changes in bone resorption to the reduction in fracture risk with risedronate. *J Bone Miner Res* **18**(6): 1051–6.

13 Randell KM *et al.* (2001) Hormone replacement therapy and risk of falling in early postmenopausal women- a population-based study. *Clin Endocrinol (Oxf)* **54**(6): 769–74.

14 Bea JW *et al.* (2011) Effect of hormone therapy on lean body mass, falls, and fractures: 6-year results from the Women's Health Initiative hormone trials. *Menopause* **18**(1): 44–52.

15 Cummings SR (1995) Risk factors for hip fracture in white women. Study of Osteoporotic Fractures Research Group. *N Engl J Med* **332**(12): 767–73.

16 Bergström I, Landgren BM, Pyykkö I (2007) Training or EPT in perimenopause on balance and flushes. *Acta Obstet Gynecol Scand* **86**(4): 467–72.

17 Naessen T, Lindmark B, Larsen HC (2007) Hormone therapy and postural balance in elderly women. *Menopause* **14**(6): 1020–4.

18 Jacobsen DE, Samson MM, Kezic S, Verhaar HJ (2007) Postmenopausal HRT and tibolone in relation to muscle strength and body composition. *Maturitas* **58**(1): 7–18.

19 Onambélé-Pearson GL (2009) HRT affects skeletal muscle contractile characteristics: a definitive answer? *J Appl Physiol* **107**(1): 4–5.

20 Kok AL *et al.* (1999) Micturition complaints in postmenopausal women treated with continuously combined hormone replacement therapy: a prospective study. *Maturitas* **31**: 143–9.

21 Freeman EE, Munoz B, Schein OD, West SK (2001) Hormone replacement therapy and lens opacities: the Salisbury Eye Evaluation Project. *Arch Ophthalmol* **119**(11): 1687–92.

22 Snow KK, Cote J, Yang W, Davis NJ, Seddon JM (2002) Association between reproductive and hormonal factors and age-related maculopathy in postmenopausal women. *Am J Ophthalmol* **134**(6): 842–8.

23 Bolscher M, Netelenbos JC, Barto R, Van Buuren LM, Van der vijgh WJ (1999) Estrogen regulation of intestinal calcium absorption in the intact and ovariectomized adult rat. *J Bone Miner Res* **14**: 1197–1202.

24 Irnaten M, Blanchard-Gutton N, Praetorius J, Harvey BJ (2009) Rapid effects of 17beta-estradiol on TRPV5 epithelial Ca2+ channels in rat renal cells. *Steroids* **74**(8): 642–9.

25 Gallagher JC, Riggs BL, DeLuca HF (1980) Effect of estrogen on calcium absorption and serum vitamin D metabolites in postmenopausal osteoporosis. *J Clin Endocrinol Metab* **51**(6): 1359–64.

26 Khosla S, Atkinson EJ, Melton LJ 3rd, Riggs BL (1997) Effects of age and estrogen status on serum parathyroid hormone levels and biochemical markers of bone turnover in women: a population-based study. *J Clin Endocrinol Metab* **82**(5): 1522–7.

27 Carrillo-López N *et al.* (2009) Indirect regulation of PTH by estrogens may require FGF23. *J Am Soc Nephrol* **20**(9): 2009–17.

28 Boucher A *et al.* (1989) Estrogen replacement decreases the set point of parathyroid hormone stimulation by calcium in normal postmenopausal women. *J Clin Endocrinol Metab* **68**(4): 831–6.

29 Wells G, Tugwell P, Shea B *et al.* (2002) Meta-analyses of therapies for post-menopausal osteoporosis. V. Meta-analysis of the efficacy of hormone replacement therapy in treating and preventing osteoporosis in postmenopausal women. *Endocr Rev* **23**(4): 529–39.

30 Jackson RD, Wactawski-Wende J, LaCroix AZ, *et al.* (2006) Effects of conjugated equine estrogen on risk of fractures and BMD in postmenopausal women with hysterectomy: results from the women's health initiative randomized trial. *J Bone Miner Res* **21**: 817–28.

31 Torgerson DJ, Bell-Syer SE (2001) Hormone replacement therapy and prevention of vertebral fractures: a meta-analysis of randomized trials. *BMC Musculoskelet Disord* **2**: 7.

32 Torgerson DJ, Bell-Syer SE (2001) Hormone replacement therapy and prevention of nonvertebral fractures: a meta-analysis of randomized trials. *JAMA* **285**(22): 2891–7. Review.

33 Ettinger B (2007) Tibolone for prevention and treatment of postmenopausal osteoporosis. *Maturitas* **57**(1): 35–8.

34 Cummings SR, Ettinger B, Delmas PD *et al.* (2008) The effects of tibolone in older postmenopausal women. *N Engl J Med* **359**(7): 697–708.

35 Riggs BL, Hartmann LC (2003) Selective estrogen-receptor modulators – mechanisms of action and application to clinical practice. *N Engl J Med* **348**(7): 618–29.

36 Ettinger B, Mitlak BH, Nickelson T, *et al.* (1999) Reduction of vertebral fracture risk in postmenopausal women with osteoporosis treated with raloxifene: results from 3-year randomized clinical trial. *JAMA* **282**: 637–45.

37 Cummings SR, Ensrud K, Delmas PD *et al.* (2010) Lasofoxifene in postmenopausal women with osteoporosis. *N Engl J Med* **362**(8): 686–96.

38 Silverman SL, Christiansen C, Genant HK *et al.* (2008) Efficacy of bazedoxifene in reducing new vertebral fracture risk in postmenopausal women with osteoporosis: results from a 3-year, randomized, placebo-, and active-controlled clinical trial. *J Bone Miner Res* **23**(12): 1923–34.

39 Ettinger B (2007) Rationale for use of lower estrogen doses for postmenopausal hormone therapy. *Maturitas* **57**(1): 81–4.

40 Peeyananjarassri K, Baber R (2005) Effects of low-dose hormone therapy on menopausal symptoms, bone mineral density, endometrium, and the cardiovascular system: a review of randomized clinical trials. *Climacteric* **8**(1): 13–23.

41 Van de Weijer PH, Mattsson LA, Ylikorkala O (2007) Benefits and risks of long-term low-dose oral continuous combined hormone therapy. *Maturitas* **56**(3): 231–48.

42 Ettinger B (2005) Vasomotor symptom relief versus unwanted effects: role of estrogen dosage. *Am J Med* **118**: 74s–78s.

43 Ettinger B, Pressman AR (1999) Effect of age on reasons for initiation and discontinuation of hormone replacement therapy. *Menopause* **6**: 282–9.

44 Lindsay R, Gallagher JC, Kleerekoper M, Pickar JH (2002) Effect of lower doses of conjugated equine estrogens with and without medroxyprogesterone acetate on bone in early postmenopausal women. *JAMA* **287**(20): 2668–76.

45 Recker RR, Davies KM, Dowd RM, Heaney RP (1999) The effect of low-dose continuous estrogen and progesterone therapy with calcium and vitamin D on bone in elderly women. A randomized, controlled trial. *Ann Intern Med* **130**(11): 897–904.

46 Prestwood KM, Kenny AM, Kleppinger A, Kulldorff M (2003) Ultralow-dose micronized 17beta-estradiol and bone density and bone metabolism in older women: a randomized controlled trial. *JAMA* **290**(8): 1042–8.

47 Lees B, Stevenson JC (2001) The prevention of osteoporosis using sequential low-dose hormone replacement therapy with estradiol-17 beta and dydrogesterone. *Osteoporos Int* **12**(4): 251–8.

48 Ettinger B, Ensrud KE, Wallace R *et al.* (2004) Effects of ultralow-dose transdermal estradiol on bone mineral density: a randomized clinical trial. *Obstet Gynecol* **104**(3): 443–51.

49 Cooper C, Stakkestad JA, Radowicki S *et al.* (1999) Matrix delivery transdermal 17beta-estradiol for the prevention of bone loss in postmenopausal women. The International Study Group. *Osteoporos Int* **9**(4): 358–66.

50 Naessen T, Berglund L, Ulmsten U (1997) Bone loss in elderly women prevented by ultralow doses of parenteral 17beta-estradiol. *Am J Obstet Gynecol* **177**(1): 115–19.

51 Canonico M, Oger E, Plu-Bureau G, Conard J *et al.* (2007) Estrogen and Thromboembolism Risk (ESTHER) Study Group. Hormone therapy and venous thromboembolism among postmenopausal women: impact of the route of estrogen administration and progestogens: the ESTHER study. *Circulation* **115**(7): 840–5.

52 Canonico M, Fournier A, Carcaillon L *et al.* (2010) Postmenopausal hormone therapy and risk of idiopathic venous thromboembolism: results from the E3N cohort study. *Arterioscler Thromb Vasc Biol* **30**(2): 340–5.

53 Delmas PD, Pornel B, Felsenberg D, *et al.* (2001) Three-year follow-up of the use of transdermal 17β-estradiol matrix patches for the prevention of bone loss in early postmenopausal women. *Am J Obstet Gynecol* **184**: 32–40.

54 Weiss SR, Ellman H, Dolker M, for the Transdermal Estradiol Investigator Group (1999) A randomized controlled trial of four doses of transdermal estradiol for preventing postmenopausal bone loss. *Obstet Gynecol* **94**: 330–6.

55 Notelovitz M, John VA, Good WR (2002) Effectiveness of Alora estradiol matrix transdermal delivery system in improving lumbar bone mineral density in healthy, postmenopausal women. *Menopause* **9**: 343–53.

56 McKeever C, McIlwain H, Greenwald M, *et al.* (2000) An estradiol matrix transdermal system for the prevention of postmenopausal bone loss. *Clin Ther* **22**: 845–57.

57 Arrenbrecht S, Boermans AJM (2002) Effects of transdermal estradiol delivered by a matrix patch on bone density in hysterectomized, postmenopausal women: a 2-year placebo-controlled trial. *Osteoporos Int* **13**: 176-83.

58 Lufkin EG, Wahner HW, O'Fallon WM, *et al.* (1992) Treatment of postmenopausal osteoporosis with transdermal estrogen. *Ann Intern Med* **117**: 1–9.

59 Michaelsson K, Baron JA, Farahmand BY, *et al.* (1998) Hormone replacement therapy and risk of hip fracture: population based case- control study. The Swedish Hip Fracture Study Group. *BMJ* **316**: 1858–63.

60 Vestergaard P, Rejnmark L, Mosekilde L (2006) Fracture reducing potential of hormone replacement therapy on a population level. *Maturitas* **54**: 285–93.

61 Al-Azzawi F, Lees B, Thompson J, Stevenson JC (2005) Bone mineral density in postmenopausal women treated with a vaginal ring delivering systemic doses of estradiol acetate. *Menopause* **12**(3): 331–9.

62 Barrett-Connor E, Wehren LE, Siris E *et al.* (2003) Recency and duration of postmenopausal hormone therapy: effects on bone mineral density and fracture risk in the National Osteoporosis Risk Assessment (NORA) study. *Menopause* **10**(5): 412–19.

63 The Writing Group for the PEPI Trial (1996) Effects of hormone therapy on bone mineral density: results from the postmenopausal estrogen/progestin interventions (PEPI) trial. *JAMA* **276**(17): 1389–96.

64 Greenspan SL, Emkey RD, Bone HG *et al.* (2002) Significant differential effects of alendronate, estrogen, or combination therapy on the rate of bone loss after discontinuation of treatment of postmenopausal osteoporosis. A randomized, double-blind, placebo-controlled trial. *Ann Intern Med* **137**(11): 875–83.

65 Trémollieres FA, Pouilles JM, Ribot C (2001) Withdrawal of hormone replacement therapy is associated with significant vertebral bone loss in postmenopausal women. *Osteoporos Int* **12**(5): 385–90.

66 Greendale GA, Espeland M, Slone S *et al.* (2002) Bone mass response to discontinuation of long-term hormone replacement therapy: results from the Postmenopausal Estrogen/Progestin Interventions (PEPI) Safety Follow-up Study. *Arch Intern Med* **162**(6): 665–72.

67 Karim R, Dell RM, Greene DF, *et al.* (2011) Hip fracture in postmenopausal women after cessation of hormone therapy: results from a prospective study in a large health management organization. *Menopause* **18**: 1172–7.

68 Yates J, Barrett-Connor E, Barlas S, Chen YT, Miller PD, Siris ES (2004) Rapid loss of hip fracture protection after estrogen cessation: evidence from the National Osteoporosis Risk Assessment. *Obstet Gynecol* **103**(3): 440–6.

69 Simon JA, Wehren LE, Ascott-Evans BH, Omizo MK, Silfen SL, Lombardi A (2006) Skeletal consequences of hormone therapy discontinuance: a systematic review. *Obstet Gynecol Surv* **61**(2): 115–24. Review.

70 Santen RJ, Allred DC, Ardoin SP *et al.* (2010) Postmenopausal Hormone Therapy: An Endocrine Society Scientific Statement. *J Clin Endocrinol Metab* **95**: S7–S66.

71 Sturdee DW, Pines A (2010) International Menopause Society Writing Group. Updated IMS recommendations on postmenopausal hormone therapy and preventive strategies for midlife health. *Climacteric* **14**(3): 302–20.

72 North American Menopause Society (2010) Estrogen and progestogen use in postmenopausal women: 2010 position statement of the North American Menopause Society. *Menopause* **17**: 242–55.

CHAPTER 9

Bisphosphonates

Paul D. Miller[1] *& Nelson B. Watts*[2]

[1] Colorado Center for Bone Research, Lakewood, CO, USA

[2] Mercy Health Osteoporosis and Bone Health Services, Cincinnati, OH, USA

Introduction

Today, forty years after their discovery, bisphosphonates are the most widely used therapy for osteoporosis [1–4]. Forty years of worldwide use of bisphosphonates for the treatment of postmenopausal osteoporosis has consistently demonstrated their exceptionally high benefit-to-risk ratio [5]. Furthermore, the past forty years has seen the registration of bisphosphonates for the treatment of many diseases (Table 9.1).

The discovery of bisphosphonates began in 1961 when Professors Bill Neuman and Herbert Fleisch, working at The University of Rochester, Rochester, NY, described pyrophosphates as the body's natural water softeners [6]. These metabolites of adenosine (ATP) breakdown do not accumulate in human tissue due to the ubiquitous presence of pyrophosphatases (e.g., alkaline phosphatase, acid phosphatase) that rapidly metabolize their P-O-P bonds. While pyrophosphates were being studied by Procter & Gamble, Inc., Cincinnati, Ohio, USA (P&G) as inhibitors to keep soap from binding to glass in dishwashing detergent, Dr. David Francis of P&G observed that substituting a carbon atom in place of the oxygen atom rendered pyrophosphates nonmetabolizable by pyrophosphatases. This new compound with a P-C-P backbone was named a disphosphonate, latter bisphosphonates, due to the presence of the two "R" side-chains [7] (Figure 9.1).

Bisphosphonates affect bone remodeling by two separate mechanisms according to the structure of the "R" side chains – a physiochemical one and a cellular one. The pharmacological features of bisphosphonates will be described in the next section.

The observations of Dr. David Francis that showed that the disphosphonate, etidronate, affected bone remodeling in distinctly different ways according to the dose: at lower doses, etidronate inhibits bone resorption, while at higher doses it inhibits bone mineralization. This landmark work

Osteoporosis: Diagnosis and Management, First Edition. Edited by Dale W. Stovall.

© 2013 John Wiley & Sons, Ltd. Published 2013 by John Wiley & Sons, Ltd.

Table 9.1 The diseases that have benefited from bisphosphonate therapy.

Bisphosphonates Have Benefited Mankind
- 1. Paget's disease
- 2. Myositis ossificans progressiva
- 3. Osteoporosis (postmenopausal, men, glucocorticoid-induced)
- 4. Drug-induced bone loss (e.g. aromatase inhibitors..)
- 4. Post-transplantation
- 5. Heterotopic ossification
- 6. Primary hyperparathyrodism
- 7. Aseptic necrosis
- 8. Metastatic cancer to bone
- 9. "Stay-Tuned" . . . .
- 10. Fibrous dysplasia
- 11. Multiple myeloma

was then extended by both in vitro and in vivo models by Dr. David Francis; Professor Herbert Fleisch, University of Berne, Switzerland; and Professor Graham Russell, at the University of Sheffield, UK [7]. Soon after these data were published, Dr. Samuel Bassett of Columbia University College of Physicians and Surgeons appealed to the US Food and Drug Administration (FDA) for permission for compassionate use of etidronate to treat a child with myositis ossificans progressiva [8]. High-dose etidronate in this child mitigated her muscle calcification. Additional understandings of the mechanisms of action of bisphosphonates were subsequently elucidated by the development of a rat in vivo model by Dr. Robert Schenk [9]. The culmination of the efforts of these early pioneers was the refinement of the understanding of the pharmacology of bisphosphonates [3, 10–12].

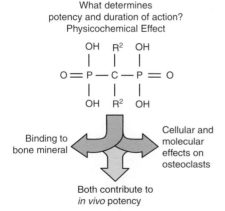

Figure 9.1 The "backbone" chemical structure of bisphosphonates. (*Source*: Bauss F and Russell RGG (2004) [92]. With kind permission from Springer Science+Business Media).

Pharmacology

Bisphosphonates are poorly absorbed when taken by mouth. On average <1% of an oral dose is absorbed. Once absorbed, bisphosphonates are quickly cleared from the circulation by attaching via a physiochemical adherence to the denuded bone calcium-phosphorus surface, exposed during the resorption phase of remodeling [10–12]. The remaining bisphosphonate that does not attach to bone in the initial phase of circulation is rapidly excreted by the kidney. Renal excretion is accomplished both by glomerular filtration and active cellular transport in the proximal tubule [13]. For any given bisphosphonate that arrives in the systemic circulation (oral or intravenous {IV}), approximately 60% becomes bound to bone tissue and the remaining 40% is excreted by the kidney [14, 15].

Bisphosphonates are not metabolized. More specifically, when a bisphosphonate that is bound to bone is subsequently detached from the bone surface and recycled back into the circulation as well as eliminated in the urine, it retains its molecular structure [15]. This persistence of the basic bisphosphonate molecular structure explains, in part, the long duration of effect on bone turnover and bone mineral density and fracture risk reduction after bisphosphonate discontinuation [16–19].

The physiochemical-binding component of the mechanism of action (MOA) of bisphosphonates explains, in part, their ability to improve bone strength. Data suggests that the bone resorption depth, osteoclast number, and remodeling space may be reduced by bisphosphonates, thereby reducing the perforation of trabecular plates ("stress-risers") [20–22]. Cortical porosity and differences in mineral distribution are reduced by bisphosphonates, which explains, in part, the improvement in cortical bone strength [23, 24]. There are differences among the bisphosphonates in the affinity for the bone surface and their detachment rate from these surfaces as well [1, 10–12] (Figures 9.2 and 9.3).

This hierarchy of affinity for the bone surface explains, in part, the ability to provide long dosing intervals. For example, the bisphosphonate with the greatest affinity for the bone surface is zoledronic acid, the same bisphosphonate that for the management of osteoporosis can be given once yearly [1, 10–12].

The second MOA of bisphosphonates in regards to the reduction of bone remodeling is a cellular one. The osteoclast, entering the basic bone remodeling unit (BMU), engulfs the bisphosphonate intracellularly. In osteoclasts, bisphosphonates inhibit the enzyme farnesyl pyrophosphate synthase, (FFPS), a key enzyme in the mevalonic acid synthesis pathway. Disruption of this pathway results in the reduction in the prenylation of specific osteoclast proteins necessary for the activity of the osteoclast to

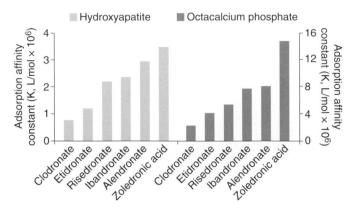

Figure 9.2 The differences of the affinity for the crystal surface among bisphosphonates. (*Source*: Nancollas GH *et al.* (2006) [10]).

resorb bone [1, 12]. Osteoclasts resorb bone by secreting hydrogen ions and enzymes into the subcellular space between the osteoclast and the bone surface. These cellular activities are inhibited by bisphosphonates that are a second explanation for the inhibition of bone remodeling that can be measured by the reduction in bone turnover markers (BTM) [25–28].

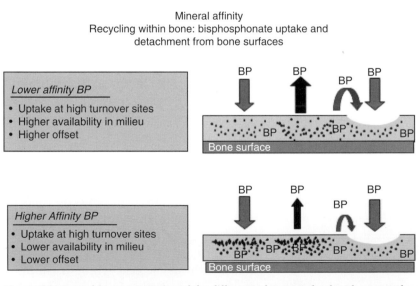

Figure 9.3 A graphic representation of the differences between the detachment and re-uptake among bisphosphonates that have low vs high affinity for the bone surface. (*Source*: Nancollas GH et al. (2006) [10]).

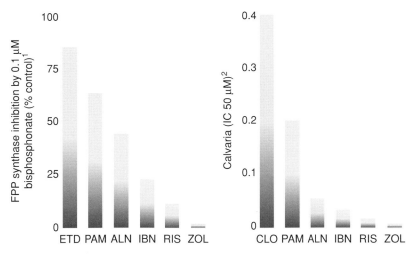

ALN, alendronate; CLO, clodronate; ETD, etidronate; IBN, ibandronate; PAM, pamidronate; RIS, risedronate; ZOL, zoledronate

Figure 9.4 The hierarchy among the bisphosphonates on the activity of osteoclast intracellular farnesyl pyrophosphate. (*Source*: Dunford JE *et al.* (2001) Structure-activity relationships for inhibition of farnesyl diphosphate synthetase in vitro and inhibition of bone resorption in vivo by nitrogen containing bisphosphonates. *J Pharmacol Exp Ther* **296**: 235–42; and Green JR *et al.* (1994) *J Bone Miner Res* **9**: 745–51).

While the activity of osteoclasts is inhibited by bisphosphonates, there is less evidence that bisphosphonates induce programmed cell death of the osteoclasts (apoptosis). In fact, in a few histomorphometric studies in patients receiving long-term alendronate and zoledronic acid, giant, multi-nucleated osteoclasts are seen [29]. It is not clear if these giant osteoclasts are metabolically active; yet, the point is that osteoclasts are seen.

Like the hierarchy that exists among bisphosphonates in regards to their affinity for the crystal surface, there is also a hierarchy among bisphosphonates on the ability to inhibit FPPS [2, 3] (Figure 9.4). Since risedronate has similar inhibitory effects on FPPS as zoledronic acid yet has far less affinity for the bone surface, it would seem that the greater effect on reduction of bone turnover and longer dosing intervals provided by zoledronic acid compared with risedronate may be more a function of their physiochemical effects as opposed to their cellular effects.

Bisphosphonate uptake and distribution into bone compartments is a function of the rate of bone remodeling and affinity characteristics of the bisphosphonates [30, 31]. Once the remodeling space is saturated with bisphosphonates, continual skeletal uptake is probably a function of the efflux of bisphosphonates from remodeling units, and the formation of new, previously resting BMUs. It is unclear if the total skeletal amount increases with continual exposure. It is clear that retained bisphosphonates undergo recycling both by release into the circulation from the bone surface and release into the circulation through trans-membrane passage from osteoclasts [1–3, 10–12]. The bisphosphonate that is released from bone has two fates: elimination from the body via renal clearance and reattachment to a different area of bone. Pharmacodynamic modeling suggests that total bone load increases with continual bisphosphonate exposure. It is estimated that the half-life of alendronate is 10 years [15]. These pharmacokinetic and pharmacodynamic models have never been validated in humans, but one can assume both from the pharmacology as well the clinical trial data that persistence of effect after discontinuation is a unique feature of the clinical pharmacology of bisphosphonates.

Clinical trial data-registration studies

The FDA requires evidence of fracture risk reduction over 3 years compared with placebo for approval of antiresorptive agents. On this basis, the daily dosing formulations of alendronate, risedronate, ibandronate, and annual intravenous zoledronic acid were registered for the treatment of postmenopausal osteoporosis [32–37]. While each of the approved bisphosphonates attained this required endpoint, there are differences among bisphosphonates in clinically important prespecified secondary endpoints, nonvertebral and hip fracture risk reduction. Some of these differences are due to the differences in study populations, sample size, or data captured in the clinical case report forms [38–40]. However, there are differences among the bisphosphonates in outcome data within each registration clinical trial (Table 9.2).

FDA registration for a particular label may differ from evidence of a benefit of any given particular bisphosphonate on reduction at a particular

Table 9.2 The clinical differences among bisphosphonates in head-to-head individual clinical trials.

Drug	Vertebral fracture	Nonvertebral fracture	Hip fracture
Ibandronate (Boniva®)	√	No effect demonstrated	No effect demonstrated
Alendronate (Fosamax®)	√	*	√
Risedronate (Actonel®, Atelvia®)	√	√	*
Zoledronic acid (Reclast®)	√	√	√

*Evidence for effect but not an FDA-approved indication.

fracture site. For example, in neither of the 2 risedronate registration clinical trials was there evidence for a statistically significant reduction in hip fracture risk [34, 35]. Nevertheless, in the separate risedronate hip fracture trial there was a significant reduction in the risk of hip fracture in the pooled risedronate doses (2.5 mg/day and 5.0 mg/day) vs placebo in a large population of patients who had osteoporosis at the femoral neck by World Health Organization (WHO) criteria [41]. Therefore, for all of the bisphosphonates, a lack of evidence may not translate into a lack of efficacy. One would need to complete a prospective, randomized head-to-head fracture trial to scientifically know if one bisphosphonate is "better" than another. Such a study has never nor will probably ever be done due to the enormous expense of such a trial at a time when patents for bisphosphonates have or are coming to an end. Choice among bisphosphonates is often based on payor coverage, patient preferences or tolerability, or physician choice based on evidence. In large observational database studies REAL, REALITY and VIBE [42] (Figure 9.5) only the REAL study suggested a greater early effect of risedronate vs alendronate to reduce the risk of nonvertebral fracture risk reduction [43].

Clinical trial evidence is limited by the strict preselection criteria for randomization while the evidence from observational data is limited by the absence of randomization. Clinical trial patients are often not real office-setting patients who often have comorbidities not reflected in the outcome data of RCTs [44]. Hence, both bodies of evidence have value as well as limitations, and use of bisphosphonates in clinical practice is often dictated by issues having little to do with the data among bisphosphonates. The one potential advantage of parenteral administration of bisphosphonates

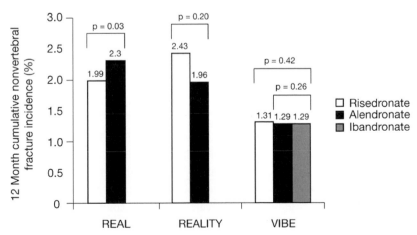

Figure 9.5 The fracture reductions among bisphosphonates from three separate observational studies.

over oral dosing is the assurance of delivery to bone. There are certainly compliance/persistence issues with oral therapy that limit their efficacy [45–47] but there are also bioavailability issues that may do the same such as diseases or prior surgery of the gastrointestinal tract that reduce the absorption of the already poorly-absorbed oral bisphosphonates. Diseases such as celiac disease (even asymptomatic) probably limit absorption. Since bisphosphonate serum levels cannot be measured in clinical practice, intravenous administration removes the uncertainty about bioavailability. In these scenarios, biochemical markers of bone turnover, as well as serial bone mineral density (BMD) measurements may provide reassurance that a positive biological effect is being achieved with oral administration [48–51]. In addition, in clinical circumstances where oral absorption is not tolerated or may not be advisable (e.g., esophageal stricture, achalasia, etc.), intravenous administration may be a safer route of administration.

One side note should be mentioned regarding the poor absorption of oral bisphosphonates: that is the abundant number of generic oral bisphosphonates on the market worldwide. While the FDA requirement for the initial registration of bisphosphonates for postmenopausal osteoporosis is very strict, registration for generic bisphosphonate is not. Generic oral bisphosphonates can become registered based on "bioequivalency," i.e., that the generic molecule has an identical molecular structure as the parent compound and the tablet contains the stated amount ±20%. For many generic drugs this requirement is acceptable. It may not be acceptable for bisphosphonates, which have fundamentally poor absorption to begin with. Due to low costs, many health plans require the use of generic oral bisphosphonates as first line therapy. In these circumstances, measurement of a BTM may provide reassurance that the oral generic bisphosphonate is being absorbed and having the proper bone biological effect, though there is little data to secure this opinion.

Clinical trial data – bridging studies

The alternate dosing regimens for postmenopausal osteoporosis (weekly alendronate, delayed-release risedronate, monthly risedronate and ibandronate, and quarterly intravenous ibandronate) received FDA registration not on the basis of any fracture reduction data but instead on BMD noninferiority endpoints. That is, for registration, the intermittent dosing schedule had to show evidence that the spine BMD by dual energy x-ray absorptiometry (DXA) increased to an equivalent level as the fracture-proven daily dosing [52]. Hence, use of these nondaily bisphosphonate dosing regimens is based on the trust that the spine BMD changes will translate into equal fracture protection. While the changes in BMD mediated by bisphosphonates have a nonlinear relationship to fracture risk reduction, and stable BMD on therapy is an acceptable clinical endpoint for pharmacological efficacy, it should be acknowledged that use of these alternative dosing regimens is not based on fracture reduction data [25, 50, 51]. The advantage of intermittent dosing regimens is better compliance/persistence, which may translate into better fracture protection than the daily dosing regimen.

The only head-to-head comparative study between alternative dosing regimens is the Fosamax-Actonel Comparator Trial (FACT) [53]. FACT was a randomized trial in treatment naïve patients between the weekly dosing regimens of these 2 oral bisphosphonates. This was not a fracture trial so the results cannot be extrapolated into how the measured endpoints (changes in BMD and BTM) translate into difference in fracture risk reduction. BMD increased more in the alendronate-treated group than the risedronate-treated group. While a substantial amount of the improvement in bone strength with antiresorptive therapy is felt to be due to reductions in bone turnover, without head-to-head fracture data, any conclusions are speculative. Addressing this point of the relationship of changes in BMD to changes in fracture risk reduction are 3 important published data:

1 The European arm of the risedronate clinical trials, 2.5 mg/day dosing regimen was as effective as the registered 5.0 mg/day dose to reduce the incidence of morphometric vertebral fracture [35].
2 In the risedronate hip fracture trial, the lower (2.5 mg/day) dose showed hip fracture risk at least as good as the higher (5.0 mg/day) regimen [41].
3 The Fracture Intervention Trial (FIT), which led to the registration of daily alendronate, used only 5.0 mg/day of alendronate for the first two years compared with 10 mg/day during the third year, yet vertebral fracture risk reduction occurred during the first two years [32, 33].

Thus, it would appear that bisphosphonates reduce fracture risk by multiple mechanisms, and that increases in BMD or reductions in BTM explain only a part of the improvement bone strength. Some of these alternative MOAs may be the preservation of horizontal trabeculae, the prevention of the accumulation of stress risers and/or a reduction in cortical porosity [20, 23, 24, 54]. It is evident, however, that the improvement in bone strength mediated by bisphosphonates is multi-factorial.

Benefit/risk

The benefit-to-risk ratio of bisphosphonates for the treatment of PMO is high [5].

Fracture risk is multifactorial as shown by the validated FRAX™ 10-year population data [55]. In the at risk population, bisphosphonates have evidence for global risk reduction, and the International Society for Clinical Densitometry (ISCD) has provided leadership in this area of risk assessment [56]. Side effects due to bisphosphonates are uncommon. The most common side effects are gastrointestinal and acute phase reactions; while musculoskeletal side effects are rare and usually transient when the dosing recommendations are followed. The risks that have received the greatest recent attention are osteonecrosis of the jaw (ONJ) and atypical mid-shaft femur fractures. Both are rare and no causality has been established for either [57, 58].

The risk for osteonecrosis of the jaw (ONJ) in the postmenopausal osteoporosis population receiving the FDA approved doses of bisphosphonates is exceedingly low (<0.7/100 000 patient years exposure) [5, 57]. Yet the perception, especially in many in the dental community, is that the risk is greater; probably related to the greater risk in the oncology population with metastatic cancer to bone requiring monthly intravenous bisphosphonates to reduce their risk for skeletal related events (SREs) [59]. SREs are fractures due to cancer in bone which induce a far greater increase in bone turnover, in part, due to the induction of a greater amount of RANK-Ligand by the cancer cells [60–62]. There are no clinical means of predicting who might and who might not develop ONJ. There is no evidence that temporary withholding of bisphosphonates has any effect on reducing the rare risk of ONJ.

Atypical mid-shaft femur fractures are spontaneous fractures of the femoral shaft below the lesser trochanter and above the femoral condyles. The American Society for Bone and Mineral Research (ASBMR) white paper on this topic has characterized features that specify the criteria for the diagnosis of bisphosphonate-associated atypical femur fractures (Table 9.3) [58]. While most fractures of the femur are "typical," occurring

Table 9.3 The American Society for Bone and Mineral Research Task Force on Atypical Femur Fractures: Provisional case definition.

- 1. Anywhere along the femur distal to the lesser trochanter and above the femur condyles.
- 2. Associated with no or minimal trauma.
- 3. Transverse of short oblique configuration.
- 4. Non-comminuted.
- 5. Complete fractures must extend through both cortices white incomplete fractures involve only the lateral cortex
- Features often present but not required: increase cortical thickness, periosteal reaction of the lateral cortex ("beaking"), prodromal pain, bilateral fractures of delayed healing.

Requires radiological confirmation; cannot be made on any ICD-9 coding
(*Source*: Shane E, Burr D, Ebeling PR et al. (2010) [58]).

in the femoral neck, intertrochanteric region or immediately below the lesser trochanter, the atypicality of these subtrochanteric fractures is not only their location in the mid-shaft of the femur but also the prodrome of constant anterior thigh pain, frequent bilaterally, and lack of trauma. These atypical fractures have been reported in patients not on bisphosphonates, though more have been reported in patients on long-term (usually 5 years or longer) bisphosphonate therapy [63, 64]. It is important to recognize that while epidemiological studies have reported the risk of bisphosphonate-associated atypical femur fractures to be 5/10 000 patient years, and, an attributable risk in untreated patients of 1/10 000 patient years, there might be underreporting of nonbisphosphonate associated fractures. Nevertheless, while these atypical fractures are rare and no causality has been established, it is important that physicians recognize that while this rare condition might be associated with the long-term use of bisphosphonates, that the benefit gained by treatment of the patient at high risk for an osteoporosis-related fracture if left untreated far exceeds the risk of these atypical fractures.

While there are no scientific data regarding management of patients on long-term bisphosphonates as it pertains to atypical femur fractures, there are a few clinical suggestions to provide guidance. Patients should be advised that the "prodrome" often described is a deep mid-thigh anterior thigh pain that may persist for weeks before the fracture, and, if reported, patients should have a femur x-ray (or even more sensitive a bone scan or MRI) to look for an early cortical thickness or "beaking" or a fracture line (Figures 9.6 and 9.7) [4, 65]. If discovered, the patients should be taken off bisphosphonates and advised to reduce the weight load to that femur. In addition, consultation with an orthopedic surgeon should be done to consider prophylactic intramedullary rod insertion [66]. The mechanism of these bisphosphonate-associated atypical femur fractures remains unknown; transiliac bone histomorphometry in small numbers of patients has shown inconsistent levels of bone remodeling. Causality has not been established.

Bisphosphonate drug-holidays

The term bisphosphonate drug-holiday has become a popular terminology in the literature [4, 5, 67–72]. The concept of a bisphosphonate "drug-holiday" has evolved in part due to the unique pharmacology of bisphosphonates and the paucity of long-term (>5 years) efficacy data where a placebo group is maintained [67–71]. The reality is that long-term data where a placebo group is maintained is unethical in higher risk populations – the type of patients required for randomization into clinical trials

Bilateral "beaking" also detected by DXA

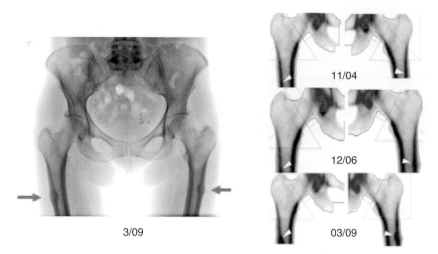

Figure 9.6 The appearance of atypical femur fracture (bilateral) by dual energy X-ray absorptiometry (DXA) showing cortical thickening and "beaking." (*Source*: McKinernan F (2010) [65]).

Subtrochanteric fractures of the femur

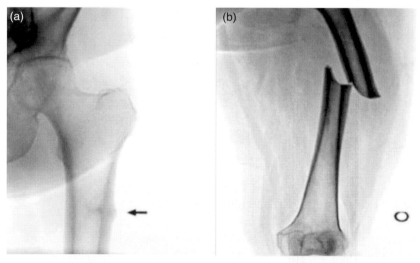

Figure 9.7 A radiograph of an early (a) and late (b) atypical femur fracture. (Courtesy of J. Lane and A. Unnanuntana, Hospital of Special Surgery, New York, NY, USA).

to achieve a fracture endpoint [72]. Despite this limitation, there are data from long-term (5 years' treatment and 5 years' placebo) alendronate and risedronate trials that fracture risk remained lower than placebo [16–19, 73], and data from the extension of the zoledronic acid registration trial that a benefit to maintain risk reduction was seen through 6 years of annual zoledronic acid [19]. This maintenance of efficacy in the FLEX and HORIZON trials was not seen in those patients who had prior vertebral fractures or femoral neck T-scores that were -2.5 or lower. Hence, it seems that for clinical management of high risk patients, continuation of therapy is advisable [5, 67–71]. What is unclear is how long discontinuation should last in those provided with a "drug-holiday" [5, 67–71], or what are the clearly defined criteria for continuing, discontinuation, or restarting therapy with either a bisphosphonate or a different pharmacological agent. It has been suggested [5, 68–71] that either a clear decline of BMD and/or increase in BTMs might indicate loss of antiresorptive effect. What is unclear is whether or not bone strength differs when BMD declines or BTMs increase after discontinuation of agents that improve bone strength versus the higher risk for fracture seen when BMD declines or BTM are elevated in treatment naïve persons. Nevertheless, it appears that the terminology of bisphosphonate drug holiday is engrained and that each patient's management should be considered on an individual patient basis.

Safety of bisphosphonates

Renal

Oral bisphosphonates are not nephrotoxic and, in fact, are effective to reduce fracture risk without any negative effect on renal function based post-hoc analyses in patients with an estimated glomerular filtration rate (eGFR) as low as 15 ml/min [5, 14, 74–79]. The FDA warnings not to use bisphosphonates in patients with an eGFR <30 or 35 ml/min (for IV zoledronic acid) is based more on the lack of data in this population and the associated case reports of negative effects of bisphosphonates on renal tissue in older literature in both animal models and human beings with the intravenous formulations. In addition, since bisphosphonates are cleared by the kidney both by glomerular filtration and proximal tubular secretion, the potential for renal effects is related to their renal pharmacokinetics. Approximately 50–60% of administered bisphosphonate is excreted unchanged by the kidneys with the remainder taken up by bone. Renal toxicity due to intravenous bisphosphonates is related to the maximum drug level achieved (Cmax) and not the area under the curve (AUC) of drug exposure.

Use of other agents that have nephrotoxic potential such as nonsteroidal anti-inflammatory drugs or diuretics, preexisting renal impairment and dehydration at the time of bisphosphonate infusion increase the risk for renal dysfunction. To avoid compromise of renal function, bisphosphonates should not be given to patients with eGFRs of ≤30 ml/min. For zoledronic acid, the threshold is <35 mL/minute; serum calcium and GFR should be assessed prior to every infusion, and drug should be administered over 15 minutes or longer. Though the FDA specifically states measuring creatinine clearance before each zoledronic acid infusion, they will accept eGFR by the Cockroft-Gault equation.

In the phase 3 HORIZON study, a small but significant number of postmenopausal women treated with zoledronic acid demonstrated mild increases in serum creatinine concentration 9–11 days after the 2nd infusion; the serum creatinine concentration returned to normal before the next infusion and there were no difference in eGFRs in drug versus placebo-treated patients over the course of the trial [19, 76]. In the 3-year extension data (6 years of zoledronic acid therapy), there were no differences in eGFR between placebo and annual zoledronic acid (Figure 9.8). Intravenous ibandronate, dosed for osteoporosis (3 mg every 3 months), has shown no significant renal toxicity if treated patients have eGFRs >30 mL/minute and no baseline renal comorbidities [79].

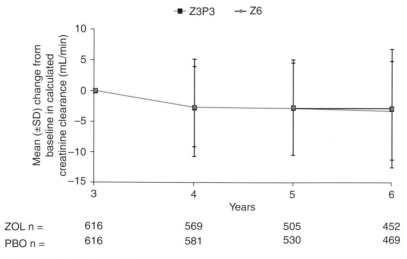

Figure 9.8 The effects of long-term (6 yr) zoledronic acid (5 mg/year) vs placebo on eGFR.

Gastrointestinal

Oral daily bisphosphonates have been associated with esophageal ulcers, esophagitis, and bleeding; however, these side-effects lessened with the advent of weekly (alendronate, risedronate) or monthly (ibandronate, risedronate) preparations [4, 5]. Concern has emerged about an association between oral bisphosphonate use and an increased risk of esophageal cancer which remains unvalidated. The bulk of evidence points away from an association between bisphosphonate and esophageal cancer [80].

Other safety concerns

Approximately 30% of patients receiving their first doses of intravenous bisphosphonate (or high dose oral) experience an acute phase reaction (fever, headache, myalgia, arthralgia, malaise) occurring within 24–36 hours and lasting up to 3 days. The incidence is reduced ~50% by acetaminophen (500–1000 mg before and for 24–48 hours postinfusion) and decreases with subsequent infusions [4, 5, 19, 37].

In the 3-year HORIZON Pivotal Fracture Trial [37], subjects treated with zoledronic acid had an increased incidence of atrial fibrillation which was recorded as a serious adverse event (1.3% with zoledronic acid versus 0.5% with placebo, $P < 0.001$). There were no significant differences in the rates of stroke, myocardial infarction, or deaths due to cardiovascular events, nor was there any relation to the timing of drug infusion, acute phase reactions, calcium levels, or electrolyte abnormalities. This report prompted additional investigation of the risk of atrial fibrillation in posthoc analyses of other bisphosphonate trials and reviews of healthcare databases. None of these studies found an association between the use of bisphosphonates and atrial fibrillation. Zoledronic acid was not associated with an increased risk of atrial fibrillation in the HORIZON Recurrent Fracture Trial [81] (subjects were older and presumably at higher risk) nor in any of the oncology trials where subjects received zoledronic acid in doses that were approximately 10 times the dose for osteoporosis (i.e., 4 mg monthly instead of the dose for osteoporosis which is 5 mg yearly). Post hoc analyses of studies with other bisphosphonates, including alendronate, risedronate, and ibandronate, did not show a statistically significant increase in the risk of atrial fibrillation [4, 5]. Population-based case-control studies are conflicting, some showing an increase in the risk of atrial fibrillation in women with past (but not current) use of alendronate, others showing no increased risk [4, 5, 82]. Besides a dearth of data associating bisphosphonates with atrial fibrillation, there is no clear biologically plausible mechanism by which this might occur. In their most recent review of these data, the FDA recommends that patients should not stop taking their bisphosphonate medication because of this theoretical concern, stating that "across all studies, no clear association between over-all bisphosphonate exposure and the rate of serious or nonserious atrial fibrillation was observed." The issue of atrial fibrillation, therefore, as being possibly associated with bisphosphonate use is generally discounted by most experts.

Possible benefits (decreased risk of breast cancer, stroke, colon cancer, mortality)

In the zoledronic acid recurrent fracture trial, there was observed a 28% reduction in all-cause mortality [81]. All-cause mortality was not a pre-specified endpoint for this trial so the mechanism(s) that might be related to this observation remained ill-defined. Nevertheless, this observation led to examination of other databases and populations examining this relationship. There are now several studies reporting on a reduction in all-cause mortality in association with bisphosphonate use [82–85]. These data, coupled with studies showing that broader bone mineral density test-ing and treatment of osteoporosis in the appropriate higher risk population reduces morbidity and is cost-effective should help promote the proper uti-lization of bisphosphonates [86–91].

Conclusions

Bisphosphonates are a highly effective and safe therapy that reduces the risk of all fractures in the postmenopausal population. Their benefit-to-risk ratio strongly favors a benefit in patients at high risk of fracture. They may be associated with side effects, though there is no established causality between bisphosphonate use and osteonecrosis of the jaw or atypical mid-shaft femur fractures. Nevertheless, continued vigilance and better science are important as we learn more about long-term bisphosphonate admin-istration. It appears that high risk patients should not only be treated but that treatment may need to be maintained to reduce further incident frac-tures. All management decisions in patients, however, need to be made on a case-by-case basis and made with shared decision-making with the patient. By using good clinical science and good clinical judgment, we should be able to reduce the mortality, morbidity and costs of this under-diagnosed and undertreated disease.

References

1 Russell RG, Watts NB, Ebetino FH, *et al.* (2008) Mechanisms of action of bisphos-phonates: similarities differences and their potential influence on clinical efficacy. *Osteoporos Int* **19**(6): 733–59.

2 Fleisch H (1998) Bisphosphonates: mechanisms of action. *Endocr Rev* **19**: 80–100.

3 Russell RG, Rogers MJ (1999) Bisphosphonates: from the laboratory to the clinic and back again. *Bone* **25**: 97–106.

4 Watts NB, Diab DL (2010) Long-term use of bisphosphonates in osteoporosis. *J Clin Endocrinol Metab* **95**(4): 1555–65.

5 Khosla S, Bilezikian JP, Dempster DW, *et al.* (2012) Benefits and risks of bisphosphonate therapy for osteoporosis, *J Clin Endocrinol Metab* **97**: as doi:10.1210/jc.2012-1027.

6 Fleisch H, Neuman W (1961) Mechanisms of calcification: role of collagen, polyphosphates, and phosphatase. *Am J Physiol* **200**: 1296–1300.

7 Fleisch H, Russell RG, Francis MD (1969) Diphosphonates inhibit hydroxyapatite dissolution in vitro and bone resorption in tissue culture and in vivo. *Science* **165**: 1262–4.

8 Bassett CAL *et al.* (1969) Diphosphonates in the treatment of myositis ossificans. *Lancet* **2**: 845.

9 Schenk R, Merz WA, Muhlbauer R *et al.* (1973) Effect of ethane-1-hydroxy-1,1-diphosphonate (EHDP) and dichloromethylene diphosphonate (Cl2MDP) on the calcification and resorption of cartilage and bone in the tibial epiphysis and metaphysis of rats. *Calcif Tissue Res* **11**: 196–214.

10 Nancollas GH, Tang R, Phipps RJ, *et al.* (2006) Novel insights into actions of bisphosphonates on bone: differences in interactions with hydroxyapatite. *Bone* **38**: 617–27.

11 Rogers MJ, Crockett JC, Coxon FP, *et al.* (2011) Biochemical and molecular mechanisms of action of bisphosphonates. *Bone* **49**: 34–41.

12 Ebetino FH, Hogan AM, Sun S, *et al.* (2011) The relationship between the chemistry and biological activity of the bisphosphonates. *Bone* **49**: 20–33.

13 Troehler U, Bonjour JP, Fleisch H (1975) Renal secretion of diphosphonates in rats. *Kidney Int* **8**: 6.

14 Miller PD (2011) The kidney and bisphosphonates. *Bone* **49**(1): 77–81.

15 Rodan G, Seedor JG, Balena R (1993) Preclinical pharmacology of alendronate. *Osteoporosis Int* (suppl) **3**: S7–12 (review).

16 Black DM, Schwartz AV, Ensrud KE, *et al.* (2006) Effects of continuing or stopping alendronate after 5 years of treatment: the Fracture Intervention Trial Long-term Extension (FLEX): a randomized trial. *JAMA* **296**: 2927–38.

17 Watts NB, Chines A, Olszynski WP, *et al.* (2008) Fracture risk remains reduced one year after discontinuation of risedronate. *Osteoporos Int* **19**: 365–72.

18 Schwartz AV, Bauer DC, Cummings SR, *et al.* (2010) Efficacy of continued alendronate for fractures in women with and without prevalent vertebral fracture: The FLEX trial. *J Bone Miner Res* **25**: 976–82.

19 Black DM, Reid I, Boonen S, *et al.* (2012) The effect of 3 versus 6 years of zoledronic acid treatment of osteoporosis: a randomized extension to the HORIZON-Pivotal Fracture Trial (PFT). *J Bone Miner Res* **27**(2): 243–54.

20 Chavassieux PM, Arlot ME, Reda C, *et al.* (1997) Histomorphometric assessment of the long-term effects of alendronate on bone quality and remodeling in patients with osteoporosis. *J Clin Invest* **100**: 1475–80.

21 Recker RR, Weinstein RS, Chesnut 3rd CH, *et al.* (2004) Histomorphometric evaluation of daily and intermittent oral ibandronate in women with postmenopausal osteoporosis: results from the BONE study. *Osteoporos Int* **15**: 231–7.

22 Recker RR, Delmas PD, Halse J, *et al.* (2008) Effects of intravenous zoledronic acid once yearly on bone remodeling and bone structure. *J Bone Miner Res* **23**: 6–16.

23 Roschger P, Rinnerthaler S, Yates J, *et al.* (2001) Alendronate increases degree and uniformity of mineralization in cancellous bone and decreases the porosity in cortical bone of osteoporotic women. *Bone* **29**: 185–91.

24 Seeman E, Delmas PD, Hanley DA, *et al.* (2010) Microarchitectural deterioration of cortical and trabecular bone: differing effects of denosumab and alendronate. *J Bone Miner Res* **25**: 1886–94.

25 Sarkar S, Reginster JY, Crans GG, *et al.* (2004) Relationship between changes in biochemical markers of bone turnover and BMD to predict vertebral fracture risk. *J Bone Miner Res* **19**: 394–401.

26 Civitelli R, Armamento-Villareal R, *et al.* (2009) Bone turnover markers: understanding their value in clinical trials and clinical practice. *Osteoporos Int.* **20**: 843–51.

27 Eastell R, Hannon RA (2008) Biomarkers of bone health and osteoporosis risk. *Proc Nutr Soc* **67**: 157–62.

28 Bauer DC *et al.* (2004) Change in bone turnover and hip, non-spine, and vertebral fracture in alendronate-treated women: the fracture intervention trial. *Journal of Bone and Mineral Research* **19**: 1250–8.

29 Jain N, Weinstein RS (2009) Giant osteoclasts after long-term bisphosphonate therapy: diagnostic challenges. *Nat Rev Rheumatol* **5**(6): 341–6.

30 Roelofs AJ, Stewart CA, Sun S, *et al.* (2012) Influence of bone affinity on the skeletal distribution of fluorescently labeled bisphosphonate in vivo. *J Bone Miner Res* **27**(4): 835–47.

31 Turek J, Ebetino FH, Lundy MW, *et al.* (2012) Bisphosphonate binding affinity affects drug distribution in both intracortical and trabecular bone of rabbits. *Calcif Tissue Int* **90**(3): 202–10.

32 Black DM, Cummings SR, Karpf DB, *et al.* (1996) Randomised trial of effect of alendronate on risk of fracture in women with existing vertebral fractures. Fracture Intervention Trial Research Group. *Lancet* **348**(9041): 1535–41.

33 Cummings SR, Black DM, Thompson DE, *et al.* (1998) Effect of alendronate on risk of fracture in women with low bone density but without vertebral fractures: results from the Fracture Intervention Trial. *JAMA* **280**(24): 2077–82.

34 Harris ST, Watts NB, Genant HK, *et al.* (1999) Effects of risedronate treatment on vertebral and nonvertebral fractures in women with postmenopausal osteoporosis: a randomized controlled trial. Vertebral Efficacy With Risedronate Therapy (VERT) Study Group. *JAMA* **282**(14): 1344–52.

35 Reginster J, Minne HW, Sorensen OH, *et al.* (2000) Randomized trial of the effects of risedronate on vertebral fractures in women with established postmenopausal osteoporosis. Vertebral Efficacy with Risedronate Therapy (VERT) Study Group. *Osteoporos Int* **11**(1): 83–91.

36 Chesnut III CH, Skag A, Christiansen C, *et al.* (2004) Effects of oral ibandronate administered daily or intermittently on fracture risk in postmenopausal osteoporosis. *J Bone Miner Res* **19**(8): 1241–9.

37 Black DM, Delmas PD, Eastell R, *et al.* (2007) Once-yearly zoledronic acid for treatment of postmenopausal osteoporosis. *N Engl J Med* **356**(18): 1809–22.

38 Miller PD (2008) Anti-resorptives in the management of osteoporosis. *Best Practice and Research Clinical Endocrinology and Metabolism* **22**(5): 849–68.

39 MacLean C, Newberry S, Maglione M, *et al.* (2008) Systematic review: comparative effectiveness of treatments to prevent fractures in men and women with low bone density or osteoporosis. *Ann Intern Med* **148**(3): 197–213.

40 Cranney A, Guyatt G, Griffith L, *et al.*, Osteoporosis Methodology Group and The Osteoporosis Advisory Research Group (2002) Meta-analyses of therapies

for postmenopausal osteoporosis. IX: Summary of meta-analyses of therapies for postmenopausal osteoporosis. *Endocr Rev* **23**(4): 570–8.

41 McClung MR, Geusens P, Miller PD, *et al.* (2001) Effect of risedronate on the risk of hip fracture in elderly women. Hip Intervention Program Study Group. *N Engl J Med* **344**(5): 333–40.

42 Silverman S (2010) Osteoporosis Therapies: Evidence from Healthcare Databases and Observational Population Studies. *Calif Tissue Int* **87**: 375–84.

43 Silverman CTI, Silverman SL, Watts NB, *et al.* (2007) Effectiveness of bisphosphonates on nonvertebral and hip fractures in the first year of therapy: the risedronate and alendronate (REAL) cohort study. *Osteoporosis Int* **18**: 25–34.

44 Dowd R, Recker RR, Heaney RP (2000) Study subjects and ordinary patients. *Osteoporos Int* **11**(6): 533–6.

45 Siris ES, Harris ST, Rosen CJ, *et al.* (2006) Adherence to bisphosphonate therapy and fracture rates in osteoporotic women: relationship to vertebral and non-vertebral fractures from 2 US claims databases. *Mayo Clinic Proc* **81**(8): 1013–22.

46 Siris ES, Pasquale MK, Wang Y, *et al.* (2011) Estimating bisphosphonate use and fracture reduction among US women aged 45 years and older, 2001–2008. *J Bone Miner Res* **26**(1): 3–11.

47 Siris ES, Selby PL, Saag KG, *et al.* (2009) Impact of osteoporosis treatment adherence on fracture rates in North America and Europe. *Am J Med* **122** (2 suppl): S3–S13.

48 Civitelli R, Armamento-Villareal R, Napoli N (2009) Bone turnover markers: understanding their value in clinical trials and clinical practice. *Osteoporos Int* **20**: 843–51.

49 Eastell R, Hannon RA (2008) Biomarkers of bone health and osteoporosis risk. *Proc Nutr Soc* **67**: 157–62.

50 Bonnick SL, Shulman L (2006) Monitoring osteoporosis therapy: bone mineral density, bone turnover markers, or both? *Am J Med* **119**(4 Suppl 1): S25–S31.

51 Lewiecki EM, Watts NB (2008) Assessing response to osteoporosis therapy. *Osteoporosis Int* **19**(10): 1363–1368.

52 Miller PD, Epstein S, Sedarati F, *et al.* (2008) Once monthly oral ibandronate comparedwith weekly alendronate: results from the head-to-head MOTION study. *Current MedicalResearch Opinion* **24**: 207–13.

53 Rosen CJ, Hochberg M, Bonnick S, *et al.* (2005) Treatment with once-weekly alendronate 70 mg compared to once-weekly risedronate 35 mg in women with postmenopausal osteoporosis: A randomized, double-blind study. *J Bone Miner Res* **20**: 141–51.

54 Borah B, Dufresne T, Nurre J *et al.* (2010) Risedronate reduces intracortical porosity in women with osteoporosis. *J Bone Miner Res* **25**(1): 41–7.

55 Kanis JA, Hans D, Cooper C, *et al.*; Task Force of the FRAX Initiative (2011) Interpretation of FRAX in clinical practice. *Osteoporos Int* **22**(9): 2395–2411.

56 Lewiecki EM, Compston JE, Miller PD, *et al.* FRAX® Position Development Conference Members (2011) Official Positions for FRAX simplification from Joint Official Positions Development Conference of The International Society for Clinical Densitometry and The International Osteoporosis Foundation on FRAX. *J Clin Densitom* **14**(3): 226–36.

57 Khosla S, Burr D, Cauley J, *et al.* (2007) Bisphosphonate-associated osteonecrosis of the jaw: report of a task force of the American Society for Bone and Mineral Research. *J Bone Miner Res* **22**(10): 1479–91.

58 Shane E, Burr D, Ebeling PR, *et al.* (2010) Atypical subtrochanteric and diaphyseal femoral fractures: Report of a task force of the American Society for Bone and Mineral Research. *J Bone Miner Res* **25**(11): 2267–94.

59 Hellstein JW, Adler RA, Edwards B, *et al.* (2011) Managing the care of patients receiving antiresorptive therapy for prevention and treatment of osteoporosis: executive summary of recommendations from the American Dental Association Council on Scientific Affairs. *J Am Dent Assoc* **142**(11): 1243–51.

60 Bilezikian, J.P., Matsumoto, T., Bellido, *et al.* (2008) Targeting bone remodeling for the treatment of osteoporosis: summary of the proceedings of an ASBMR workshop. *J Bone Miner Res* **24**: 373–85.

61 Ortiz A, Lin SH (2012) Osteolytic and osteoblastic bone metastases: two extremes of the same spectrum. *Recent Results Cancer Res* **192**: 225–33 (review).

62 Stopeck AT, Lipton A, Body JJ, *et al.* (2010) Denosumab compared with zoledronic acid for the treatment of bone metastases in patients with advanced breast cancer: a randomized, double-blind study. *J Clin Oncol* **28**: 5132–9.

63 Giusti A, Hamdy NA, Papapoulos SE (2010) Atypical fractures of the femur and bisphosphonate therapy: A systematic review of case/case series studies. *Bone* **48**(5): 966–71.

64 Schilcher J, Michaelsson K, Aspenberg P (2011) Bisphosphonate use and atypical fractures of the femoral shaft. *N Engl J Med* **364**(18): 1728–37.

65 McKinernan F (2010) Atypical femur disphyseal fractures documented by serial DXA. *J Clin Densitom* **13**(1): 102–3.

66 Paul O, Barker JU, Lane JM, *et al.* (2012) Functional and radiographic outcomes. *J Orthop Trauma* **26**(3): 148–54.

67 Whitaker M, Guo j, Kehoe T, Benson G (2012) Bisphosphophonates for osteoporosis: Where do we go from here? *New Engl J Med* **366**(22): 2048–51.

68 Bonnick SL (2011) Going on a drug holiday? *J Clin Densit* **14**(2): 1–7.

69 Compston JE, Bilezikian JP (2012) Bisphosphoante therapy for osteoporosis: the long and short of it. *J Bone Miner Res* **27**(2): 240–2. (editorial).

70 Boonen S, Ferrari S, Miller PD, *et al.* (2012) Postmenopausal osteoporosis treatment with antiresorptives: effects of discontinuation or long term continuation on bone turnover and fracture risk – a perspective. *J Bone Miner Res* **27**(12): 963–74.

71 Black DM, Bauer DC, Schwartz AV, Cummings SR, Rosen CJ (2012) Continuing bisphosphonate treatment for osteoporosis; for whom and for how long? *N Engl J Med* **366**(22): 2051–3.

72 Bone HG, Hosking D, Devogelaer JP, *et al.* (2004) Ten years' experience with alendronate for osteoporosis in postmenopausal women. *N Engl J Med* **350**(12): 1189–99.

73 Mellstrom DD, Sorensen OH, Goemaere S, *et al.* (2004) Seven years of treatment with risedronate in women with postmenopausal osteoporosis. *Calcif Tissue Int* **75**(6): 462–8.

74 Miller PD, Roux C, Boonen S, *et al.* (2005) Safety and efficacy of risedronate in patients with age-related reduced renal function as estimated by the Cockcroft and Gault method: a pooled analysis of nine clinical trials. *J Bone Miner Res* **20**: 2105–15.

75 Jamal SA, Bauer DC, Ensrud KE, *et al.* (2007) Alendronate treatment in women with normal to severely impaired renal function: an analysis of the fracture intervention trial. *J Bone Miner Res* **22**: 503–8.

76 Boonen S, Sellmeyer DE, Lippuner K, *et al.* (2008) Renal safety of annual zoledronic acid infusions in osteoporotic postmenopausal women. *Kidney Int* **74**: 641–8.

77 Miller PD (2005) Treatment of osteoporosis in chronic kidney disease and end-stage renal disease. *Curr Osteoporos Rep* **3**(1): 5–12.

78 Miller PD (2009) Fragility fractures in chronic kidney disease: an opinion-based approach. *Cleve Clin J Med* **76**(12): 715–23. Review.

79 Miller PD, Ragi-Eis S, Mautalen C, *et al.* (2011) Effects of intravenous ibandronate injection on renal function in women with postmenopausal osteoporosis at high risk for renal disease – the DIVINE study. *Bone* **49**: 1317–22.

80 Abrahamsen B, Pazianas M, Eiken P, *et al.* (2012) Esophageal and gastric cancer incidence and mortality in alendronate users. *J Bone Miner Res* **27**(3): 679–86.

81 Lyles KW, Colon-Emeric CS, Magaziner JS, *et al.* (2007) Zoledronic acid and clinical fractures and mortality after hip fracture. *N Engl J Med* **357**(18): 1799–1809.

82 Center JR, Bliuc D, Nguyen ND, *et al.* (2011) Osteoporosis medication and reduced mortality risk in elderly women and men. *J Clin Endocrinol Metab* **96**(4): 1006–14.

83 Sambrook PN, Cameron ID, Chen JS, *et al.* (2011) Oral bisphosphonates are associated with reduced mortality in frail older people: a prospective five-year study. *Osteoporos Int* **22**(9): 2551–6.

84 Beaupre LA, Morrish DW, Hanley DA, *et al.* (2011) Oral bisphosphonates are associated with reduced mortality after hip fracture. *Osteoporos Int* **22**(3): 983–91.

85 Bolland MJ, Grey AB, Gamble GD, *et al.* (2010) Effect of osteoporosis treatment on mortality: a meta-analysis. *J Clin Endocrinol Metab* **95**(3): 1174–81.

86 Nevitt MC, Thompson DE, Black DM, *et al.* (2000) Effect of alendronate on limited-activity days and bed-disability days caused by back pain in postmenopausal women with existing vertebral fractures. Fracture Intervention Trial Research Group. *Arch Intern Med* **160**(1): 77–85.

87 Dell R, Greene D (2010) Is osteoporosis disease management cost effective? *Curr Osteoporos Rep* **8**(1): 49–55.

88 Newman ED, Ayoub WT, Starkey RH, *et al.* (2003) Osteoporosis disease management in a rural health care population: hip fracture reduction and reduced costs in postmenopausal women after 5 years. *Osteoporos Int* **14**(2): 146–51.

89 King AB, Fiorentino DM (2011) Medicare payment cuts for osteoporosis testing reduced use despite tests' benefit in reducing fractures. *Health Aff (Millwood)* **30**: 2362–70.

90 Curtis JR, Adachi JD, Saag KG (2009) Bridging the osteoporosis quality chasm. *J Bone Miner Res* **24**: 3–7.

91 Lewiecki EM, Laster A, Miller PD, Bilezikian JP (2012) More bone density testing is needed, not less. *J Bone Miner Res* **27**(4): 739–42.

92 Bauss F, Russell RGG (2004) Ibandronate in osteoporosis: preclinical data and rationale for intermittent dosing. *Osteoporosis Internat* **15**: 423–33.

CHAPTER 10

Denosumab

Michael A. Bolognese
Bethesda Health Research, Bethesda, MD, USA

Introduction

Postmenopausal osteoporosis is a chronic, progressive disease leading to loss of bone mass and strength which results in an increased fracture risk [1]. Osteoporosis is the most common bone disease in humans, representing a growing major public health problem in the United States. Data from the 2005–2006 National Health and Nutrition Examination Survey revealed, >34 million US adult age 50 or older, had osteopenia, as evidenced by a low bone mineral density (BMD) of the femoral neck [2]. An estimated 10 million US adults 50 or older, had osteoporosis, with >5 million having osteoporosis of the femoral neck, including 4.5 million women and 800 000 men [2, 3] and thus are at a higher risk for fracture.

Drug therapies for osteoporosis aim to prevent further bone loss and thus reduce fracture risk. Changes in lifestyle such as adequate calcium, vitamin D and weight-bearing exercise are adjuncts to pharmacotherapy [1].

Clinical pharmacology

Denosumab is a subcutaneously administered fully human monoclonal RANKL-specific IgG2 antibody developed for the treatment of osteoporosis in postmenopausal women who are at a high risk for fracture or who are refractory to or cannot tolerate other therapies for osteoporosis [4].

In postmenopausal women, estrogen levels are decreased and this results in an increase in rank ligand expression (RANKL) [1]. RANKL is an essential mediator for osteoclast formation, function, and survival [2]. There are three major molecular components to the RANKL pathway, which all have an effect on the osteoclast.

Osteoporosis: Diagnosis and Management, First Edition. Edited by Dale W. Stovall.
© 2013 John Wiley & Sons, Ltd. Published 2013 by John Wiley & Sons, Ltd.

1 RANKL is a protein that is expressed by osteoblast lining cells and by binding to a receptor on the osteoclast called RANK.
2 RANK, the RANKL promotes osteoclast differentiation, activity, and prolongs the lifespan of the osteoclast which results in increased bone resorption.
3 Osteoprogerin (OPG) is secreted by osteoblasts/bone lining cells and is a natural inhibitor of RANKL which results in balancing bone remodeling (Figure 10.1) [5,6].

Estrogen may indirectly inhibit the expression of RANKL and stimulate the expression of OPG. Denosumab (Prolia, Amgen Inc., Thousand Oaks, CA) is a fully human IgG2 antibody that binds to RANKL with very high specificity and is the first RANKL inhibitor that has been approved by the FDA. This is a different antiresorptive and is not a bisphosphonate. Prolia thus inhibits osteoclast formation, function, and survival and thus decreases bone resorption. This results in an increased bone mass and strength that occurs in both cortical and trabecular bone.

A phase I, three Phase II and 4 Phase III studies have assessed the efficacy of denosumab in reducing bone resorption in postmenopausal osteoporosis. Markers of bone metabolism, BMD T scores, and the prevalence of new vertebral fractures were used as outcome measures (Tables 10.1 and 10.2).

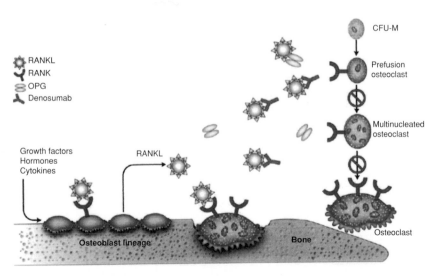

Figure 10.1 Mechanism of action of denosumab. Denousumab reduces osteoclast differentiation and activity by binding to the receptor activator of nuclear factor κB ligand (RANKL). CFU-M, CFU-macrophage; OPG, osteoprotegerin. (*Source*: Bridgeman MB, Pathak R (2011) [33]).

Table 10.1 Study of the efficacy of denosumab in reducing bone resorption in postmenopausal osteoporosis: phases 1 and II.

Authors and study	Phase	Number and mean age	Characteristics	Duration	Primary endpoints	Efficacy findings	Safety profile
Bekker et al. [29]	I	49 healthy postmenopausal females, 59.6 years	Randomized, double-blind, single dose-escalation study	6 or 9 mos.	Bone antiresorptive activity and safety	Dose-dependent rapid and sustained decrease in bone turnover	No related SAE's: no meaningful lab changes
McClung et al. [7]	II	412 postmenopausal females with low BMD, 63 years	Randomized, placebo-controlled, dose-ranging study, with alendronate group, once-weekly	12 mos.	The % change from baseline in BMD	Increased BMD and decreased BTMs vs.placebo	No significat differences in adverse events in denosumab, placebo and ALN groups
Miller et al. [8]	II	412 postmenopausal females with low BMD, 63 years	Extension of (7), study review, dosing of denosumab modified; ALN group was stop for 23 mos extension	48 mos.	The % change from baseline in BMD at LS; changes in BTMs; endpoints – effects of discontinuing and reinitiating denosumab on BMD and remodeling	Significant increases in BMD and sustained suppression of BTMs. Discontinuing therapy for 24 mos decreased BMD to baseline levels. Re-treatment for 12 months increased BMD similar to initial gains.	Similar AEs, more infections as SAEs with denosumab
McClung et al. [9]	II	200 postmenopausal women with low BMD, 63 years	Extension of (7)all patients now on denosumab, some 8 years depending on initial treatment	96 mos.	The % change from baseline of IS and total hip, effect on BTMs	Significant increases in BMD of Spine and BTMs over the 8 years	Similar AEs, consistent with an aging population
Seeman et al. [18]	II	247 osteopenic and osteoporotic postmenopausal women, 60.6 years	Double-blind pilot study; subjects randomized to SC, denosumab, oral ALN, or placebo	12 mos.	Evaluation of the effects of denosumab and alendronate on cortical and trabecular micro-architecture with pQCT	Better favorable effects of denosumab than ALN on the examined variables	AEs were similar between groups

Table 10.2 Study of the efficacy of denosumab in reducing bone resorption in postmenopausal osteoporosis: phase III.

Authors and study	Number and mean age of subjects	Characteristics	Duration	Primary end points	Efficacy findings	Safety profile
Bone HG et al. [32]	332 osteopenic postmenopausal women, 59.4 years	Randomized, double blind, placebo-controlled trial; Denosumab vs Placebo Prevention of PMO DEFEND Trial	24 mos	% change from baseline in LS BMD	Increased BMD vs. placebo	Overall rates of infection similar; greater incidence of local rashes and increased incidence of hospitalized infections in denosumab group
Cummings et al. [10]	7868 osteoporotic women, 72.3 years	Randomized, pivotal international study, largest phase III study, denosumab vs placebo, treatment of PMO, Freedom Trial	36 mos	Reduction in incidence of morphometric vertebral facture	Denosumab decreased risk of vertebral, non-vertebral (hip) fractures	Similar AEs and SAEs vs placebo
Brown et al. [16]	1189 postmenopausal women with low BMD, 64.4 years	A multi-center, double blind non-inferiority study (DECIDE), head to head comparison denosumab vs. ALN	12 mos	changes in BMD at total hip, femoral neck,LS and distal radius from baseline	Greater increases in BMD at all measured sites in denosumab group	Overall rates of AEs and SAEs balanced in both groups
Kendler et al. [19]	504 osteopenic osteoporotic postmenopausal women, 67.6 years	A multi-center, international, randomized, double-blind trial switch from ALN to denosumab (Stand Trial)	12 mos	Total hip BMD, bone remodelling and safety at 12 months	Transition to denosumab increased BMD and decreased BTMs to greater extent than continued ALN therapy	Overall rates of AEs and SAEs balanced in both groups
Genant et al. [17]	332 osteopenic postmenopausal women, 59.4 years	Randomized, double-blind, placebo-controlled trial; Denosumab vs. placebo; prevention of PMO	24 mos	% change from baseline in vBMD, vBMC, cortical structural parameters and PMI of distal radius with QCT	Positive effect of denosumab on both cortical and trabecular bone compartments	Overall rates of infection similar; greater incidence of local rashes and increased incidence of hospitalized infections in denosumab group

Phase II trials

A phase 2 dose-ranging study included eight double blind groups and one open-label treatment group (Figure 10.2). A total of 412 postmenopausal women with lumbar spine BMD T-scores of −1.8 to −4.0 or femoral neck/total hip T-scores of −1.8 to −3.5 from 29 study centers in the United States were randomly assigned to receive denosumab SC either every three months (doses were 6, 14 or 30 mg) or every six months (doses were 14, 60, 100, or 210 mg), open-label alendronate was given once a week (at a dose of 70 mg), or placebo [7,8]. Denosumab treatment for twelve months resulted in an increase in BMD at the lumbar spine of 3.0 to 6.7% (as compared with an increase of 4.6% with alendronate and a loss of 0.8% with placebo), at the total hip of 1.9 to 3.6% (as compared with an increase of 2.1% with alendronate and a loss of 0.6% with placebo) and at the distal third of the radius of 0.4 to 1.3% (as compared with decreases of 0.5% with alendronate and 2.0% with placebo). The increased BMD at the distal radius, which is composed mainly of cortical bone, differentiated the response to denosumab from alendronate at this site. Near-maximal reductions in mean levels of serum C-teleopeptide from baseline were evident three days after the administration of denosumab [7].

In this phase 2 study [9] after 24 months, patients receiving denosumab either continued treatment at 60 mg Q6M for an additional 24 months, discontinued therapy or discontinued treatment for 12 months and then re-initiated denosumab (60 mg Q6M) for 12 months. The placebo cohort was maintained. Alendronate-treated patients discontinued alendronate and were followed. Changes in BMD and BTMs as well as safety outcomes

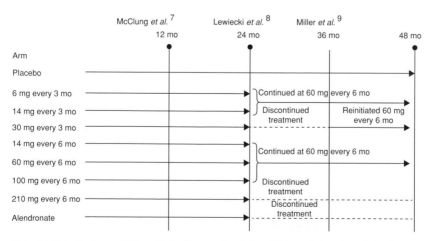

Figure 10.2 Designs of Phase II studies: study of the efficacy of denosumab in the prevention and treatment of postmenopausal osteoporosis.

were evaluated. Overall, 262/412 (64%) of patients completed 48 months. Continuous, long-term denosumab treatment increased BMD at the lumbar spine (9.4% to 11.8%) and total hip (4.0% to 6.1%). BTMs were consistently suppressed over 48 months. Discontinuation of denosumab was associated with a BMD decrease of 6.6% at the lumbar spine and 5.3% at the total hip within the first 12 months of treatment discontinuation. Retreatment with denosumab increased lumbar spine BMD by 9% from the original baseline values. Levels of BTM increased upon discontinuation and decreased with retreatment. Adverse events were similar between treatment groups. Thus in postmenopausal women with low BMD, long-term treatment with denosumab led to gains in BMD and decreases in BTMs throughout the course of the study. The effects on bone turnover were fully reversible with discontinuation and restored with subsequent retreatment. Thus it became apparent that Prolia would need to be given every 6 months and that it would be more like estrogen in that, once it is stopped, the effect is short lived.

We now have eight-year data in this phase 2 study [10]. The parent study was extended for an additional four years. All subjects in the extension study received open-label denosumab 60 mg every 6 months (Q6m). The results focused on those subjects who received denosumab treatment for 8 years total in the parent and extension studies, and those subjects who received placebo for 4 years in the parent study followed by denosumab for 4 years in the extension.

Out of the 262 subjects who completed the parent study, 200 enrolled in the extension study and of these, 138 (69%) completed the 4 year extension study. Out of the 88 subjects who received 8 years of continuous denosumab treatment, BMD increased on average by 16.5% at the lumbar spine, 6.8% at the total hip, and 1.3% at the 1/3 radius compared with their parent study baseline. Out of the 12 subjects in the previous placebo group, 4 years of denosumab therapy resulted in gains in BMD comparable with those observed during the first 4 years of 60 mg Q6M in the parent study. Reductions in the bone turnover markers (BTMs) of resorption, CTX, and of bone formation, BSAP, were sustained over the duration of continuous denosumab treatment. At year 8, median reductions from the parent study baseline in CTX and BSAP were −65% and −44%, respectively. Reductions in BTMs were also observed when the placebo group transitioned to densoumab therapy. The adverse event profile was similar to prior reports and consistent with an aging population. There were no cases of atypical fractures or ostenecrosis of the jaw (ONJ).

Denosumab is absorbed in the serum very quickly with the median time to maximum concentration being 10 days and then there was a decline down to six months. The serum CTx (a marker of osteoclastic bone resorption) was decreased 85% within 3 days and then there was an attenuation of the CTx at the end of six months reflecting the reversibility of prolia as the serum denosumab levels diminish.

Phase III trials

The pivotal fracture study [11] was an international, randomized double blind, placebo-controlled phase 3 study investigating Prolia (denosumab). The primary endpoint was vertebral fracture at 36 months. Secondary end-points included times to first nonvertebral and hip fracture.

Women were eligible between age 60–91 years, with a T score <2.5 at the lumbar spine or total hip but not <−4 at these sites and there were other inclusion criteria.

Baseline characteristics in the study included overall T scores of −2.8 at the lumbar spine and −1.9 at the total hip with 23% of patients having had a prevalent vertebral fracture.

7868 women were enrolled. Subjects in the active arm (n = 3902) received prolia 60 mg SC every 6 months; subjects in the placebo arm (n = 3906) received SC placebo injections every 6 months. All subjects received daily calcium (>1 g) and vitamin D (>400 IU) supplementation.

Baseline characteristics were similar between treatment groups with over 80% in each group completing the study.

An open-label, 7-year extension to this pivotal fracture study is under-way in 4550 subjects with a planned total exposure of up to 10 years. All patient are receiving Prolia S.C. every 6 months.

There was a relative risk reduction of new vertebral fractures at three years of 68%. There also was a relative risk reduction of hip fractures by 40% and nonvertebral fractures of 20%.

Also noted was an increased bone mineral density at 3 years of 8.8% in the lumbar spine, 6.4% in the total hip, and 5.2% in the femoral neck.

In an extension study of a phase three prevention trial in post-menopausal women with low bone mass [12], Prolia demonstrated reversibility of bone turnover markers and BMD upon discontinuation fol-lowing 24 months of treatment (last dose at 18 months). Following discon-tinuation of Prolia, levels of serum CTx increased to levels 40–60% above pretreatment levels, but returned to baseline levels within 12 months.

Substudies in the original Freedom trial

In one of the substudies [13], Austin and colleagues evaluated the relation-ship between bone mineral density changes with denosumab treatment and risk reduction for vertebral and nonvertebral fractures. They found that gains in total hip BMD explained a large proportion of the fracture risk reductions observed with denosumab. It appears that previous studies may underestimate the value of change in DXA BMD as a surrogate marker for the effect of treatment on fracture risk or the relationship may be unique to denosumab.

In another substudy of the Freedom trial, McClung *et al.* did a subgroup analysis prospectively planned before study unblinding to evaluate the effect of denosumab on new vertebral and nonvertebral fractures across various subgroups [14]. Subgroups were nine on new vertebral fracture and five on nonvertebral fracture. The subgroups of age, BMI, femoral neck BMD T-score, prevalent vertebral fracture, and prior nonvertebral fracture were included in the assessment of denosumab treatment on both new vertebral and nonvertebral fracture. Subgroups based on estimated creatinine clearance, geographic region, race, and prior use of osteoporosis medications were also evaluate for new vertebral fracture. The effect of denosumab decreasing new vertebral and nonvertebral fractures in these nine subgroups was no different than in the overall 3 year study. The 20% reduction in nonvertebral fractures in the study cohort over 3 year was statistically significant in women with a baseline femoral neck BMD T-score = to or <−2.5 but not in those with a T-score >−2.5; in those with a body mass index (BMI) <25 kg/m2 but not = to or >25 kg/m2; and in those without but not with a prevalent vertebral fracture. These differential treatment effects were not explained by difference in BMD responses to denosumab. Denosumab 60 mg administered every 6 months for 3 years in women with osteoporosis reduced the risk of new vertebral fractures to a similar degree in all subgroups. Estimated creatinine clearance, BMI and history of previous osteoporosis therapy were not predictors of new vertebral fracture risk. Older age, lower femoral neck BMD, and a history of prior vertebral or nonvertebral fractures were associated with a higher risk of new vertebral fractures.

The effect of denosumab on total BMD of the hip appears to be different than the responses to other anti-resorptive agents [15, 16].

A continued increase in hip BMD has also been observed in the six year extension of the Freedom trial [17].

Cortical BMD has not been observed with other antiresorptive agents for osteoporosis, and its effect has also been confirmed and further characterized with quantitative computed tomography (QCT) and HRpQCT imaging techniques [18, 19]. These QCT techniques demonstrated that the cortical BMD gains observed with DXA were associated with increased cortical thickness, increased cortical bone mineral content, decreased cortical porosity, and improved estimated strength in response to denosumab treatment.

In conclusion, denosumab treatment in women with postmenopausal osteoporosis in Freedom led to significant and clinically meaningful increases in BMD throughout the trabecular and cortical skeleton, and these increases were observed early and progressed over the 36 months of therapy.

Seventy percent of eligible women from the pivotal phase 3 fracture study enrolled in the study extension study; 2343 women continued to receive Prolia® treatment (long-term group), and 2207 transitioned from placebo to Prolia (crossover group). The long-term group experienced significant mean increases in BMD for cumulative 6-year gains of 15.2 percent at the lumbar spine and 7.5 percent at the total hip [17]. Fracture incidence remained low in the long-term group. During the first three years of the extension study, the crossover group had significant mean gains of 9.4 percent at the lumbar spine and 4.8 percent at the total hip; yearly incidence of new vertebral and nonvertebral fractures were lower than in the pivotal phase 3 fracture study placebo group.

In order to determine if prolia could be used after a bisphosphonate and what a comparison would be, a phase 3 Transition Study, the Stand Trial (Study of Transitioning from Alendronate to Denosumab) was done [20]. The inclusion criteria were postmenopausal women who were previously treated with alendronate 70 mg QW or equivalent for 6 or more months. The mean treatment with alendronate was 3 years and overall T-scores were −2.6 at the lumbar spine and −1.8 at the total hip. The primary endpoint was change in total hip BMD over 1 year and the secondary endpoints were BMD at the lumbar spine, femoral neck, and 1/3 radius at 12 months along with changes in bone turnover markers (sCTX-1, PINP) over 12 months. 253 patient were in the transitioning group to Prolia and 251 patients remained on alendronate 70 mg QW.

There was a 1.2 percent increase in BMD at the spine, 0.8% at the total hip, 1 percent at the femoral neck and 0.7 percent at the distal 1/3 radius. All these changes were significantly different from alendronate. These data were not intended to imply relative fracture risk reduction with Prolia® versus alendronate and no comparative fracture data have been conducted thus far.

A somewhat similar trial, DECIDE (Determining Efficacy: Comparison of Initiating Denosumab vs. Alendronate) [21]) included women who had limited exposure to oral bisphosphonates. At a one-year follow-up assessment, denosumab increased BMD more than oral alendronate at all measured sites.

As part of the trial, patients were given a questionnaire after 12 months of treatment to gauge preference on mode of administration as well as satisfaction with frequency of dosing of twice-yearly denosumab vs weekly oral tablets. More than 3/4 of patients in both study arms preferred subcutaneous injection over oral pills (77% vs 23%, p < .0001. In addition, significantly more patients were satisfied with twice-yearly dosing compared to weekly dosing.

Newer indications for Prolia®

Prolia® has been approved to increase bone mass in men at high risk for fracture receiving androgen deprivation therapy for nonmetastatic prostate cancer where Prolia® also reduced the incidence of vertebral fracture [22].

Also, Prolia® is indicated as a treatment to increase bone mass in women at high risk for fracture receiving adjuvant aromatase inhibitor therapy for breast cancer [23].

XGEVA®, which is the 120 mg dose of Prolia®, has approval for men with metastatic prostate cancer to bone [24] and for women with metastatic breast cancer to bone [25]. XGEVA demonstrated superior efficacy vs zolendroic acid, reducing the risk of first skeletal related event (SRE) and first and subsequent SREs in patients with breast cancer or prostate cancer. Hypocalcemia and ONJ were more frequent in patients on XGEVA and the most common serious adverse reaction was dyspnea.

Studies are ongoing in men with osteoporosis, The ADAMO Trial (**A**, randomized, double-blind, placebo-controlled study to compare the efficacy and safety of **D**enosum**A**b 60 mg every 6 months versus placebo in **M**ales with **O**steoporosis) is a two-year study with men on either placebo or denosumab for the first 12 months and then all subjects on denosumab for the second year. The primary endpoint is the percent change in lumbar spine BMD at month 12 with secondary endpoints being % change in total hip, femoral neck, trochanter and 1/3 radius BMD at month 12. They qualify with a T score of = or <−2.0 and = or <−3.5 at the lumbar spine or femoral neck or had a prior major osteoporotic fracture and a T score = to or <−1 and = or >−3.5. This multicenter study will report one-year data at the ISCD meeting in Los Angeles [26].

Clinical safety of Prolia®

In the Freedom trial, 3876 women exposed to placebo and 3886 exposed to Prolia. Seventy subjects (1.8%) died in the Prolia® group and 90 (2.3%) in the placebo group. The average age at the start of the study was 72.3 years. The most common fatal AE's were myocardial infarction (6 placebo vs 7 prolia), pancreatic cancer (3 placebo vs 4 Prolia®), cardiogenic shock (2 placebo vs 4 Prolia®), lung neoplasm (5 placebo vs 3 Prolia®). The overall incidence of infection were balanced between treatment groups.

Adverse events occurring in at least 2% of subjects and with a significant difference between groups included:

- Eczema: 3% of subjects in the Prolia® group and 1.7% in the placebo group (P < 0.001)
- Falls not associated with a fracture: 4.5% in the Prolia® group and 5.7% in the placebo group (P = 0.02)

- Flatulence: 2.2% of subjects in the Prolia® group and 1.4% in the placebo group (P = 0.008).

The most common adverse reactions (>5% and more than placebo) were:

- back pain, pain in the extremity, musculoskeletal pain, hypercholesterolemia, and cystitis;
- epidermal and dermal adverse events such as dermatitis, eczema and rashes occurred at a significantly higher rate in the Prolia® group (10.8%) compared to the placebo group. And most of these reactions were not specific to the injection site;
- pancreatitis was reported in 4 subjects (0.1%) in the placebo and 8 (0.2%) in the Prolia groups; of these, 1 subject in the placebo group and all 8 subjects in the Prolia® group had serious events, including one death in the Prolia® group;
- the overall incidence of new malignancies was 4.3% in the placebo and 4.8% in the Prolia® groups; a causal relationship to drug exposure has not been established.

Serious adverse events included 12 subjects (0.3%) in the Prolia® group and 1 subject (<0.1%) in the placebo group reported serious adverse events of cellulitis (P = 0.002) [10]. In addition to skin infections, the following serious infections leading to hospitalization:

- abdomen (0.7% placebo vs 0.9% Prolia®)
- urinary tract (0.5% placebo vs 0.7% Prolia®)
- ear (0.0% placebo vs 0.1% Prolia®)

Three subjects treated with prolia had adverse events of endocarditis or endocarditis bacterial.

Two were reported as SAEs:

- causative pathogen not identified in either case;
- diagnosis made clinically (e.g., echocardiography) in both cases.

No increased risk of sepsis or death was observed.

Hypocalcemia would be a contraindication to the use of Prolia® [4].

The most common adverse reactions leading to discontinuation of Prolia® are breast cancer, back pain and constipation.

Prolia® is not cleared through the kidney and therefore dose adjustments are not required for Prolia®.

If the creatinine clearance <30 mL/min or patient is receiving dialysis, the risk for hypocalcemia is greater [4].

In addition to expression in bone, RANKL and RANK are expressed by cells of the immune system including activated T lymphocytes, B cells [27, 28, 29], and dendritic cells suggesting that immune cells might alter immune function. However, in a dose ranging study of denosumab in healthy postmenopausal women, no clinically meaningful differences in overall lymphocyte counts, T cells, or B cells were observed in patients treated with denosumab [30].

In a recent article by Dr. Nelson Watts [31], he evaluated the infections in postmenopausal women with osteoporosis treated with denosumab or placebo to see if this was coincidence or a causal association. He concluded that serious adverse events had a heterogeneous etiology, with no clear pattern to suggest a relationship to time or duration of exposure to denosumab. The benefit/risk profile of denosumab continues to be evaluated in ongoing trials, including the open-label extension of the Freedom Trial which continues for a total of 10 years.

The safety profile of denosumab up to six years in the Open-label extension trial [16] revealed the incidences of adverse events and serious adverse events did not increase over time with Prolia® treatment. Four subjects developed osteonecrosis of the jaw (ONJ) during the extension study that healed without further complications. One of these subjects continued Prolia®, and one subject discontinued. Follow-up is ongoing for the other two subjects. No atypical femoral fractures were reported in either group.

Prolia® did result in significant suppression of bone remodeling as evidenced by markers of bone turnover and bone histomorphometry [4]. The significance of these findings and the effect of long-term treatment are unknown and patients continue to be monitored for consequences, including ONJ, atypical fractures, and delayed fracture healing. Compared to placebo, Prolia® was not associated with increased occurrence of delayed fracture healing in the Freedom Trial.

The Prolia® Postmarketing Active Surveillance Program is available to collect information from prescribers on specific adverse events.

Drug–drug interactions

A literature search on studies of the potential for denosumab to affect the metabolism of other pharmacologic agents were not identified. However, because of the serious infections associated with the use of denosumab, the simultaneous use of immunosuppresants, including corticosteroids, chemotherapeutic agents, and immune modulators, could increase the risk of infection [32].

Administration of Prolia®

All patients should receive calcium 1000 mg daily and at least 400 IU vitamin D daily. Because of the half-life of Prolia®, if a dose is missed, administer the injection as soon as the patient is available.

Prolia® is supplied in a single-use prefilled syringe with a safety guard or in a single-use vial. The recommended dose of Prolia® is 60 mg administered as a single subcutaneous injection once every six months. It is administered in the upper arm the upper thigh, or the abdomen by a healthcare provider in the office [4].

References

1 North American Menopause Society (2010) The management of osteoporosis in postmenopausal women: 2010 Position Statement of the North American Menopause Society. *Menopause* **17**: 25–54.

2 Looker AC, Melton LJ, Harris TB, *et al.* (2010) Prevalence and trends in low femur bone density among older US Adults: NHANES 2005–2006 compared with NHANES III, *J Bone Miner Res* **20**: 64–71.

3 National Osteoporosis Foundation. Fast Facts. (Accessed Jan 9, 2011).

4 Prolia (denosumab) (prescribing information). Thousand Oaks, Calif: Amgen Inc: 2010.

5 Boyle WJ, Simonet WS, Lacey DL (2003) Osteoclast differentiation and activation. *Nature* **423**: 337–42.

6 Kosternuik PJ (2005) Osteoprogerin and RANKL regulate bone resorption, density, geometry and strength. *Curr Opin Pharmacol* **5**: 618–25.

7 McClung MR, Lewiecki EM, Cohen SB, *et al.* (2006) Denosumab in postmenopausal women with low bone mineral density. *N Engl J Med* **354**: 821–31.

8 Lewiecki EM, Miller PD, McClung MR, *et al.* (2007) Two-year treatment with denosumab (AMG) 162) in a randomized phase 2 study of postmenopaausal women with low bone mineral density. *J Bone Miner Res* **22**: 1832–41.

9 Miller, PD, Bolognese MA, Lewiecki EM, *et al.* (2008) Effect of denosumab on bone density and turnover in postmenopausal women with with low bone mass after long term continued, discontinued, and restarting of therapy: A randomized blinded phase II clinical trial. *Bone* **43**: 222–9.

10 McClung MR, Lewiecki EM, Bolognese MA, *et al.* (2010) 233 8-year abstract. *ISCD* March.

11 Cummings SR, *et al.* (2009) Denosumab for prevention of fractures in postmenopausal women with osteoporosis. *N Eng J Med* **361**: 756–65.

12 Bone HG, Bolognese MA, Yuen CK, *et al.* (2011) Effects of densoumab treatment and discontinuation on bone mineral density and bone turnover markers in postmenopausal women with low bone mass. *J Clin Endocriol Metab* **96**: 972–80.

13 Austin M, Yang Y-C, Vittinghof E, *et al.* (2011) Relationship between bone mineral density changes with denosumab treatment and risk reduction for vertebral and nonvertebral fractures, *J Bone Miner Res*. Published online as doi: 10.1002/jbmr.1472.

14 McClung MR, Boonen S, Torring O, *et al.* (2012) Effect of denosumab treatment on ther risk of fractures in subgroups of women with postmenopausal osteoporosis. *J Bone Miner Res* **10**: 27211–18.

15 Bone HG, Hosking D, Devogelaer, *et al.* (2004) Ten years experience with alendronate for osteoporosis in postmenopausal women. *N Engl J Med* **350**: 1189–99.

16 Mellstrom DD, Sorensen OH, Goemoeres, *et al.* (2004) Seven years of treatment with risedronate in women with postemenopausal osteoporosis, *Calcif Tissue Int* **75**: 462–8.

17 Brown JP (2011) Open-label extension trial showed continued increase in BMD over six years with similar safety profile observed in original fracture trial. *Am Coll Rheum*. Annual Scientific Meeting.

18 Genant HK, Engleke K, Hanley DA, *et al.* (2010) Denosumab improves density and strength parameters as measured by QCT of the radius in in postmenopausal women with low bone mineral density. *Bone* **47**: 131–9.

19 Seeman E, Delmas PD, Hanley DA, *et al.* (2010) Microarchitectural deterioration of cortical and trabecular bone: differing effects of denosumab and alendronate. *J Bone Miner Res* **25**: 1886–94.

20 Kendler DL, *et al.* (2010) Effects of denosumab on bone mineral density and bone-turnover in postmenopausal women transitioning from alendronate therapy. *J Bone Miner Res* **25**: 728–81.

21 Brown JP, Prince RL, Deal C, *et al.* (2009) Comparison of the effect of denosumab and alendroante on BMD and BMTs in postmenopausal women with low bone mass: a randomized blinded, phase 3 trial. *J Bone Miner Res* **24**: 153–61.

22 Saith MR, *et al.* (2009) Denosumab Halt Prostate Cancer Study Group. Denosumab in men receiving androgen-deprivation therapy for prostate cancer. *N Eng J Med* **301**: 745–55.

23 Ellis GK, *et al.* (2008) Randomized trial of denosumab in patients receiving aromatase inhibitors for nonmetastatic breast cancer. *J Clin Oncol* **26**: 4875–82.

24 Fizazi K, *et al.* (2011) Densosumab versus zolendroic acid for treatment of bone metastases in men with castration-resistant prostate cancer: a randomized double-blind study. *Lancet* **377**: 812–22.

25 Stopek AT, *et al.* (2011) Denosumab compared with zolendroic acid for the treatment of bone metastases in patients with advanced breast cancer; a randomized double-blind study (ex or multiple myeloma). *J Clin Oncol*: **29**: 1125–32.

26 Orwell E, *et al.* (2012) Adamo Study Poster *ISCD* Los Angeles, CA.

27 Kong YY, Yoshida H, Saros, I, *et al.* (1999) OPGL is a key regulator of osteoclastogenesis, lymphocyte development and lymph-node organogenesis. *Nature* **397**: 315–23.

28 Anderson DM, Muraskovsky E, Billingsley WL, *et al.* (1997) A homologue of the tNF receptor and its ligand enhance T-cell growth and dendritic-cell function. *Nature* **390**: 175–9.

29 Bachman MF, Wong BR, Josien R *et al.* (1999) TRANCE, a tumor necrosis factor family member critical for CD40 ligand-independent T helper cell activation. *J Exp Med* **189**: 1025–31.

30 Bekker PJ, Holloway DL. Rasmussen AS, *et al.* (2004) A single-dose placebo-controlled study of dmab(162), a fully human monoclonal antibody to RANKL, in postemenopausal women. *J Bone Miner Res* **19**: 1059–66.

31 Watts NB, *et al.* (2012) Infections in postmenopausal women with osteoporosis treated with denosumab or placebo: coincidence or causal association? *Osteoporosis Int* **23**: 327–37.

32 Bone HG, Bolognese MA, Yuen Ck, *et al.* (2008) Effects of denosumab on bone mineral density and bone turnover in postmenopausal women. *J Clin Endocrinol Metab* **93**: 2149–57.

33 Bridgeman MB, Pathak R (2011) Denosumab for the reduction of bone loss in post-menopausal osteoporosis: a review. *Clinical Therapeutics* **33**: 1547–59.

CHAPTER 11

Parathyroid Hormone: Anabolic Treatment of Osteoporosis

Erik Fink Eriksen

Oslo University Hospital, Oslo, Norway

Contrary to anti-resorptive agents, which reduce fracture incidence by reducing bone turnover and stabilize bone mass, anabolic treatments actually increase bone turnover and build new bone. In contrast to the anti-resorptive drugs, which mainly target osteoclasts and removal of bone, anabolic agents target the osteoblast. By stimulating bone formation to a greater extent and earlier than bone resorption, anabolic agents have the potential to positively affect a number of skeletal properties besides bone density. These include bone size, microarchitecture and rejuvenation of bone matrix. They thus have the potential to reconstruct the skeleton, an endpoint not shared by any of the anti-resorptive agents. The anabolic agents to be discussed in this review include the recombinant PTH (1-34), which is currently available in most countries as teriparatide, and recombinant intact PTH (1-84), which has been approved for use in some European countries.

Parathyroid hormone as an anabolic agent

In primary hyperparathyroidism (PHPT), characterized by chronic, continuous secretion of excess PTH, catabolic effects, primarily at cortical sites such as the distal 1/3 radius, are common in the more severe cases. In milder cases, however, cortical bone loss is low, and trabecular bone architecture is actually preserved [1]. The pronounced anabolism of intermittent administration of the hormone hinges on the attainment of a narrow peak of PTH in the circulation. The peak should not exceed 3 hours in width, otherwise the catabolic effects seen in chronic hyper secretion tend to predominant [2].

When comparing the bone response to intermittent versus chronically elevated levels of PTH, several significant differences emerge:

1 The genes that are turned on differ profoundly with little overlap between intermittent and chronic excess [3].

2 Intermittent administration causes up-regulation of osteoprotegrin (OPG) and down-regulation of RANK Ligand which promotes a reduction in osteoclastic activity, while chronic elevated levels of PTH induce the opposite changes thus favoring bone resorption [4].

3 At the tissue level, intermittent administration causes overfilling of resorption lacunae (Figure 11.1) [5, 6].

4 Intermittent administration causes increased osteoblastic activity without increasing cell proliferation, which likely results in a dedifferentiation of bone lining cells into a more active bone forming phenotype. This leads to deposition of bone without previous resorption and the formation of smooth cement lines. These changes are are not seen with chronically elevated PTH levels (Figure 11.1) [7].

5 Intermittent administration of PTH inhibits sclerostin expression, causing less inhibition of bone formation, and stimulates Wnt signaling, which favors differentiation of osteoblasts at the expense of other cell types [8].

6 Intermittent administration of PTH induces increases in IGFs and other anabolic growth factors (BMPs, cbfa1) at the tissue level [3, 6].

In humans, intermittent administration of teriparatide leads to a rapid increase in bone formation markers followed sometime (usually about 3

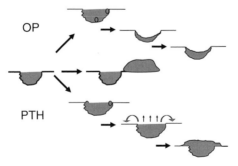

Figure 11.1 Effects of PTH treatment on bone remodeling in osteoporosis (OP). PTH reverses the negative bone balance at each remodeling site, which is the hallmark of osteoporosis (upper panel), into a positive balance leading ot overfilling of resorption lacunae (lower panel). Early during PTH therapy, but waning over time, bone formation on quiescent bone surfaces, without previous resorption, may take place (modeling bone formation)(middle panel). (*Source*: Derived from Dempster *et al.* (2001) [5] and Ma *et al.* (2006) [6]).

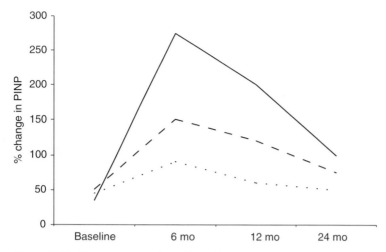

Figure 11.2 Changes in a marker of bone formation (PINP) after initiation of therapy with PTH(1-34) in 3 patients. Note the peak at 6 mo.

months) thereafter by increases in bone resorption markers. This sequence of events has led to the concept of the "anabolic window," a period of time when the actions of PTH are maximally anabolic. Bone formation markers peak at 6 months, then they gradually return towards baseline over a period of 3 years [9] (Figure 11.2). Bone histomorphometric analysis after therapy with PTH reveals increased remodeling mimicking the changes seen in bone markers with increased bone turnover as reflected in increased osteoid synthesis, mineralization of bone surfaces, and increased osteoblastic vigor as reflected by an increased distance between double tetracycline labels [10]. The increased bone formation eventually results in pronounced improvements in cancellous and well as cortical bone. Cancellous bone volume increases by an average of 35% and trabecular connectivity, which is reduced in osteoporosis, is improving as well. Also, trabecular number increases and trabecular morphology returns to a more plate like appearance as seen in younger individuals and different from the more rod-like shape of osteoporotic bone (Figure 11.3). Cortical thickness and cortical cross sectional area also increase, which is an effect never seen with anti-resorptive treatments [11] (Figure 11.3). These improvements in cancellous and cortical bone structure have also been corroborated in vivo by quantitative CT (QCT) [12, 13].

Bone matrix formed during PTH treatment exhibits less mineralization and less collagen crosslinks typical of younger bone [14]. Another effect seen after treatment with PTH, which has not been seen with anti-resorptive agents, is an increase in bony dimensions. Peripheral QC

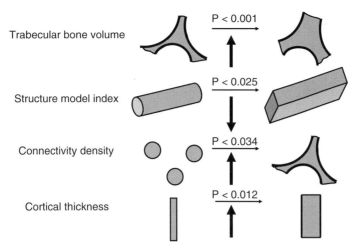

Figure 11.3 Quantitative assessment by μCT of bone structure after PTH treatment in 51 biopsies obtained before and after PTH therapy in the pivotal trial (ref. [17]). Prior to treatment the biopsies exhibited a structure typical of osteoporosis with reduced bone mass, trabecular connectivity and cortical thickness. Trabeculae also exhibited the rod like appearance typical for osteoporosis. PTH treatment significantly reversed these changes after a median treatment period of 19 months. (*Source*: Jiang Y, Zhao JJ, Mitlak BH (2003) [11]).

measurements and analyses of hip DXA scans have demonstrated a dose dependent increase in bone perimeter in the forearm and hip after PTH treatment [15, 16].

The stimulation of bone formation causes a dose dependent increase in BMD amounting to 6–9% over placebo in the spine and 3–6% at the hip with 20 and 40 μg daily dosing after a median treatment period of 21 months [17]. At certain sites rich in cortical bone, such as the distal 1/3 of the radius, PTH typically does not increase bone density. In fact, there may be a small decline in BMD. Early BMD assessment at the hip may reveal a decrease too, which then gradually reverses into an increase. This is mainly caused by an increase in cortical porosity accompanying the increase in overall bone turnover and to a lesser extent the formation of new, less mineralized bone together with dimensional changes. However, the transient reduction of BMD does not translate into decreased bone strength because the increased porosity occurs only in the inner one third of bone, where the mechanical effect is minimal. Even more importantly, however, is the fact that changes in bone geometry and microarchitecture, more than compensate for any potential adverse effects of increased cortical porosity on bone strength [18].

PTH as monotherapy in postmenopausal osteoporosis

In the pivotal PTH trial by Neer *et al.*, women with severe osteoporosis were treated with subcutaneous injections of placebo, 20 or 40 μg of teriparatide [17]. The average number of fragility fractures per patient was over 2, defining the population as high risk. Over a follow-up period of 21 months, BMD increased by an average of 10–14% (Figure 11.4). Femoral neck BMD also improved, but more slowly and to a lesser extent (approximately 3%). The incidence of new vertebral fractures was reduced by 65% with the 20 μg dose. The overall incidence of new nonvertebral fractures was reduced by 35% with the 20 μg dose. When examining nonvertebral low trauma fragility fractures separately, a reduction of 53% was demonstrable. The higher, 40 ug dose, used in the trial did not further enhance the anti-fracture efficacy. Hip fracture incidence was not analyzed separately because the study was not sufficiently powered to examine this endpoint [17]. When evaluating these results it is worth noting, however, that the effect sizes emerging were the result of an incomplete trial as the trial was stopped abruptly due to the increased risk of osteosarcoma identified in a long-term toxicology study in rats. The true potential of the drug was shown in a post-hoc analysis by Lindsay *et al.* [19], where patients receiving more than 18 months of treatment with teriparatide revealed a 90% relative risk reduction in vertebral fractures and a 75–80% relative risk reduction in nonvertebral fractures (Figure 11.5). The latter effect should be compared to the 20–25% reduction of nonvertebral fractures seen in the trials using the newer parenterally administered antiresorptives like zoledronic acid and

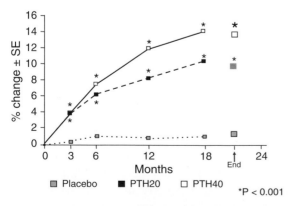

Figure 11.4 Increases in BMD in postmenopausal women treated with either placebo (Ca+D supplementation), 20 and 40 μg of PTH(1-34) after a median treatment duration of 19 months. (*Source*: Adapted from Neer *et al.* (2001) [17]).

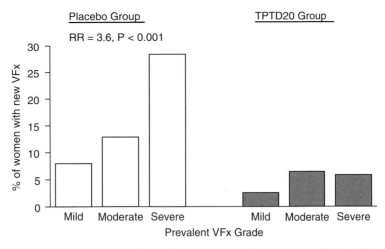

Figure 11.5 Distribution of vertebral compression fractures classified as either mild (20–25% compression(SQ1)), moderate (25–40% compression (SQ2)) and severe (>40% compression (SQ3)). (*Source*: Based on data from Neer *et al.* (2001) [17]).

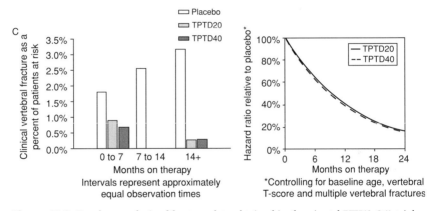

Figure 11.6 Post hoc analysis of fracture data obtained in the pivotal PTH(1-34) trial by Neer *et al.* (2001) *N Engl J Med.* **344**: 1434–41). Vertebral fractures (left panel) and nonvertebral fractures (right panel) were analyzed according to duration of treatment in the trial. With increasing duration the reduction of both fractures were reduced progressively. (*Source*: Lindsay R, Miller P, Pohl G *et al.* (2009) [19]. With kind permission from Springer Science+Business Media).

denosumab [20, 21]. The pronounced effects of teriparatide on severe vertebral compression fractures (Figure 11.6) is probably the main reason behind the significant reduction in back pain demonstrated in several studies [17].

Further post-hoc analyses revealed, that the reduction in fracture incidence due to teriparatide was not related to the number, severity, or site of previous fractures [22] and was largely independent of age and initial BMD [23, 24].

PTH (1-84) in postmenopausal osteoporosis

PTH (1-84) has been the object of a limited number of studies. In a preliminary clinical trial, preparatory to the definitive clinical trial, subjects were administered placebo, or 1 of 3 doses of PTH (1-84): 50, 75, or 100 μg for 12 months [25]. These data demonstrated both time- and dose-related increases in lumbar spine BMD. Similar to the teriparatide studies, bone turnover markers rose quickly. Histomorphometric analyses of bone biopsy specimens confirmed an anabolic response to PTH (1-84) with an increase in bone formation and improvements in cancellous bone architecture [26]. PTH (1-84) was found to reduce the risk for new or worsening vertebral fractures by 40% [27]. Contrary to the results obtained in the teriparatide trial, no reduction of nonvertebral fractures was seen with PTH (1-84), however. This study used a higher overall dose of PTH (100 ug PTH (1-84)), which on a molar basis is equivalent to 40 ug of PTH (1-34). Not surprisingly this higher dose also resulted in far more adverse events and discontinuations due to hypercalcemia [27]. Moreover, the population tested in this study also had a lower overall risk of osteoporotic fracture than patients in the PTH(1-34) trial. In contrast to the study by Neer *et al.* in which the average number of fragility fractures in subjects at baseline was >2, the incidence in the PTH (1-84) study was only 19%. This difference in baseline fracture status, together with the higher dose may have contributed to the lack of demonstrable effects on nonvertebral fractures.

Teriparatide in men with osteoporosis

In the first study that evaluated the effects of PTH in men, Kurland *et al.* randomized 23 men to 400 U/day of teriparatide (equivalent to 25 μg/day) or placebo for 18 months [28]. The men treated with teriparatide demonstrated a13.5% increase in lumbar spine BMD and a 2.9% increase in femoral neck BMD. Cortical bone density at the distal radius did not change as compared to placebo. In a larger trial of 437 men by Orwoll *et al.* [29], BMD increased significantly in the 20 μg treatment group by 5.9% at the lumbar spine and by 1.5% at the femoral neck independent of gonadal status. The magnitude and time course of BMD increases at the lumbar spine and hip over the 11 months of the study, were superimposable on the time course seen in the postmenopausal women studied by Neer *et al.* [17]. In a follow-up observational period of 30 months, 279 men from the original cohort had lateral spine X-rays 18 months after treatment was stopped. When combining fracture assessment in the combined treatment groups (20 μg and 40 μg), the risk of vertebral fracture was reduced nonsignificantly by 51% (p = 0.07), but when only moderate or severe fractures were considered, significant fracture risk reductions were found (6.8% vs. 1.1%; p < 0.02) [30]. When evaluating these fracture reductions, one has to keep in mind that a substantial number (25–30%) of study subjects reported use of antiresorptive agents during the follow-up period.

PTH in secondary osteoporosis

In secondary osteoporosis characterized by severe impairment of bone formation such as in glucocorticoid-induced osteoporosis (GIO), PTH should be more effective than anti-resorptive agents, because it more specifically targets the primary defect of these diseases. This was indeed shown to be the case in a recent study. Saag *et al.* [31] compared teriparatide with alendronate in 428 women and men with GIO (22–89 years of age) and glucocorticoid treatment for at least 3 months (dose ≥5 mg prednisolone equivalents daily or more). Patients received either teriparatide (20 μg /day) or alendronate (10 mg/day) for 18 months. In the teriparatide group the increase in BMD was higher than in the alendronate group (7.2 ± 0.7% vs. 3.4 ± 0.7%, P < 0.001). Although the trial was not powered to assess differences in fracture rates, pronounced differences in vertebral fracture incidence were demonstrable. Patients in the teriparatide group suffered fewer vertebral fractures than patients treated with alendronate (0.6% vs. 6.1%, P = 0.004), while the incidence of nonvertebral fractures was similar in the two groups (5.6% vs. 3.7%, P = 0.36).

Indications for Parathyroid hormone

Teriparatide is used in postmenopausal women and men with osteoporosis who are at high risk for fracture. It is an injectable drug, so patients have to be able to self-administer a daily subcutaneous pen injection. However, the technique of administration of teriparatide has been successfully taught to elderly patients. Patients with prevalent osteoporotic fractures before treatment are good candidates for therapy as they carry a much higher risk of fracture as compared to patients without fractures and a T-score below −2.5. Moreover, this risk increases progressively with both the number and severity of fractures. Thus, teriparatide is clearly indicated in severe manifest osteoporosis with multiple prevalent low energy fractures.

A very low T-score on its own (e.g., < −3.5), even without an osteoporotic fracture, also confers a high risk for fracture. Patient age is also important as for any T-score, the older the patient the greater the risk. Certainly, patients who fracture while on anti-resorptive therapy are good candidates for teriparatide. Other potential candidates for teriparatide include patients for whom one might consider a bisphosphonate, but who cannot tolerate the drug, and finally, severe osteoporosis in younger individuals in the thirties or forties also may constitute an indication for PTH therapy. These individuals have a long life ahead of them, and it seems logical to add bone to the skeleton to reduce their future risk of fracture, instead of just preserving bone mass and stabilizing the skeleton with anti-resorptive regimen.

Monitoring PTH therapy

Assessment of bone mass by DXA in the early phases will lead to under-estimation of new bone formed due to the relative hypomineralization of newly formed bone [10, 32]. The increase in turnover and porosity, which reaches its maximum at 6 months [10], will also contribute to a decreased DXA response early on. Therefore, DXA measurements should not be performed before at least one year after initiation of therapy. Later DXA measurements will suffer less from the biases associated with the early phases of PTH therapy and are therefore useful after 1 year of therapy as well as during sequential treatment with anti-resorptive agents.

Assessment of bone markers is more informative than DXA in the early phases of PTH therapy. PINP (Type I procollagen N-terminal propeptide) has emerged as the most dynamic and specific bone turnover marker for monitoring PTH effects in vivo, but markers like bone specific alkaline phosphatase and osteocalcin will also increase significantly [33]. Further supporting the use of bone markers is the fact the initial increases between 1 and 6 months in bone markers, in particular PICP and PINP, predict subsequent improvements in bone structure [34] and BMD increases [35, 36].

Sequential and combination therapy with teriparatide and an antiresorptive agent

Previous use of anti-resorptive drugs

As a substantial number of patients who are candidates for anabolic treatment have previously been treated with bisphosphonates or other anti-resorptive agents, it is important to consider whether such treatment affects the bone forming effects of PTH.

In a short 6-month clinical trial in postmenopausal women, Deal *et al.* reported superior effects on BMD for a combination of teriparatide and raloxifene over monotherapy with teriparatide alone [37]. Bone formation markers increased similarly in both groups. Bone resorption markers, however, were reduced in the combination group. BMD increased to a similar extent in the lumbar spine and femoral neck in both groups, but the increase in total hip BMD was significantly greater in subjects treated with both teriparatide and raloxifene. Cosman *et al.* treated postmenopausal women, previously given estrogen for at least 1 year, with teriparatide [38]. Lumbar spine BMD increased in a linear fashion during the entire 3-year study. Ettinger *et al.* studied the influence of two other anti-resorptive drugs, raloxifene and alendronate, prior to treatment with teriparatide [39]. In this study, 59 postmenopausal women with T-scores $\leq$ -2.0 who had been treated for an average of 28 months either with raloxifene or alendronate were evaluated. As seen for estrogen in the study of Lindsay *et al.*, raloxifene did not blunt the anabolic effects of teriparatide. In contrast, alendronate caused a delayed BMD response in the lumbar spine. After 18 months of treatment with teriparatide, lumbar spine BMD increased by 10.2% in the prior raloxifene-treated group compared to only 4.1% after prior alendronate treatment (p $<$ 0.05). The alendronate-treated group showed an initial decline in hip BMD at 6 months but at 18 months, mean total hip BMD was not different from baseline. During teriparatide treatment, bone markers in prior alendronate patients increased later and peaked at levels about 30% lower than seen in the raloxifene-treated patients. A different response to prior alendronate therapy was seen in another study where postmenopausal women who also had previously received alendronate for the same period of time responded to teriparatide with rapid increases in BMD [40].

In the Eurofors trial postmenopausal women with established osteoporosis were randomized to receive open-label teriparatide 20 µg/day for the first year. In a post-hoc analysis, their BMD-response was assessed according to previous osteoporosis treatment as follows: (a) treatment-naïve; (b) prior treatment with an anti-resorptive drug with adequate response; and (c) prior anti-resorptive treatment with inadequate response (inadequate AR-responders) (n = 421). BMD was measured by dual energy x-ray absorptiometry. In all three groups BMD increased significantly from baseline, but differed slightly between treatment-naïve patients (8.4%), patients treated adequately with anti-resorptive drug (7.1%), and inadequate responders to anti-resorptive therapy (6.2%). The same trend was seen for total hip BMD, which increased only in treatment-naive patients (1.8%), while remaining unchanged in the two other groups. Thus the blunting after prior alendronate therapy previously observed in other trials was demonstrable, but less pronounced.

These results imply that the potency of the anti-resorptive regimen to control bone turnover can determine the early response to teriparatide. To account for these differences, it is important to note that the baseline bone turnover markers prior to the initiation of teriparatide therapy were markedly different in the two studies. In the study by Ettinger *et al.*, bone turnover markers were almost completely suppressed, while the women in the study by Cosman *et al.*, exhibited less suppression. Thus, it may not be the specific anti-resorptive agent used prior to teriparatide which determines the subsequent skeletal response but rather the extent to which bone turnover is reduced by this agent. To support this idea, the response to teriparatide has been shown to be a function of the level of baseline bone turnover, with higher turnover levels achieving more robust densitometric responses [28].

Concomitant use of anabolic and anti-resorptive therapy

The initial decreases in BMD seen early after the initiation of PTH therapy at sites rich in cortical have not been associated with increased skeletal fragility at these sites [41]. These findings, however, have lead some clinicians to consider combination therapy with anti-resorptive agents as more beneficial than monotherapy given that their mechanisms of action are quite different from each other. Also theoretically, if bone resorption were inhibited by an anti-resorptive regimen while bone formation is being stimulated, combination therapy might give better results than with either agent alone. Several trials exploring this concept have, however, yielded important data to the contrary [42, 43]. Two groups published trials using a form of PTH (1-34) or PTH (1-84) alone, alendronate alone, or the combination of a PTH form and alendronate. Black *et al.* studied postmenopausal women treated with 100 µg of PTH (1-84)/day. The study by Finkelstein *et al.* treated men with 40 µg/day of teriparatide. Both studies used both DXA and QCT to measure areal and volumetric BMD. Much to the surprise of proponents of combination therapy, the gains in BMD in patients treated with PTH alone exceeded densitometric gains seen with either combination therapy or alendronate alone at the lumbar spine (Figure 11.7). Measurement by QCT, in fact, showed that combination therapy was associated with substantially smaller increases in cancellous bone BMD as compared to monotherapy with PTH. Bone turnover markers exhibited the expected increases and decreases for PTH and alendronate, respectively. Subjects treated with combination therapy, however, revealed bone marker levels in between the two regimens, indicating a blunting of the bone forming effect of the anabolic agent.

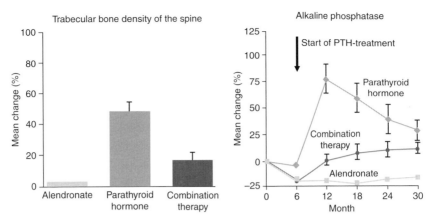

Figure 11.7 Trabecular bone density of lumbar vertebrae as assessed by quantitative computerized tomography (QCT) and bone formation as reflected in serum levels of bone specific alkaline phosphatase. Note the reduced BMD and he blunted marker response in the combination group treated with PTH + Alendronate.
(*Source*: Finkelstein JS, Hayes A, Hunzelman JL *et al.* (2003) [43]. Copyright Massachusetts Medical Society).

It seems, however, that the mode of administration of the bisphosphonate also plays a role. Cosman *et al.* compared the BMD and bone marker response to combined therapy with once yearly Zoledronic acid (5 mg) and daily PTH(1-34) with the response seen in patients treated with either agent alone [44]. Contrary to the findings of the studies using orally administered bisphosphonate, the combination of intravenous bisphosphonate and PTH yielded superior BMD responses at the hip and spine over those seen in patients treated with either agent alone (Figure 11.8). Bone markers revealed an initial reduction of formation markers as seen with oral bisphoshonates, but over time these markers increased and approached markers levels in patients treated with PTH alone within a year; much different from the constant suppression of bone formation seen in the combination group with PTH and oral bisphosphonates.

Consequences of discontinuing PTH therapy

After discontinuation of PTH, bone mass will return to levels close to baseline within a 2-year period [41, 45] (Figure 11.9). Several studies have suggested that this loss of bone mass after discontinuation can be offset by anti-resorptive treatment with either bisphosphonate [45, 46], estrogen [47] or raloxifene [37, 48].

The PaTH study provided further prospective data to address this issue [49]. In this study, postmenopausal women who had received PTH (1-84)

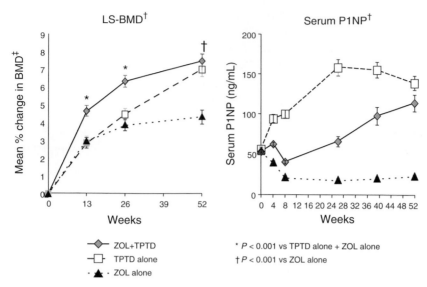

Figure 11.8 Changes in lumbar spine BMD (LS-BMD) and bone formation as reflected in the bone marker PINP in patients treated with a 15 min. infusion of the bisphosphonate zoledronic acid (ZOL)(5 mg) at day 1 followed by 1 year of daily injections with PTH(1-34)(20 μg/Day). Contrary to what was seen in the trials testing the combination PTH + Alendronate, ZOL did not blunt the BMD response in the combination group (PTH+ZOL). After an initial decrease, bone formation in the combination group picked up and reached the level seen in patients treated with PTH alone. (*Source*: Cosman F *et al.* (2011) [44]).

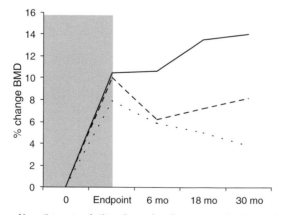

Figure 11.9 Change in Bone Mineral Density (BMD) in 3 groups after discontinuation following therapy with PTH(1-34) (shaded area): (1) no antiresoprtive after discontinuation (lower line); (2) initiation of antiresorptive treatment 6 months after discontinuation (middle line); initiation of antiresorptive immediately after discontinuation (upper line). (*Source*: Data from Lindsay *et al.* (2004) [41]).

for 12 months were randomly assigned to 12 additional months of therapy with 10 mg of alendronate daily or placebo. In subjects who received alendronate, BMD at the lumbar spine increased further by 4.9% while those who received placebo experienced a substantial decline in BMD. By QCT analysis, the net increase over 24 months in cancellous bone BMD among those treated with alendronate after PTH (1-84) was 30%. In those who received placebo after PTH (1-84), the net change was only 13%. There were similar differences in hip BMD, with patients treated with alendronate exhibiting a 13% increase vs. a 5% increase in patients on placebo.

Prince *et al.*, studied a cohort of patients for 30 months following the pivotal PTH trial. After discontinuation of PTH (1-34), subjects were given the option of switching to a bisphosphonate or not taking any further medications following teriparatide. A majority (60%) of patients were treated with anti-resorptive therapy after PTH discontinuation [50]. Gains in bone density were maintained in those who chose to begin anti-resorptive therapy immediately after teriparatide. Reductions in BMD were progressive throughout the 30-month observational period in subjects who elected not to follow teriparatide with any therapy. In a group who did not begin anti-resorptive therapy until 6 months after discontinuation of teriparatide, major reductions in BMD were seen during these first 6 months but no further reductions were observed after initiation of anti-resorptive regimens [41]. Despite the loss of bone mass in a substantial proportion of patients after the discontinuation of teriparatide, vertebral and nonvertebral fracture rates remained reduced for as long as 31 months after discontinuation in women previously treated with PTH (with or without a bisphosphonate) as compared with those treated with placebo (with or without a bisphosphonate; $p < 0.03$).

Following the initial trial testing the effect of PTH (1-34) in estrogen treated postmenopausal women, 52 women were randomly assigned to remain on hormone therapy (HT) alone or continue PTH+HT. Women continuing PTH + HT showed an increase in bone mass over baseline after 3 years by 13.4% in the spine and by 4.4% in the total hip. In women discontinuing PTH, but continuing HT, bone density did not increase, but remained stable for 1 year after discontinuation without any significant loss, as did bone markers. PTH + HT reduced vertebral fractures from 37.5% to 8.3% ($p < 0.02$).

Raloxifene and estrogen also preserve bone mass after discontinuation of PTH. In the Eurofors study, Eastell *et al.* reported a preservation of bone mass after discontinuation of PTH therapy for 1 year, while patients receiving calcium + D supplementation alone lost 2.8% at the spine and 2% at the hip in year 2 [48]. Based on these results it has become routine to institute treatment with antiresorptive drugs, mainy bisphosphonates, after discontinuation of PTH after 2 years.

Safety of PTH

Overall, PTH is well tolerated. The main side effects of PTH (1-34) and PTH (1-84) are usually mild nausea, vertigo and headache, which appear early after initiation of treatment and usually resolves over a few weeks [17]. Hypercalcemia is rarely seen, but is more prevalent with PTH (1-84) [27]. A toxicity that appears to be unique to rodents and not applicable to human subjects is osteosarcoma. The pivotal trial of PTH (1-34) was terminated early by the finding of increased risk osteosarcoma in Fisher rats given very high doses of PTH (1-34) with a treatment duration close to the lifespan of a rat (2 years) [51]. It is unlikely that this animal toxicity is related to human skeletal physiology [52], and no increased risk has ever been demonstrable in humans. The risk of osteosarcoma after treatment of more than 1 million patients with PTH remains at the background level of 1/250 000. With anabolic treatment changing bony dimensions, concerns regarding compression symptoms have also been raised, but no increase in such adverse effects have been demonstrable, and spinal canal diameter remains unchanged. In fact, small increases in spinal canal diameter have been reported [53].

PTH and the future

Less frequent administration of PTH, such as once weekly, has been considered as a treatment option, but the skeletal response is generally inferior, and whether the excellent vertebral and nonvertebral anti-fracture efficacy is preserved with this regimen remains unclear [54, 55].

Other modes of administration such as nasal and transdermal administration have also been considered, but large-scale clinical trials that evaluate these options have not emerged.

Parathyroid hormone-related protein (PTHrP), which is elevated in humoral hypercalcemia of malignancy, has also been studied as an anabolic skeletal agent. In a small sample of postmenopausal women, subcutaneous administration of PTHrP resulted in a 4.7% increase in lumbar spine density after only 3 months of treatment [56], but trials with fracture endpoints have not been published so far.

Cyclical 3-month courses of teriparatide during continued alendronate use has been reported by Cosman *et al.* [40]. In comparison to regular, uninterrupted teriparatide use, the cyclic administration of teriparatide was associated with similar densitometric gains. Due to the small size of these studies, no fracture endpoints were assessed.

Calcilytics which induce increases in short-term boosts of endogenous PTH from the parathyroids by interacting with the calcium receptor have also been subjected to early phase testing [57], but to date, no phase III trials have been performed using these agents.

Conclusion

Intermittent administration of PTH elicits pronounced changes in bone structure in patients with osteoporosis, and constitutes the only anabolic regimen currently available for the treatment of osteoporosis. The fragile bone quality of osteoporotic bone characterized by reduced cortical thickness and impaired cancellous bone structure and reduced mass is improved by PTH therapy and a significant, albeit variable amount of new bone is added to the skeleton. These changes results in a pronounced reduction in the risk of vertebral and in particular nonvertebral fractures. PTH treatment also reduces back pain more than other osteoporosis treatments. Due to price and mode of administration, PTH is generally reserved for patients with the most severe osteoporosis including those with multiple fractures and very low bone mass. In a comparator trial PTH was superior to alendronate in increasing bone mass and reducing vertebral fractures in GIO. While sequential therapy with anti-resorptive drugs following discontinuation of PTH is considered necessary to preserve bone mass, concomitant therapy is rarely indicated. Moreover, if oral bisphosphonates are administered concomitantly, varying degrees of blunting of the anabolic effect may occur.

References

1 Dempster DW, Parisien M, Silverberg SJ, *et al.* (1999) On the mechanism of cancellous bone preservation in postmenopausal women with mild primary hyperparathyroidism. *J Clin Endocrinol Metab* **84**(5): 1562–6.

2 Dobnig H, Turner RT (1997) The effects of programmed administration of human parathyroid hormone fragment (1-34) on bone histomorphometry and serum chemistry in rats. *Endocrinology* **138**(11): 4607–12.

3 Onyia JE, Helvering LM, Gelbert L, *et al.* (2005) Molecular profile of catabolic versus anabolic treatment regimens of parathyroid hormone (PTH) in rat bone: an analysis by DNA microarray. *Journal of Cellular Biochemistry* **95**(2): 403–18.

4 Ma YL, Cain RL, Halladay DL, *et al.* (2001) Catabolic effects of continuous human PTH (1–38) in vivo is associated with sustained stimulation of RANKL and inhibition

of osteoprotegerin and gene-associated bone formation. *Endocrinology* **142**(9): 4047–54.

5 Dempster DW, Cosman F, Kurland ES, *et al.* (2001) Effects of daily treatment with parathyroid hormone on bone microarchitecture and turnover in patients with osteoporosis: a paired biopsy study. *J Bone Miner Res* **16**(10): 1846–53.

6 Ma YL, Zeng Q, Donley DW, Ste-Marie LG, Gallagher JC, Dalsky GP, *et al.* (2006) Teriparatide increases bone formation in modeling and remodeling osteons and enhances IGF-II immunoreactivity in postmenopausal women with osteoporosis. *J Bone Miner Res* **21**(6): 855–64.

7 Dobnig H, Turner RT (1995) Evidence that intermittent treatment with parathyroid hormone increases bone formation in adult rats by activation of bone lining cells. *Endocrinology* **136**(8): 3632–8.

8 Keller H, Kneissel M (2005) SOST is a target gene for PTH in bone. *Bone* **37**(2): 148–58.

9 Lindsay R, Nieves J, Formica C, *et al.* (1997) Randomised controlled study of effect of parathyroid hormone on vertebral-bone mass and fracture incidence among postmenopausal women on oestrogen with osteoporosis. *Lancet* **350**(9077): 550–5.

10 Arlot M, Meunier PJ, Boivin G, *et al.* (2005) Differential effects of teriparatide and alendronate on bone remodeling in postmenopausal women assessed by histomorphometric parameters. *J Bone Miner Res* **20**(7): 1244–53.

11 Jiang Y, Zhao JJ, Mitlak BH (2003) Recombinant human parathyroid hormone (1-34) [teriparatide] improves both cortical and cancellous bone structure. *J Bone Miner Res* **18**(11): 1932–41.

12 Graeff C, Timm W, Nickelsen TN, *et al.* (2007) Monitoring teriparatide-associated changes in vertebral microstructure by high-resolution CT in vivo: results from the EUROFORS study. *J Bone Miner Res* **22**(9): 1426–33.

13 Borggrefe J, Graeff C, Nickelsen TN, *et al.* (2010) Quantitative computed tomographic assessment of the effects of 24 months of teriparatide treatment on 3D femoral neck bone distribution, geometry, and bone strength: results from the EUROFORS study. *J Bone Miner Res* **25**(3): 472–81.

14 Paschalis EP, Glass EV, Donley DW, *et al.* (2005) Bone mineral and collagen quality in iliac crest biopsies of patients given teriparatide: new results from the fracture prevention trial. *J Clin Endocrinol Metab* **90**(8): 4644–9.

15 Uusi-Rasi K, Semanick LM, Zanchetta JR, *et al.* (2005) Effects of teriparatide [rhPTH (1-34)] treatment on structural geometry of the proximal femur in elderly osteoporotic women. *Bone* **36**(6): 948–58.

16 Zanchetta JR, Bogado CE, Ferretti JL, *et al.* (2003) Effects of teriparatide [recombinant human parathyroid hormone (1-34)] on cortical bone in postmenopausal women with osteoporosis. *J Bone Miner Res* **18**(3): 539–43.

17 Neer RM, Arnaud CD, Zanchetta JR, *et al.* (2001) Effect of parathyroid hormone (1-34) on fractures and bone mineral density in postmenopausal women with osteoporosis. *N Engl J Med* **344**(19): 1434–41.

18 Burr DB, Hirano T, Turner CH, *et al.* (2001) Intermittently administered human parathyroid hormone (1-34) treatment increases intracortical bone turnover and porosity without reducing bone strength in the humerus of ovariectomized cynomolgus monkeys. *J Bone Miner Res* **16**(1): 157–65.

19 Lindsay R, Miller P, Pohl G, *et al.* (2009) Relationship between duration of teriparatide therapy and clinical outcomes in postmenopausal women with osteoporosis. *Osteoporos Int* **20**(6): 943–8.

20 Black DM, Delmas PD, Eastell R, *et al.* (2007) Once-yearly zoledronic acid for treatment of postmenopausal osteoporosis. *N Engl J Med* **356**(18): 1809–22.

21 Cummings SR, San MJ, McClung MR, *et al.* (2009) Denosumab for prevention of fractures in postmenopausal women with osteoporosis. *N Engl J Med* **361**(8): 756–65.

22 Gallagher JC, Genant HK, Crans GG, *et al.* (2005) Teriparatide reduces the fracture risk associated with increasing number and severity of osteoporotic fractures. *J Clin Endocrinol Metab* **90**(3): 1583–7.

23 Marcus R, Wang O, Satterwhite J, *et al.* (2003) The skeletal response to teriparatide is largely independent of age, initial bone mineral density, and prevalent vertebral fractures in postmenopausal women with osteoporosis. *J Bone Miner Res* **18**(1): 18–23.

24 Lyritis G, Marin F, Barker C, *et al.* (2010) Back pain during different sequential treatment regimens of teriparatide: results from EUROFORS. *Curr Med Res Opin* **26**(8): 1799–1807.

25 Hodsman AB, Hanley DA, Ettinger MP, *et al.* (2003) Efficacy and safety of human parathyroid hormone-(1-84) in increasing bone mineral density in postmenopausal osteoporosis. *J Clin Endocrinol Metab* **88**(11): 5212–20.

26 Fox J, Miller MA, Recker RR, *et al.* (2005) Treatment of postmenopausal osteoporotic women with parathyroid hormone 1-84 for 18 months increases cancellous bone formation and improves cancellous architecture: a study of iliac crest biopsies using histomorphometry and micro computed tomography. *J Musculoskeletal & Neuronal Interactions* **5**(4): 356–7.

27 Greenspan SL, Bone HG, *et al.* (2007) Effect of recombinant human parathyroid hormone (1-84) on vertebral fracture and bone mineral density in postmenopausal women with osteoporosis: a randomized trial. *Ann Intern Med* **146**(5): 326–39.

28 Kurland ES, Cosman F, McMahon DJ, Rosen CJ, Lindsay R, Bilezikian JP (2000) Parathyroid hormone as a therapy for idiopathic osteoporosis in men: effects on bone mineral density and bone markers. *J Clin Endocrinol Metab* **85**(9): 3069–76.

29 Orwoll ES, Scheele WH, Paul S, *et al.* (2003) The effect of teriparatide [human parathyroid hormone (1-34)] therapy on bone density in men with osteoporosis. *J Bone Miner Res* **18**(1): 9–17.

30 Kaufman JM, Orwoll E, Goemaere S, *et al.* (2005) Teriparatide effects on vertebral fractures and bone mineral density in men with osteoporosis: treatment and discontinuation of therapy. *Osteoporosis International* **16**(5): 510–16.

31 Saag KG, Shane E, Boonen S, *et al.* (2007) Teriparatide or alendronate in glucocorticoid-induced osteoporosis. *N Engl J Med* **357**(20): 2028–39.

32 Misof BM, Roschger P, Cosman F, *et al.* (2003) Effects of intermittent parathyroid hormone administration on bone mineralization density in iliac crest biopsies from patients with osteoporosis: a paired study before and after treatment. *J Clin Endocrinol Metab* **88**(3): 1150–6.

33 McClung MR, San MJ, Miller PD, *et al.* (2005) Opposite bone remodeling effects of teriparatide and alendronate in increasing bone mass. *Arch Intern Med* **165**(15): 1762–8.

34 Dobnig H, Sipos A, Jiang Y, *et al.* (2005) Early changes in biochemical markers of bone formation correlate with improvements in bone structure during teriparatide therapy. *J Clin Endocrinol Metab* **90**(7): 3970–7.

35 Chen P, Miller PD, Recker R, *et al.* (2007) Increases in BMD correlate with improvements in bone microarchitecture with teriparatide treatment in postmenopausal women with osteoporosis. *J Bone Miner Res* **22**(8): 1173–80.

36 Blumsohn A, Marin F, Nickelsen T, *et al.* (2011) Early changes in biochemical markers of bone turnover and their relationship with bone mineral density changes after 24 months of treatment with teriparatide. *Osteoporosis International* **22**(6): 1935–46.

37 Deal C, Omizo M, Schwartz EN, *et al.* (2005) Combination teriparatide and raloxifene therapy for postmenopausal osteoporosis: results from a 6-month double-blind placebo-controlled trial. *J Bone Miner Res* **20**(11): 1905–11.

38 Cosman F, Nieves J, Woelfert L, *et al.* (2001) Parathyroid hormone added to established hormone therapy: effects on vertebral fracture and maintenance of bone mass after parathyroid hormone withdrawal. *J Bone Miner Res* **16**(5): 925–31.

39 Ettinger B, San Martin J, Crans J, *et al.* (2004) Differential effects of teriparatide on BMD after treatment with raloxifene or alendronate. *J Bone Miner Res* **19**(5): 745–51.

40 Cosman F, Nieves J, Zion M, *et al.* (2005) Daily and cyclic parathyroid hormone in women receiving alendronate. *N Engl J Med* **353**(6): 566–75.

41 Lindsay R, Scheele WH, Neer R, *et al.* (2004) Sustained vertebral fracture risk reduction after withdrawal of teriparatide in postmenopausal women with osteoporosis. *Archives of Internal Medicine* **164**(18): 2024–30.

42 Black DM, Greenspan SL, Ensrud KE, *et al.* (2003) The effects of parathyroid hormone and alendronate alone or in combination in postmenopausal osteoporosis. *N Engl J Med.* **349**(13): 1207–15.

43 Finkelstein JS, Hayes A, Hunzelman JL, *et al.* (2003) The effects of parathyroid hormone, alendronate, or both in men with osteoporosis. *N Engl J Med* **349**(13): 1216–26.

44 Cosman F, Eriksen EF, Recknor C, *et al.* (2011) Effects of intravenous zoledronic acid plus subcutaneous teriparatide [rhPTH(1-34)] in postmenopausal osteoporosis. *J Bone Miner Res* **26**(3): 503–11.

45 Prince R, Sipos A, Hossain A, *et al.* (2005) Sustained nonvertebral fragility fracture risk reduction after discontinuation of teriparatide treatment. *N Engl J Med* **20**(9): 1507–13.

46 Kurland ES, Heller SL, Diamond B, *et al.* (2004) The importance of bisphosphonate therapy in maintaining bone mass in men after therapy with teriparatide [human parathyroid hormone(1-34)]. *Osteoporos Int* **15**(12): 992–7.

47 Lane NE, Sanchez S, Modin GW, *et al.* (2000) Bone mass continues to increase at the hip after parathyroid hormone treatment is discontinued in glucocorticoid-induced osteoporosis: results of a randomized controlled clinical trial. *J Bone Miner Res* **15**(5): 944–51.

48 Eastell R, Nickelsen T, Marin F, *et al.* (2009) Sequential treatment of severe postmenopausal osteoporosis after teriparatide: final results of the randomized, controlled European Study of Forsteo (EUROFORS). *J Bone Miner Res* **24**(4): 726–36.

49 Black DM, Bilezikian JP, Ensrud KE, *et al.* (2005) One year of alendronate after one year of parathyroid hormone (1-84) for osteoporosis. *J Bone Miner Res* **353**(6): 555–65.

50 Prince R, Sipos A, Hossain A, *et al.* (2005) Sustained nonvertebral fragility fracture risk reduction after discontinuation of teriparatide treatment. *J Bone Miner Res* **20**(9): 1507–13.

51 Vahle JL, Long GG, Sandusky G, *et al.* (2004) Bone neoplasms in F344 rats given teriparatide [rhPTH(1-34)] are dependent on duration of treatment and dose. *Toxicologic Pathology* **32**(4): 426–38.

52 Tashjian AH, Jr., Gagel RF (2006) Teriparatide [human PTH(1-34)]: 2.5 years of experience on the use and safety of the drug for the treatment of osteoporosis. *J Bone Miner Res* **21**(3): 354–65.

53 Schnell R, Graef C, Krebs A *et al.* (2010) *Calcif Tissue Int* **87**: 130–6.

54 Nakamura Y (2012) Parathyroid hormone as a Bone anabolic agent. Evidence of osteoporosis treatment with weekly teriparatide injection. *Clinical Calcium* **22**(3): 407–13.

55 Fujita T, Inoue T, Morii H, *et al.* (1999) Effect of an intermittent weekly dose of human parathyroid hormone (1-34) on osteoporosis: a randomized double-masked prospective study using three dose levels. *Osteoporosis International* **9**(4): 296–306.

56 Horwitz MJ, Tedesco MB, Garcia-Ocana A, *et al.* (2010) Parathyroid hormone-related protein for the treatment of postmenopausal osteoporosis: defining the maximal tolerable dose. *J Clin Endocrinol Metab* **95**(3): 1279–87.

57 Gowen M, Stroup GB, Dodds RA, *et al.* (2000) Antagonizing the parathyroid calcium receptor stimulates parathyroid hormone secretion and bone formation in osteopenic rats. *J Clin Investigation* **105**(11): 1595–1604.

CHAPTER 12

Optimum Calcium and Vitamin D for the Prevention and Treatment of Osteoporosis

Michael F. Holick

Boston University Medical Center, Boston, MA, USA

Sources of vitamin D

The major source of vitamin D for most children and adults is exposure to sunlight [1, 2]. When sunlight that contains ultraviolet B (UVB; 315 nm) radiation enters the skin, it is absorbed by 7-dehydrocholesterol that is present in the keratinocyte plasma membrane resulting in its transformation into previtamin D_3. Previtamin D_3 is thermodynamically unstable and at body temperature over a period of a few hours it is converted to vitamin D_3 [3]. Once formed vitamin D_3 is ejected out of the skin cell into the extra vascular space. By diffusion vitamin D_3 enters the dermal capillary bed where it is bound to the vitamin D binding protein. Once in the bloodstream vitamin D_3 can either enter fat cells to be stored or travel to the liver for its first metabolism. Excessive exposure to sunlight can cause sunburning but will not lead to the overproduction of vitamin D_3. The reason is that during exposure to sunlight any excess previtamin D_3 and vitamin D_3 are converted to a variety of photoproducts that have no activity on calcium and bone metabolism (Figure 12.1) [1].

Very few foods naturally contain vitamin D. They include oily fish including salmon, herring and mackerel, liver oils from some fish including cod liver oil, and mushrooms exposed to sunlight or ultraviolet radiation [1] (Table 12.1). Some countries, including the United States, Canada, Finland and Sweden, fortify dairy products including milk, cheese and yogurt with vitamin D. In the United States some orange juices, cereals and bread are fortified with vitamin D. In Europe vitamin D fortification was banned in the 1950s because of the belief that infants who developed hypercalcemia and had altered facial features did so due to the over fortification of milk with vitamin D [4]. Although this was never proven and it has been suggested that these children actually suffered from the rare genetic

Osteoporosis: Diagnosis and Management, First Edition. Edited by Dale W. Stovall.
© 2013 John Wiley & Sons, Ltd. Published 2013 by John Wiley & Sons, Ltd.

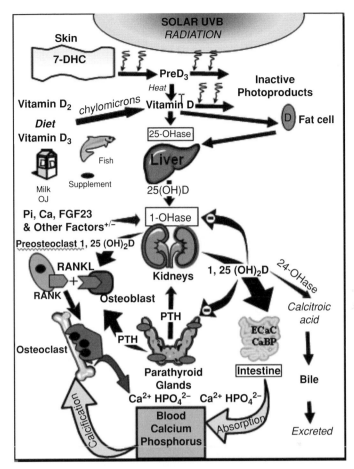

Figure 12.1 Schematic representation of the synthesis and metabolism of vitamin D for regulating calcium, phosphorus and bone metabolism. During exposure to sunlight 7-dehydrocholesterol in the skin is converted to previtamin D_3. PreD$_3$ immediately converts by a heat dependent process to vitamin D_3. Excessive exposure to sunlight degrades previtamin D_3 and vitamin D_3 into inactive photoproducts. Vitamin D_2 and vitamin D_3 from dietary sources is incorporated into chylomicrons, transported by the lymphatic system into the venus circulation. Vitamin D (D represents D_2 or D_3) made in the skin or ingested in the diet can be stored in and then released from fat cells. Vitamin D in the circulation is bound to the vitamin D binding protein which transports it to the liver where vitamin D is converted by the vitamin D-25-hydroxylase to 25-hydroxyvitamin D [25(OH)D]. This is the major circulating form of vitamin D that is used by clinicians to measure vitamin D status (although most reference laboratories report the normal range to be 20–100 ng/ml, the preferred healthful range is 30–60 ng/ml). It is biologically inactive and must be converted in the kidneys by the 25-hydroxyvitamin D-1α-hydroxylase (1-OHase) to its biologically active form 1,25-dihydroxyvitamin D [1,25(OH)$_2$D].

disorder, Williams syndrome, which is now known to also be associated with a hypersensitivity to the calcemic action of vitamin D, most European countries still forbid the fortification of dairy products with vitamin D. They, however, do permit margarine and some cereals to be fortified with vitamin D. The amount of vitamin D is limited to 100 IUs of vitamin D per serving, that is, 8 ounces of milk or orange juice are fortified with 100 IUs of vitamin D.

There are two major forms of vitamin D. Vitamin D_2 (ergocalciferol) is made by plants and is obtained commercially by exposing yeast to ultraviolet radiation. It is also produced in mushrooms exposed to sunlight and ultraviolet radiation. Vitamin D_3 (cholecalciferol) is produced in the skin as a result of sun exposure. Commercially it is produced from cholesterol present in lanolin. It is also the form of vitamin D found in fish and cod liver oil. Although there has been some controversy as to whether vitamin D_2 is as effective as vitamin D_3 in maintaining a person's vitamin D status [5, 6], most evidence suggests that at least at physiologic doses they are equally effective [7–9]. It should also be noted that vitamin D_2 is the only pharmaceutical form of vitamin D available in the United States because it was grandfathered by the FDA. Vitamin D_2 has been used for more than 80 years for the treatment and prevention of vitamin D deficiency in both children and adults.

Factors that influence vitamin D status

There are a variety of environmental, exogenous and endogenous factors that can greatly influence the cutaneous production of vitamin D as well as vitamin D absorption and metabolism. Melanin is an effective natural

Figure 12.1 (*Continued*) Serum phosphorus, calcium fibroblast growth factors (FGF-23) and other factors can either increase (+) or decrease (−) the renal production of $1,25(OH)_2D$. $1,25(OH)_2D$ feedback regulates its own synthesis and decreases the synthesis and secretion of parathyroid hormone (PTH) in the parathyroid glands. $1,25(OH)_2D$ increases the expression of the 25-hydroxyvitamin D-24-hydroxylase (24-OHase) to catabolize $1,25(OH)_2D$ to the water soluble biologically inactive calcitroic acid which is excreted in the bile. $1,25(OH)_2D$ enhances intestinal calcium absorption in the small intestine by stimulating the expression of the epithelial calcium channel (ECaC) and the calbindin 9K (calcium binding protein; CaBP). $1,25(OH)_2D$ is recognized by its receptor in osteoblasts causing an increase in the expression of receptor activator of NFκB ligand (RANKL). Its receptor RANK on the preosteoclast binds RANKL which induces the preosteoclast to become a mature osteoclast. The mature osteoclast removes calcium and phosphorus from the bone to maintain blood calcium and phosphorus levels. Adequate calcium and phosphorus levels promote the mineralization of the skeleton. (Holick copyright 2007).

Table 12.1 Sources of vitamin D_2 and vitamin D_3 (*Source*: Holick MF (2007), [1]. Copyright © (2007) Massachusetts Medical Society. Reprinted with permission).

Source	Vitamin D Content IU = 25 ng
Natural Sources	

Vitamin D_2 (Ergocalciferol)   Vitamin D_3 (Cholecalciferol)

Source	Vitamin D Content
Cod liver oil	~400–1,000 IU/tsp vitamin D_3
Salmon, fresh wild caught	~600–1,000 IU/3.5 oz vitamin D_3
Salmon, fresh farmed	~100–250 IU/3.5 oz vitamin D_3, vitamin D_2
Salmon, canned	~300–600 IU/3.5 oz vitamin D_3
Sardines, canned	~300 IU/3.5 oz vitamin D_3
Mackerel, canned	~250 IU/3.5 oz vitamin D_3
Tuna, canned	236 IU/3.5 oz vitamin D_3
Shiitake mushrooms, fresh	~100 IU/3.5 oz vitamin D_2
Shiitake mushrooms, sun dried	~1,600 IU/3.5 oz vitamin D_2
Egg yolk	~20 IU/yolk vitamin D_3 or D_2
Sunlight/UVB radiation	~20,000 IU equivalent to exposure to 1 minimal erythemal dose (MED) in a bathing suit. Thus, exposure of arms and legs to 0.5 MED is equivalent to ingesting ~3,000 IU vitamin D_3.
Fortified Foods	
Fortified milk	100 IU/8 oz usually vitamin D_3
Fortified orange juice	100 IU/8 oz vitamin D_3
Infant formulas	100 IU/8 oz vitamin D_3
Fortified yogurts	100 IU/8 oz usually vitamin D_3
Fortified butter	56 IU/3.5 oz usually vitamin D_3
Fortified margarine	429/3.5 oz usually vitamin D_3
Fortified cheeses	100 IU/3 oz usually vitamin D_3
Fortified breakfast cereals	~100 IU/serving usually vitamin D_3
Pharmaceutical Sources in the United States	
Vitamin D_2 (Ergocalciferol)	50,000 IU/capsule
Drisdol (vitamin D_2) liquid	8000 IU/cc
Supplemental Sources	
Multivitamin	400, 500, 1000 IU vitamin D_3 or vitamin D_2
Vitamin D_3	400, 800, 1000, 2000, 5,000, 10,000, and 50,000 IU

*Designated calciferol which usually means vitamin D_2.

sunscreen that efficiently absorbs solar UVA and UVB radiation. Therefore an increase in skin pigmentation reduces the efficiency of sunlight to produce vitamin D_3. When Caucasian and African American adults were exposed to the same amount of simulated sunlight in a tanning bed the Caucasian adults raised their blood level of vitamin D_3 by more than 60 fold whereas there was no significant change in the blood levels of vitamin D_3 in African American adults. When the same African American adults were exposed to ~6 times the amount of simulated sunlight they raised their blood level by about 30-fold [10]. This is similar to a Caucasian wearing sunscreen with a sun protection factor (SPF) of 10–15. The topical application of a sunscreen with an SPF of 15 absorbs approximately 90% of solar UVB radiation and thus reduces the production of vitamin D_3 by the same amount, that is, 90%. A sunscreen with an SPF of 30 reduces the synthesis of vitamin D_3 by more than 97%. Aging also influences the cutaneous production of vitamin D_3. A 20-year-old adult exposed to the same amount of simulated sunlight as a 70-year-old adult can make 2–3 times more vitamin D_3 due to the fact that there is a significant decline of more than 75% of the skin concentrations of 7-dehydrocholesterol, the precursor for vitamin D_3, in the 70 year old [11, 12].

The solar zenith angle of the sun has a dramatic influence on the cutaneous production of previtamin D_3. Only about 0.5–1% of solar UVB radiation is able to reach the earth's surface in the summer at noon. The reason for this is that ozone in the stratosphere efficiently absorbs most of the solar UVB radiation before it can reach the earth's surface. As the zenith angle of the sun increases, the UVB radiation has a longer path length to transit through the ozone layer and thus more of the vitamin D producing UVB radiation is absorbed. This is the explanation for why exposure to winter sunlight results in little if any vitamin D production in the skin [13]. In those individuals who live either above or below ~33° latitude, essentially no vitamin D is produced during the winter. Time of day is also influenced by the zenith angle of the sun. Early morning and late afternoon the zenith angle is more oblique similar to winter sunlight and thus essentially no vitamin D is produced in the skin before 10 am and after 3 pm even in the summertime [14] (Figure 12.2).

Vitamin D is fat-soluble and is stored in body fat. More importantly, it is now recognized that vitamin D deficiency is more common in obese children and adults due to the fact that the vitamin D is sequestered in body fat. In a study of healthy adults who were either normal weight or who had a BMI >30 and who received either the same amount of vitamin D as a single oral dose or who were exposed to the same amount of simulated sunlight, these individuals were only able to raise their blood level of vitamin D_3 by ~45% as compared to adults with a BMI <30 [15]. This is the explanation for why obese adults require at least 2–3 times more vitamin D to both treat and prevent vitamin D deficiency.

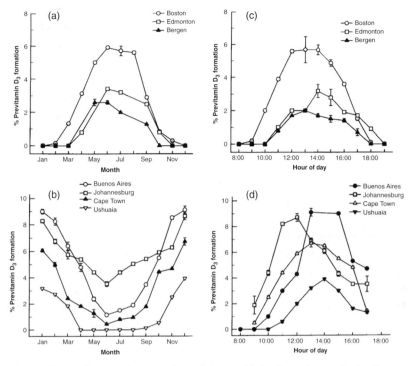

Figure 12.2 Influence of season, time of day, and latitude on the synthesis of previtamin D3 in Northern (a, c) and southern hemispheres (b, d). The hour indicated in C and D is the end of the 1-hr exposure time. (Holick copyright 1998).

There are a variety of medications that can alter the metabolism of vitamin D including antiseizure medications, glucococorticoids and medications used to treat AIDS; and thus these medications can influence a person's vitamin D status and vitamin D requirement which is usually increased 2–3-fold [1, 2].

Malabsorption syndromes including active and quiescent inflammatory bowel disease can markedly reduce both calcium and vitamin D absorption. Furthermore, an often silent cause of both vitamin D deficiency and calcium malabsorption is celiac disease. Often the diagnosis of celiac disease is made in patients who present with vitamin D deficiency and who do not respond to vitamin D therapy [16].

Vitamin D metabolism for regulating calcium and phosphorus homeostasis

Once vitamin D_3 is made in the skin it enters the circulation. When vitamin D_2 or vitamin D_3 (D represents either vitamin D_2 or vitamin D_3)

is ingested, it is incorporated into chylomicrons which are absorbed into the lymphatic system and then deposited into the venous blood supply. Once in the blood, vitamin D travels to the liver and is converted to 25-hydroxyvitamin D [25(OH)D] (Figure 12.1). 25(OH)D is the major circulating form of vitamin D and is measured to determine a patient's vitamin D status. 25(OH)D, however, is biologically inactive in regards to calcium and phosphorus metabolism and requires an additional hydroxylation in the kidneys on carbon-1 by the mitochondrial 25-hydroxyvitamin D-1-hydroxylase (cyp27B1) to form 1,25–dihydroxyvitamin D [1,25(OH)$_2$D]. 1,25(OH)$_2$D is considered to be the biologically active form of vitamin D that is responsible for maintaining blood calcium and phosphorus levels in the normal range [1, 17].

There are a variety of factors that enhance the renal production of 1,25(OH)$_2$D including PTH, low serum calcium and low serum phosphorus levels. Both fibroblast growth factor 23 (FGF-23) and a high serum phosphorus level will reduce renal production of 1,25(OH)$_2$D [1] (Figure 12.1).

1,25(OH)$_2$D is bound to vitamin D binding protein and is transported to the small intestine where it enters the enterocyte. Once inside the enterocyte, vitamin D travels to the cell nucleus where it interacts with the vitamin D receptor (VDR). This complex binds to the retinoic acid X receptor (RXR) which in turn acts as a transcription factor and interacts with vitamin D responsive elements within the genes that help regulate intestinal absorption of calcium including an epithelial calcium channel, calcium binding protein and calcium-dependent ATP-ase [1, 17] (Figure 12.1). In a vitamin D deficient patient only about 10–15% of dietary calcium is absorbed. In a vitamin D sufficient patient the absorption of calcium is enhanced two-fold to approximately 30–40%. 1,25(OH)$_2$D also enhances intestinal phosphate absorption from approximately 60% (passively absorbed in a vitamin D deficient patient) to approximately 80% [1].

A low dietary intake of calcium results in a transient decrease in ionized calcium which in turn is recognized by the calcium sensor in the parathyroid glands resulting in an increase in the expression, production and release of PTH into the circulation. Besides increasing renal tubular reabsorption of calcium, PTH stimulates the kidneys to produce 1,25(OH)$_2$D. When intestinal calcium absorption is insufficient to sustain normal ionized calcium concentrations, 1,25(OH)$_2$D travels to the skeleton and interacts with the VDR in the osteoblast to increase the expression of receptor activator of NFkB (RANK) ligand (RANKL). The RANK on the monocytic pre-osteoclast binds the RANKL which results in its transformation into a mature osteoclast [1, 18] (Figure 12.1). The mature osteoclast releases HCl and collagenases which in turn removes the mineral and matrix respectively releasing precious calcium into the circulation to maintain neuromuscular activity and a wide variety of metabolic functions. Thus the major function of vitamin D is to maintain serum calcium and phosphorus in a physiologically functional range. When there is enough calcium coming from intestinal calcium absorption to maintain serum calcium levels the resulting calcium-phosphate product is then adequate to mineralize newly laid down collagen matrix to maintain and enhance bone mineral density.

Definitions of vitamin D deficiency and vitamin D insufficiency

Both the Institute of Medicine (IOM)[19] and the Endocrine Society[2] have defined vitamin D deficiency as a 25(OH)D < 20 ng/mL. The Endocrine Society also defined vitamin D insufficiency as a 25(OH)D of 21–29 ng/mL [2]. These recommendations are based on the findings of several studies. In one of these studies, Malabanan *et al.* [20] gave healthy adults who had a serum 25(OH)D level of 11–25 ng/mL, calcium supplementation along with 50 000 IUs of vitamin D_2 once a week for 8 weeks and measured blood levels of 25(OH)D, calcium and PTH at baseline and at the end of the study. They observed an average decline of 35% in PTH levels in adults who had blood levels of 25(OH)D < 20 ng/mL. No significant change was observed in the adults who had serum 25(OH)D levels above 20 ng/mL. A study of French postmenopausal women that correlated the study participant's serum 25(OH)D concentrations to their PTH levels, suggested that PTH levels plateaue with serum 25(OH)D levels between 30 and 40 ng/mL [21]. Several other studies also made the same observation including one conducted in the United States in over 1500 postmenopausal women who were taking a bone active drug for their osteoporosis [22]. Not only did that study demonstrate that PTH was at its plateau in women who had a serum 25(OH)D level > 30 ng/mL, it also revealed that women with an average serum 25(OH)D level of 21 ng/mL had a 2-fold higher risk of having secondary hyperparathyroidism (Figure 12.3). Still further, in support of a physiologic benefit of maintaining serum 25(OH)D >30 ng/mL was the observation that postmenopausal women who raised their blood levels of 25(OH)D from 20 ng/mL to on average 32 ng/mL increased their intestinal calcium absorption by approximately 65% [23].

The IOM reported that a review of a study of 675 German motor vehicle accident victims' blood, 25(OH)D and bone biopsy for evidence of vitamin D deficiency osteomalacia revealed that 99% had no evidence of osteomalacia if their blood level of 25(OH)D was >20 ng/mL [19, 24]. However,

(a)

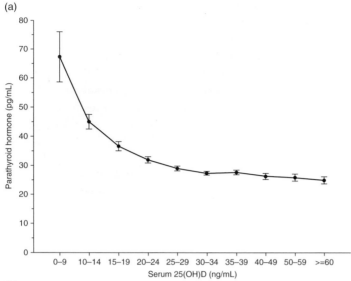

(b)

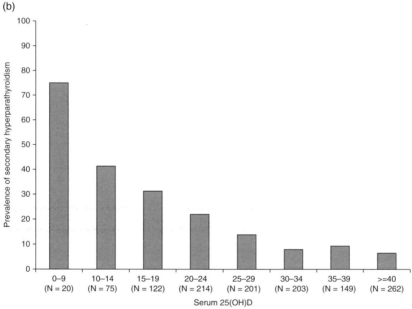

Figure 12.3 (a). Mean (±SE) serum PTH (picograms per milliliter) by serum 25(OH)D subgroups. Subject PTH concentrations (picograms per milliliter) relative to serum 25(OH)D concentrations sorted by subgroups delineated by predefined cutoffs for analyses of 25(OH)D inadequacy. Serum PTH values began to increase with 25(OH)D concentrations less than 29.8 ng/ml. (b). Percent of subjects with secondary hyperparathyroidism by 25(OH)D level. The percent of subjects with secondary hyperparathyroidism (PTH > 40 pg/ml) sorted by subgroups with serum 25(OH)D concentrations delineated by predefined cutoffs for analyses of 25(OH)D inadequacy. (*Source*: Holick MF, Siris ES, Binkley N *et al.* (2005) [22]. Copyright 2005, The Endocrine Society).

a more careful analysis of the study revealed an error in the calculation and that 8.5% of these otherwise healthy adults had clear evidence of osteomalacia [25]. In addition, the authors of the study revealed that more than 30% of the adults had evidence of either osteomalacia or osteoidosis, that is, evidence of unmineralized osteoid buried within mineralized bone [24]. The authors of the study concluded that to guarantee no evidence of osteomalacia blood levels of 25(OH)D should be >30 ng/mL. It was based on this evidence as well as observations associating a serum 25(OH)D level of >30 ng/mL with a plateauing of the PTH levels that the Endocrine Society defined vitamin D insufficiency as a 25(OH)D level of 21–29 ng/mL and stated that to maximize bone health a blood level of at least 30 ng/mL should be maintained [2]. They also reported that the safe upper limit could be as high as 100 ng/mL. Vitamin D toxicity is usually not seen until a 25(OH)D is >150 ng/mL and is associated with hypercalcemia, hyperphosphatemia and a suppressed PTH level. However patients with granulomatous disorders such as sarcoidosis have a hypersensitivity to vitamin D and as a result their blood levels of 25(OH)D should be maintained between 20–30 ng/mL. Higher blood levels are usually associated with hypercalciuria and hypercalcemia [2, 26].

Prevalence of vitamin D deficiency in osteoporotic women and men

Vitamin D deficiency and insufficiency is one of the most common medical problems worldwide in children and adults [1]. This is especially true in men and women who have osteopenia and osteoporosis [27–33]. Middle-aged and older adults are at high risk because of poor dietary intake either because of a lactase deficiency or lack of interest in consuming dairy products, inadequate sun exposure, use of a sunscreen and an age-related decrease in vitamin D synthesis [1, 34]. Gaugris *et al.* [35] reviewed 30 studies and concluded that postmenopausal women, especially those with osteoporosis and a history of fracture, had a high prevalence of vitamin D deficiency. A cross-sectional observational study conducted at 61 sites across North America revealed that 52% of postmenopausal receiving an expensive therapy for osteoporosis had 25(OH)D levels that were <30 ng/mL [22] (Figure 12.2). Even women who took a vitamin D supplement containing 400 IUs of vitamin D were vitamin D deficient or insufficient. Similar observations have been made in postmenopausal women and in older men in Canada, United States, Europe and Central and South America [1, 27–37].

Consequences of vitamin D deficiency on skeletal health

It is well known that vitamin D deficiency results in the bone-deforming disease rickets in children [38]. However, it is not often appreciated that in adults, vitamin D deficiency not only can cause and exacerbate both osteopenia and osteoporosis but also causes a painful bone disease osteomalacia [1, 37, 39–41]. Vitamin D deficiency results in decreased efficiency of the small intestine to absorb dietary calcium. This results in a decrease in ionized calcium which is a signal to the parathyroid glands to produce and secrete more PTH. PTH, like $1,25(OH)_2D$, stimulates osteoblasts to produce RANKL which stimulates the formation of mature bone resorbing osteoclasts. These osteoclasts remove both mineral and matrix and thus decrease bone mineral density leading to osteopenia and osteoporosis. In addition PTH causes phosphaturia which in turn lowers serum phosphorus levels. As a result there is an inadequate calcium-phosphate product in the circulation and extracellular space. Thus, the newly laid down collagen matrix by osteoblasts cannot be mineralized. This unmineralized matrix not only does not provide any structural support resulting in increased risk for fracture but also causes throbbing aching and bone pain which is often misdiagnosed as fibromyalgia or chronic fatigue syndrome [40, 41]. The likely cause for this unusual pain syndrome is the unmineralized collagen matrix which is essentially gelatin hydrates and pushes upward underneath the periosteal covering which is heavily innervated with sensory fibers resulting in the sensation of throbbing aching bone pain. Furthermore, the gelatin matrix provides little structural support and any pressure on the periosteum causes deformation and induces sensory fibers to elicit acute bone pain. The diagnosis can easily be made by palpation of the sternum or anterior tibia with a forefinger or thumb with minimum-to-moderate pressure. If the patient winces in pain it is likely they have periosteal bone pain and osteomalacia rather than a trigger point for making the diagnosis of fibromyalgia [41].

Vitamin D and calcium for fracture prevention

Worsening of osteopenia and osteoporosis with or without osteomalacia increases one's risk for a skeletal fracture. Chapuy *et al.* [42] reported that elderly French women who ingested 1200 mg of calcium and 800 IUs of vitamin D_3 daily reduced their risk of hip fracture by 51% and nonvertebral fracture incidents by 32%. A study in elderly Bostonian men and women who received both 500 mg of calcium and 700

IUs of vitamin D_3 revealed that these individuals had a 58% reduction in nonvertebral fractures [43]. Similarly, in a study of community-dwelling men and women who received 1000 mg of calcium and 400 IUs of vitamin D_3 daily, a 15% reduction in the risk of fracture was demonstrated [44].

However, there have been a few large randomized controlled trials that have concluded that calcium and vitamin D supplementation does not influence fracture risk. Furthermore, it has been suggested that vitamin D and calcium supplementation could have detrimental effects including an increased risk for developing kidney stones and cardiovascular disease [1] Porthouse *et al.* [45] followed elderly women who were given either a placebo (a leaflet providing general advice about the fall prevention and sources of dietary calcium and vitamin D) or 1000 mg of calcium and 800 IUs of vitamin D_3 daily plus the leaflet for 25 months. There was no significant difference in the risk of fracture in either group. Similarly, in the RECORD (Randomized Evaluation of Calcium or Vitamin D) study, over 5000 elderly men and women (>70 years of age) with a history of a previous low trauma fracture received in a double-blind controlled fashion calcium alone, vitamin D alone or combined calcium and vitamin D. In this trial, there was no significant difference in new low trauma fractures in any of the groups studied [46]. In the United States a large randomized controlled trial (Women's Health Initiative; WHI) revealed no significant reduction in the risk of hip and nonvertebral fractures in women who were asked to take 1000 mg of calcium and 400 IUs of vitamin D_3 daily for 7 years. Furthermore, it was suggested that women who ingested 1000 mg of calcium and 400 IUs of vitamin D_3 had a 15% higher risk for developing kidney stones [47]. These studies and others were recently reviewed by the United States Preventative Services Task Force (USPSTF) and they too came to the same conclusion that calcium and vitamin D provided no benefit for reducing risk for fracture and possibly increased risk for kidney stones [48].

However, all three of these studies had serious deficiencies that call into question their conclusion that calcium and vitamin D supplementation do not reduce the risk for fracture [34]. These studies were confounded by the simple fact that there was poor compliance. More specifically, the community dwellers who participated in the studies were <60% compliant in taking their calcium and vitamin D. A subanalysis of the WHI study revealed that women who took their calcium and vitamin D at least 80% of the time, had a statistically significant (29%) reduction in the risk of hip fracture [49]. Furthermore, none of these studies controlled for the study participants' calcium and vitamin D intake. In the WHI study, 64% of women in the placebo group had a daily calcium intake from diet and supplements of at least 800 mg at baseline and 42% had a daily vitamin

D intake of at least 400 IUs a day [47]. Still further, most of the women in the WHI study were vitamin D deficient at the initiation of the trial and they only received 400 IUs of vitamin D daily which the IOM now recognizes was inadequate for maximum bone health [19]. Finally, there was no determination of blood levels of 25(OH)D at the end of the trial and it is very likely that after 7 years of therapy with 400 IUs of vitamin D, that the women remained vitamin D deficient. Also, no determination of PTH was made in any of the participants.

However, what is likely is that some women who were taking 1000 mg of calcium daily, in addition to another 1000 mg of calcium that they were taking at baseline, were ingesting up to 2000 mg of calcium daily which could explain for why the WHI reported a 15% increase in the risk for developing kidney stones in women who ingested calcium and vitamin D. There is, however, no evidence as reviewed by the IOM [19] and Endocrine Society [2] to suggest that ingesting calcium and vitamin D at the recommended levels increases one's risk for developing kidney stones.

There have been several meta-analyses that have concluded that ingesting 1000 mg of calcium along with at least 800 IUs of vitamin D will not only reduce one's risk of fracture but will also improve muscle strength and reduce the risk of falls [50–52]. Patients who received 400 IUs of vitamin D_3 daily showed no benefit in fracture reduction whereas a higher dose of 700–800 IUs of vitamin D_3 daily reduced risk of hip fracture by 26% and nonvertebral fracture by 23% (Figure 12.3). These results are consistent with the observation that elderly men and women who received 100 000 IUs of vitamin D_3 every 4 months (equivalent to 833 IUs of vitamin D_3 daily) had a 33% reduced risk of developing a fracture of the hip, wrist, forearm or vertebra [53].

Intermittent high dose vitamin D as a method of improving vitamin D status in the elderly and reducing the risk of fracture was recently challenged in a study of elderly Australians (>70 years) who received 500 000 IUs of vitamin D_3 and who were observed to have an increased risk for fracture [54]. What is unknown is whether these elderly subjects who were likely vitamin D deficient had muscle weakness, fatigue and bone pain associated with osteomalacia. After receiving vitamin D they likely had significant improvement in all of these symptoms as well as in their feeling of well-being and thus were more active; and therefore, more likely to fall thereby increasing their risk for fracture of their osteoporotic skeleton. A study conducted in Scandinavia observed that elderly men and women who received an intramuscular injection of 150 000–300 000 IUs of vitamin D_3 yearly had a reduced risk of fracture by 25% [55].

Vitamin D and fall prevention

It is well known that vitamin D deficiency causes proximal muscle weakness in children and adults [1, 38, 40, 51, 52, 56–60]. There is a VDR in skeletal muscle and aging appears to decrease VDR in skeletal muscle [61]. An evaluation of the NHANES (National Health and Nutrition Examination Survey) database revealed that muscle strength as measured by the amount of time it takes to stand from a sitting position or to walk 8 feet continued to improve until blood levels of 25(OH)D reached approximately 44 ng/mL [62]. Several meta-analyses of randomized controlled trials revealed that vitamin D supplementation reduced the risk of falling by as much as 22% [52, 63]. Muscle performance was found to be maximal when 25(OH)D levels were > 28 ng/mL in healthy elderly subjects, but in a randomized controlled trial it was observed that men and women in a nursing home who received either placebo, 200, 400 or 600 IUs of vitamin D_3 daily for 5 months had no significant effect on fall reduction [59, 60, 64]. However, men and women who received 800 IUs of vitamin D_3 daily for 5 months had a dramatic, 72%, reduced risk for falling. Since falls markedly increased risk for fracture it is therefore not surprising that patients who are vitamin D deficient are at higher risk for fractures due to decreased muscle strength and increased swaying [59, 60].

Treatment and prevention of calcium and vitamin D deficiency

It is recommended by the IOM that all adults up to 50 years of age consume a total of 1000 mg of calcium from diet and supplements, and adults 50 years of age and older should increase their calcium intake to 1200 mg a day [19]. Often patients believe that if they had been calcium deficient in the past that taking more calcium than what is recommended will improve their bone density. Unfortunately, not only will this not work but it increases their risk for kidney stones and cardiovascular calcifications. It has been suggested that because the elderly are more likely to suffer from achlorhydria that they cannot absorb calcium carbonate and should take calcium citrate. However, it was observed that achlorhydric patients were able to absorb calcium carbonate if they took it with a meal [65]. The reason is that if you ingest a calcium carbonate pill which is basically a piece of chalk on an empty stomach and have no stomach acid the piece of chalk will not dissolve and will pass through the intestines and not be absorbed. However, if taken with a meal as the food is being ground up over a period of 2–4 hours in the stomach, so too is the calcium carbonate pill. Therefore, calcium carbonate is a perfectly good source of calcium even for patients with achlorhydria or who are on proton pump inhibitor if it is taken with a meal. The additional advantage is that when calcium is taken with a meal it will bind dietary oxalate and reduce one's risk for developing kidney stones. This is the explanation for why it was observed that people who have an adequate calcium intake have a reduced risk for developing kidney stones. For those patients with calcium oxalate kidney stones, they should be receiving calcium supplementation in the form of calcium citrate with their meals.

The IOM made its recommendations for vitamin D intake based on a population model, not a medical model. This Institute recommended that for the population as a whole, adults up to the age of 70 need 600 IUs of vitamin D daily while adults over age 70 years need 800 IUs of vitamin D daily [19]. The Endocrine Society reviewed the literature and used a medical model for its recommendations for the prevention and treatment of vitamin D deficiency [2, 66] (Table 12.2). They recommended that one strategy to treat vitamin D deficiency is to give 50 000 IUs of vitamin D_2 or vitamin D_3 once a week (equivalent to 6600 IUs of vitamin D daily) for 8 weeks. To prevent recurrence of vitamin D deficiency they recommended either 50 000 IUs of vitamin D once every 2 weeks (equivalent to 3300 IUs of vitamin D daily) or taking a supplement containing 1500–2000 IUs of vitamin D daily [2]. Although there has been concern that taking this much vitamin D could potentially build up in the body fat and ultimately lead to vitamin D intoxication, a recent study revealed that after taking 50 000 IUs of vitamin D_2 once every 2 weeks for up to 6 years, patients maintained their blood levels of 25(OH)D between 40 and 60 ng/mL with no evidence of toxicity [67] (Figure 12.4). This is consistent with a previous observation that healthy adult men who ingested 10 000 IUs of vitamin D_3 daily for 5 months had no change in either their 24-hour urinary calcium excretion or their serum calcium level [68].

There continues to be a concern about osteoporotic men and women who were placed on an osteoporotic medication who do not respond to the therapy. It is now recognized that in order for these medications to be maximally effective that the patient also needs to take an adequate amount of calcium and vitamin D.

Conclusion

Adequate calcium and vitamin D intake throughout life is essential for the maintenance of muscle and bone health. It is estimated that on average, young and middle aged adults lose 0.25–0.5% of their skeletal mass yearly because of inadequate calcium and vitamin D intake. Although these

Table 12.2 Vitamin D intakes recommended by the IOM and the Endocrine Practice Guidelines Committee.

| Life Stage Group | IOM recommendations | | | | Committee recommendations for patients at risk for vitamin D deficiency | |
	AI	EAR	RDA	UL	Daily Allowance (IU/d)	UL (IU)
Infants						
0 to 6 mo	400 IU (10 μg)	–	–	1000 IU (25 μg)	400–1000	2000
6 to 12 mo	400 IU (10 μg)	–	–	1500 IU (38 μg)	400–1000	2000
Children						
1–3 y	–	400 IU (10 μg)	600 IU (15 μg)	2500 IU (63 μg)	600–1000	4000
4–8 y	–	400 IU (10 μg)	600 IU (15 μg)	3000 IU (75 μg)	600–1000	4000
Males						
9–13 y	–	400 IU (10 μg)	600 IU (15 μg)	4000 IU (100 μg)	600–1000	4000
14–18 y	–	400 IU (10 μg)	600 IU (15 μg)	4000 IU (100 μg)	600–1000	4000
19–30 y	–	400 IU (10 μg)	600 IU (15 μg)	4000 IU (100 μg)	1500–2000	10 000
31–50 y	–	400 IU (10 μg)	600 IU (15 μg)	4000 IU (100 μg)	1500–2000	10 000
51–70 y	–	400 IU (10 μg)	600 IU (15 μg)	4000 IU (100 μg)	1500–2000	10 000
>70 y	–	400 IU (10 μg)	800 IU (20 μg)	4000 IU (100 μg)	1500–2000	10 000

(continued)

Table 12.2 *(Continued)*

Life Stage Group	IOM recommendations				Committee recommendations for patients at risk for vitamin D deficiency	
	AI	EAR	RDA	UL	Daily Allowance (IU/d)	UL (IU)
Females						
9–13 y	–	400 IU (10 μg)	600 IU (15 μg)	4000 IU (100 μg)	600–1000	4000
14–18 y	–	400 IU (10 μg)	600 IU (15 μg)	4000 IU (100 μg)	600–1000	4000
19–30 y	–	400 IU (10 μg)	600 IU (15 μg)	4000 IU (100 μg)	1500–2000	10 000
31–50 y	–	400 IU (10 μg)	600 IU (15 μg)	4000 IU (100 μg)	1500–2000	10 000
51–70 y	–	400 IU (10 μg)	600 IU (15 μg)	4000 IU (100 μg)	1500–2000	10 000
>70 y	–	400 IU (10 μg)	800 IU (20 μg)	4000 IU (100 μg)	1500–2000	10 000
Pregnancy						
14–18 y	–	400 IU (10 μg)	600 IU (15 μg)	4000 IU (100 μg)	600–1000	4000
19–30 y	–	400 IU (10 μg)	600 IU (15 μg)	4000 IU (100 μg)	1500–2000	10 000
31–50 y	–	400 IU (10 μg)	600 IU (15 μg)	4000 IU (100 μg)	1500–2000	10 000
Lactation*						
14–18 y	–	400 IU (10 μg)	600 IU (15 μg)	4000 IU (100 μg)	600–1000	4000
19–30 y	–	400 IU (10 μg)	600 IU (15 μg)	4000 IU (100 μg)	1500–2000	10 000
31–50 y	–	400 IU (10 μg)	600 IU (15 μg)	4000 IU (100 μg)	1500–2000	10 000

*Mother's requirement 4000–6000 (mother's intake for infant's requirement if infant is not receiving 400 IU/d).

NOTE: AI, Adequate Intake; EAR, Estimated Average Requirement; IU, International Units; RDA, Recommended Dietary Allowance; UL, Tolerable Upper Intake Level.

(*Source:* Holick M (2011) [2]. Copyright 2011, The Endocrine Society).

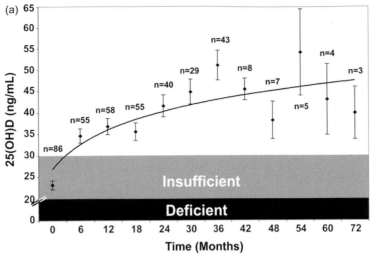

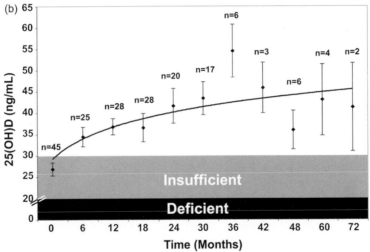

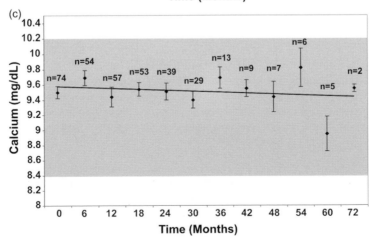

Figure 12.4 (*Continued*)

numbers appear to be insignificant, when multiplied by 2 or 3 decades a substantial amount of bone is lost and therefore increases one's risk for developing osteopenia and osteoporosis earlier in life. Also bone mass is heavily dependent on muscle mass and muscle loading of the skeleton. Thus exercise, especially walking at least 3–5 miles a week, will help maintain and possibly improve both hip and lower spinal bone density.

A potential additional advantage to increasing one's vitamin D intake is that there have been a large number of association studies and a few randomized controlled trials suggesting that improvement in children's and adults' vitamin D status reduces risk for autoimmune diseases including multiple sclerosis, type 1 diabetes, rheumatoid arthritis, Crohn's disease, several cancers, cardiovascular disease, infectious diseases and cognitive disorders [1, 69–72]. There is no downside to ingesting an adequate amount of calcium as recommended by the IOM and an adequate amount of vitamin D as recommended by Endocrine Society.

Acknowledgements

This work is supported in part by the UV Foundation, the Mushroom Council and the NIH CTSI Grant # UL1-RR025771.

Figure 12.4 (*Continued*) (a) Mean serum 25-hydroxyvitamin D [25(OH)D] levels in all patients: Includes patients treated with 50 000 IU vitamin D2 every 2 weeks (maintenance therapy, N = 81), including those patients with vitamin D insufficiency who were initially treated with 8 weeks of 50 000 IU vitamin D2 weekly prior to maintenance therapy (N = 39). Error bars represent standard error of the mean, mean result over 5 years shown. Time 0 is initiation of treatment, results shown as mean values averaged for 6 month intervals. When mean 25(OH)D in each 6 month group was compared to mean initial 25(OH)D, p < 0.001 up until month 43; p < 0.001 when all remaining values after month 43 were compared to mean initial 25(OH)D. (b) Mean serum 25(OH)D levels in patients receiving maintenance therapy only: Levels for 37 patients who were vitamin D insufficient (25[OH]D levels <30 ng/mL) and 5 patients who were vitamin D sufficient (25[OH]D levels ≥30 ng/ml) who were treated with maintenance therapy of 50 000 IU vitamin D2 every two weeks. Error bars represent standard error of the mean, mean result over 5 years shown. Time 0 is initiation of treatment, results shown as mean values averaged for 6 month intervals. When mean 25(OH)D in each 6 month group were compared to mean initial 25(OH)D, p < 0.001 up until month 37; p < 0.001 when all remaining values after month 43 were compared to mean initial 25(OH)D. (c) Serum calcium levels: Results for all 81 patients who were treated with 50 000 IU of vitamin D2. Error bars represent standard error of the mean. Time 0 is initiation of treatment, results shown as mean values averaged for 6 month intervals. Normal serum calcium: 8.5–10.2 mg/dL. (*Source*: Pietras SM, Obayan BK, Cai MH *et al.* (2009) [67]. Copyright 2009, American Medical Association).

References

1 Holick MF (2007) Vitamin D deficiency. *N Eng J Med* **357**: 266–81.

2 Holick MF, Binkley NC, Bischoff-Ferrari HA, *et al.* (2011) Evaluation, treatment, and prevention of vitamin D deficiency: an Endocrine Society Clinical Practice Guideline. *J Clin Endocrinol Metab* **96**(7): 1911–30.

3 Tian XQ, Chen TC, Matsuoka LY, *et al.* (1993) Kinetic and thermodynamic studies of the conversion of previtamin D_3 in human skin. *J Biol Chem* **268**: 14888–92.

4 BPA (1964) A British Paediatric Association Report: Infantile hypercalcaemia, nutritional rickets, and infantile scurvy in Great Britain. *Br Med J* **1**: 1659–61.

5 Heaney RP, Recker RR, Grote J, *et al.* (2011) Vitamin D_3 is more potent than vitamin D_2 in humans. *J Clin Endocrinol Metab* **152**(2): 741.

6 Tang HM, Cole DEC, Rubin LA, *et al.* (1998) Evidence that vitamin D_3 increases serum 25-hydroxyvitamin D more efficiently than does vitamin D_2. *Am J Clin Nutr* **68**: 854–8.

7 Holick MF, Biancuzzo RM, Chen TC, *et al.* (2008) Vitamin D_2 is as effective as vitamin D_3 in maintaining circulating concentrations of 25-hydroxyvitamin D. *J Clin Endocrinol Metab* **93**(3): 677–81.

8 Biancuzzo RM, Cai MH, Winter MR, *et al.* (2010) Fortification of orange juice with vitamin D_2 or vitamin D_3 is as effective as an oral supplement in maintaining vitamin D status in adults. *Am J Clin Nutr* **91**: 1621–6.

9 Gordon CM, Williams AL, Feldman HA, *et al.* (2008) Treatment of hypovitaminosis D in infants and toddlers. *J Clin Endocrinol Metab* **93**(7): 2716–21.

10 Clemens TL, Henderson SL, Adams JS *et al.* (1982) Increased skin pigment reduces the capacity of skin to synthesis vitamin D_3. *Lancet* **1**(8263): 74–6.

11 Holick MF, Matsuoka LY, Wortsman J (1989) Age, vitamin D, and solar ultraviolet. *Lancet* **334**: 1104–5.

12 MacLaughlin J, Holick MF (1985) Aging decreases the capacity of human skin to produce vitamin D_3. *J Clin Invest* **76**: 1536–8.

13 Webb AR, Kline L, Holick MF (1988) Influence of season and latitude on the cutaneous synthesis of vitamin D_3: Exposure to winter sunlight in Boston and Edmonton will not promote vitamin D_3 synthesis in human skin. *J Clin Endocrinol Metab* **67**: 373–8.

14 Holick MF (2003) Vitamin D: A millennium perspective. *J Cell Biochem* **88**: 296–307.

15 Wortsman J, Matsuoka LY, Chen TC, *et al.* (2000) Decreased bioavailability of vitamin D in obesity. *Am J Clin Nutr* **72**: 690–3.

16 Farraye F, Nimitphong H, Stucchi A, *et al.* (2011) The use of a novel vitamin D bioavailability test demonstrates that vitamin D absorption is decreased in patients with quiescent Crohn's disease. *Inflamm Bowel Dis* **17**: 2116–21.

17 Christakos S, Dhawan P, Liu Y, *et al.* (2003) New insights into the mechanisms of vitamin D action. *J Cell Biochem* **88**: 695–705.

18 Khosla S (2001) The OPG/RANKL/RANK system. *Endocrinol* **142**(12): 5050–5.

19 IOM (Institute of Medicine) (2011) *Dietary Reference Intakes for Calcium and Vitamin D. Committee to Review Dietary Reference Intakes for Calcium and Vitamin D.* Washington DC: The National Academies Press. Institute of Medicine.

20 Malabanan A, Veronikis IE, Holick MF (1998) Redefining vitamin D insufficiency. *Lancet* **351**: 805–6.

21 Chapuy MC, Preziosi P, Maaner M, *et al.* (1997) Prevalence of vitamin D insufficiency in an adult normal population. *Osteopor Int* **7**: 439–43.

22 Holick MF, Siris ES, Binkley N, *et al.* (2005) Prevalence of vitamin D inadequacy among postmenopausal North American women receiving osteoporosis therapy. *J Clin Endocrinol Metab* **90**: 3215–24.

23 Heaney RP, Dowell MS, Hale CA, *et al.* (2003) Calcium absorption varies within the reference range for serum 25-hydroxyvitamin D. *J Am Coll Nutr* **22**(2): 142–6.

24 Priemel M, von Domarus C, Klatte TO, *et al.* (2010) Bone mineralization defects and vitamin D deficiency: histomorphometric analysis of iliac crest bone biopsies and circulating 25-hydroxyvitamin D in 675 patients. *J Bone Miner Res* **25**(2): 305–12.

25 Maxmen A (2011) The vitamin D-lemma. *Nature* **475**: 23–5.

26 Demetriou ETW, Pietras SM, Holick MF (2010) Hypercalcemia and soft tissue calcification owing to sarcoidosis: The sunlight-cola connection. *J Bone Miner Res* **25**(7): 1695–9.

27 Lips P, Duong T, Okeksik A, *et al.* (2001) A global study of vitamin D status and parathyroid function in postmenopausal women with osteoporosis: baseline data from the multiple outcomes of raloxifene evaluation clinical trial. *J Clin Endocrinol Metab* **86**: 1212–21.

28 Souberbielle J-C, Lawson-Body E, Hammadi B, *et al.* (2003) The use in clinical practice of parathyroid hormone normative values established in vitamin D-sufficient subjects. *J Clin Endocrinol Metab* **88**(8): 3501–4.

29 Kyriakidou-Himonas M, Aloia JF, Yeh JK (1999) Vitamin D supplementation in postmenopausal black women. *J Clin Endocrinol Metab* **84**: 3988–90.

30 Isaia G, Giorgino R, Rini GB, *et al.* (2003) Prevalence of hypovitaminosis D in elderly women in Italy: clinical consequences and risk factors. *Osteoporos Int* **14**: 577–82.

31 McKenna MJ (1992) Differences in vitamin D status between countries in young adults and the elderly. *Am J Med* **93**: 69–77.

32 Bakhtiyarova S, Lesnyak O, Kyznesova N, *et al.* (2006) Vitamin D status among patients with hip fracture and elderly control subjects in Yekaterinburg, Russia. *Osteoporos Int* **17**: 441–6.

33 Gloth FM, Gundberg CM, Hollis BW, *et al.* (1995) Vitamin D deficiency in homebound elderly persons. *JAMA* **274**: 1683–6.

34 Holick MF (2007) Optimal vitamin D status for the prevention and treatment of osteoporosis. *Drugs & Aging* **24**(12): 1017–29.

35 Gaugris S, Heaney RP, Boonen S, *et al.* (2005) Vitamin D inadequacy among postmenopausal women: a systematic review. *Q J Med* **98**: 667–76.

36 Beard MK, Lips P, Holick MF, *et al.* (2005) Vitamin D inadequacy is prevalent among postmenopausal osteoporotic women. *Climacteric* **8**(Suppl 2): 199–200.

37 Aaron JE, Gallagher JC, Anderson J, *et al.* (1974) Frequency of osteomalacia and osteoporosis in fractures of the proximal femur. *Lancet* **1**: 229–33.

38 Holick MF (2006) Resurrection of vitamin D deficiency and rickets. *J Clin Invest* **116**(8): 2062–72.

39 Malabanan AO, Turner AK, Holick MF (1998) Severe generalized bone pain and osteoporosis in a premenopausal black female: Effect of vitamin D replacement. *J Clin Densitometr* **1**: 201–4.

40 Plotnikoff GA, Quigley JM (2003) Prevalence of severe hypovitaminosis D in patients with persistent, nonspecific musculoskeletal pain. *Mayo Clin Proc* **78**: 1463–70.

41 Holick MF (2003) Vitamin D deficiency: What a pain it is. *Mayo Clin Proc* **78**(12): 1457–59.

42 Chapuy MC, Arlot ME, Duboeuf F, *et al.* (1992) Vitamin D$_3$ and calcium to prevent hip fractures in elderly women. *N Engl J Med* **327**: 1637–42.

43 Dawson-Hughes B, Harris SS, Krall EA, *et al.* (1997) Effect of calcium and vitamin D supplementation on bone density in men and women 65 years of age or older. *N Engl J Med* **337**: 670–6.

44 Larsen ER, Mosekilde L, Foldspang A (2004) Vitamin D and calcium supplementation prevents osteoporotic fractures in elderly community dwelling residents: a pragmatic population-based 3-year intervention study. *J Bone Miner Res* **19**: 370–8.

45 Porthouse J, Cockayne S, King C, *et al.* (2005) Randomized controlled trial of supplementation with calcium and cholecalciferol (vitamin D$_3$) for prevention of fractures in primary care. *BMJ* **330**: 1003–6.

46 Grant AM, Avenell A, Campbell MK, *et al.* (2005) Oral vitamin D$_3$ and calcium for secondary prevention of low trauma fractures in elderly people (randomized evaluation of calcium or vitamin D, RECORD): a randomized placebo controlled trail. *Lancet* **365**: 1621–8.

47 Jackson RD, LaCroix AZ, *et al.* (2006) Calcium plus vitamin D supplementation and the risk of fractures. *N Engl J Med* **354**(7): 669–83.

48 Chung, M, Lee, J, Terasawa, T, *et al.* (2011) Vitamin D with or without calcium supplementation for prevention of cancer and fractures: An updated meta-analysis for the U.S. Preventive Services Task Force. *Ann Intern Med* **155**(12): 827–38.

49 Terris S, Lesser GT, Dawson-Hughes B (2006) Calcium plus vitamin D and the risk of fractures. *N Engl J Med* **354**(21): 2285–6.

50 Bischoff-Ferrari HA, Giovannucci E, Willett WC, *et al.* (2006) Estimation of optimal serum concentrations of 25-hydroxyvitamin D for multiple health outcomes. *Am J Clin Nutr* **84**: 18–28.

51 Bischoff-Ferrari HA, Dawson-Hughes B, Staehelin HB, *et al.* (2009) Fall prevention with supplemental and active forms of vitamin D: a meta-analysis of randomised controlled trials. *BMJ* **339**: b3692.

52 Murad HM, Elamin KB, Abu Elnour, *et al.* (2011) The effect of vitamin D on falls: A systematic review and meta-analysis. *J Clin Endocrinol Metab* **96**(10): 2997–3006.

53 Trivedi DP, Doll R, Khaw KT (2003) Effect of four monthly oral vitamin D$_3$ (cholecalciferol) supplementation on fractures and mortality in men and women living in the community: Randomized double blind controlled trial. *BMJ* **326**: 469–75.

54 Sanders KM, Stuart AL, Williamson EJ, *et al.* (2010) Annual high-dose oral vitamin D and falls and fractures in older women. A randomized controlled trial. *JAMA* **303**(18): 1815–22.

55 Heikinheima RJ, Inkovaara JA, Harju EJ, *et al.* (1992) Annual injection of vitamin D and fractures of aged bones. *Calcif Tissue Int* **51**: 105–10.

56 Glerup H, Middelsen K, Poulsen L, *et al.* (2000) Hypovitaminosis D myopathy without biochemical signs of ostemalacia bone involvement. *Calcif Tissue Int* **66**: 419–24.

57 Hess AF (1929) *Rickets Including Osteomalacia and Tetany*. Pennsylvania: Lea J. Febiger.

58 Schott G, Wills M (1976) Muscle weakness in osteomalacia. *Lancet* **2**: 626–9.

59 Pfeifer M, Begerow B, Minne HW, *et al.* (2001) Vitamin D status, trunk muscle strength, body sway, falls, and fractures among 237 postmenopausal women with osteoporosis. *Exp Clin Endocrinol Diabetes* **109**: 87–92.

60 Pfeifer M, Begerow B, Minne H, *et al.* (2000) Effects of a short-term vitamin D and calcium supplementation on body sway and secondary hyperparathyroidism in elderly women. *J Bone Min Res* **15**: 1113–18.

61 Bischoff-Ferrari HA, Borchers M, Gudat, F, *et al.* (2004) Vitamin D receptor expression in human muscle tissue decreases with age. *J Bone Miner Res* **19**(2): 265–9.

62 Bischoff-Ferrari HA, Dietrich T, Orav EJ, *et al.* (2004) Higher 25-hydroxyvitamin D concentrations are associated with better lower-extremity function in both active and inactive persons aged ≥60 y. *Am J Clin Nutr* **80**: 752–8.

63 Bischoff-Ferrari HA, Dawson-Hughes B, Willett WC, *et al.* (2004) Effect of vitamin D on falls: a meta-analysis. *JAMA* **291**: 1999–2006.

64 Broe KE, Chen TC, Weinberg J, *et al.* (2007) A higher dose of vitamin D reduces the risk of falls in nursing home residents: a randomized, multiple-dose study. *J Am Geriatr Soc* **55**(2): 234–9.

65 Recker RR (1985) Calcium absorption and achlorhydria. *N Engl J Med* **313**: 70–3.

66 Holick MF, Binkley NC, Bischoff-Ferrari HA, *et al.* (2012) Controversy in clinical endocrinology: Guidelines for preventing and treating vitamin D deficiency and insufficiency revisited. *J Clin Endocrinol Metab* **97**: 1153–8.

67 Pietras SM, Obayan BK, Cai MH, *et al.* (2009) Vitamin D_2 treatment for vitamin D deficiency and insufficiency for up to 6 years. *Arch Intern Med* **169**: 1806–8.

68 Heaney RP, Davies KM, Chen TC, *et al.* (2003) Human serum 25-hydroxycholecalciferol response to extended oral dosing with cholecalciferol. *Am J Clin Nutr* **77**: 204–10.

69 Holick, MF (2011) Health benefits of vitamin D and sunlight: A D-bate. *Nat Rev Endocrinol* **7**: 73–5.

70 Holick, MF (2011) Vitamin D: Evolutionary, physiological and health perspectives. *Current Drug Targets* **12**: 4–18.

71 Adams JS, Hewison M (2010) Update in vitamin D. *J Clin Endocrinol Metab* **95**(2): 471–8.

72 Bikle DD (2009) Nonclassic actions of vitamin D. *J Clin Endocrinol Metab* **94**(1): 26–34.

CHAPTER 13

The Use of Combination Therapy in the Treatment of Postmenopausal Osteoporosis

Juliet Compston

Cambridge University Hospitals NHS Foundation Trust, Cambridge, UK

Introduction

Pharmacological interventions to prevent fragility fractures act by a variety of mechanisms. Anti-resorptive drugs are most commonly used; these include the bisphosphonates (alendronate, risedronate, ibandronate and zoledronic acid), raloxifene, and denosumab, a humanized monoclonal antibody to receptor activator of NFκB ligand (RANKL). Anabolic skeletal agents are available in the form of parathyroid hormone (PTH) peptide PTH (1-34) (teriparatide) and PTH (1-84). Finally, strontium ranelate acts by mechanisms that are incompletely understood; its effects on bone remodeling are relatively weak [1,2] and alteration of bone material properties may be mainly responsible for its beneficial effects on bone strength and fracture reduction [3].

Combination therapy might be used for several reasons [4]. First, synergistic effects of interventions with different modes of action or additive effects of drugs with a similar mechanism of action might result in greater fracture reduction than the use of a single agent. Secondly, since anabolic agents are only approved for a total of 24 months duration of therapy and as BMD declines following withdrawal of treatment, other drugs may be required to maintain their beneficial effects. Thirdly, particularly with potent anti-resorptive agents, it may be desirable to limit the duration of therapy for a period of 3–5 years and to continue treatment with other drugs in individuals who remain at high risk of fracture. Finally, in patients who become intolerant to a treatment and need to switch to an alternative drug, it is important to know whether the response is affected by the initial treatment. For the purposes of this review combination therapy includes the use of more than one treatment either contemporaneously or in sequence.

Combination anti-resorptive therapy

Studies evaluating the use of combinations of anti-resorptive agents in postmenopausal osteoporosis have included: concurrent use of hormone therapy (HT) and bisphosphonates [5–11], raloxifene and alendronate, HT and calcitonin, and estrogen and methyltestosterone [12–14]. In most of these studies, larger increases in BMD have been seen with combination than with monotherapy, but the studies have not been powered to demonstrate differences in fracture risk reduction. In view of the greater cost of combination therapy, the potential for more side effects, and lack of evidence of improved anti-fracture efficacy, simultaneous use of two anti-resorptive drugs is not generally recommended.

Sequential treatment with anti-resorptive drugs: alendronate followed by denosumab

Switching treatment from one to another anti-resorptive drug is common in clinical practice. The effect of switching from alendronate to denosumab has been studied in postmenopausal women who had received treatment with alendronate 70 mg once weekly for at least 6 months and were then randomized to continue with alendronate or switch to denosumab 60 mg sc every 6 months [15]. In women who switched to denosumab, increases in BMD in the lumbar spine and hip were significantly greater at 6 and 12 months and there was also greater suppression of bone turnover markers than in women continuing on alendronate. These data thus indicate that in patients who need to stop bisphosphonate therapy, switching to denosumab results in further increases in BMD, although the effects on fracture rate are unknown.

Sequential therapy with bisphosphonates and strontium ranelate

A recent study provides evidence that prior bisphosphonate therapy results in blunting and delay of the BMD response to strontium ranelate. In a prospective study in postmenopausal women with osteoporosis, 56 bisphosphonate-naïve women and 52 women treated with an oral bisphosphonate for at least one year, who had stopped bisphosphonate therapy within the last month, were given strontium ranelate 2 g daily, together with calcium and vitamin D supplements [16]. After 1 year of treatment, BMD in the lumbar spine had increased by 5.6% in bisphosphonate-naïve women and by 2.1% in women previously treated with bisphosphonates;

at both 6 and 12 months the BMD increase in the former group was significantly less than in the latter. At the total hip there was no significant change in BMD at one year in the bisphosphonate pretreated women compared to an increase of 3.4% in the treatment naive group. In an extension of this study, it was shown that BMD in the spine in pretreated women increased in parallel with treatment naïve women from 6 months onwards, whereas some blunting of the BMD response at the hip was still observed after 2 years of treatment [17]. The most likely mechanism to explain these effects is that bisphosphonates inhibit the uptake of strontium into bone because of suppression of bone turnover and the consequent reduction in newly formed bone.

Combined anabolic and anti-resorptive therapy

The different mechanisms of action of anabolic and anti-resorptive drugs provide a possible rationale for combination therapy, since simultaneous stimulation of bone formation and inhibition of bone resorption might be expected to result in greater efficacy than the use of either alone. However, as an alternative, it is also possible that suppression of remodeling by anti-resorptives could prevent or reduce the increase in remodeling rate required for anabolic skeletal effects of PTH peptides [18].

Deal *et al.* [19] compared the effects of combination teriparatide and raloxifene therapy to teriparatide alone in postmenopausal women with osteoporosis. Similar increases in lumbar spine BMD after 6 months of treatment were observed in the two groups (6.19% in the combination group, 5.19% in the teriparatide alone group) whilst combination therapy was associated with a significantly greater increase in total hip BMD.

In the Parathyroid Hormone and Alendronate study (PATH), 238 postmenopausal women with low BMD were randomised to PTH (1-84) 100 μg/d, alendronate 10 mg/d or both [20]. After one year of treatment, spine areal BMD had increased in all treatment groups and to a similar extent in the combination and PTH alone treatment groups. Volumetric BMD, measured by quantitative computed tomography (QCT), was almost two-fold greater in the PTH alone group than that observed in either of the other treatment groups. In the proximal femur, areal BMD did not change significantly in the PTH alone group but increased in the other two groups, and the increase in the combination group was significantly greater than that in the PTH alone group. Volumetric BMD in the total hip decreased significantly in the PTH group, did not change significantly in the combination group and increased slightly in the alendronate group. Conversely, cortical bone volume increased significantly at the total hip and femoral neck in the PTH group, but did not change significantly in the other two groups. Based on the changes in spine volumetric BMD and hip cortical volume, the authors concluded that concurrent use of alendronate blunted the anabolic effects of PTH. Two other studies investigating the effects of PTH (1-34) alone or in combination with alendronate in men with low BMD [21] and in postmenopausal women [22] reported similar findings.

In a recent study, combination therapy with intravenous zoledronic acid and teriparatide was compared to treatment with teriparatide alone [23]. Postmenopausal women with osteoporosis were randomized to one of three treatment groups: a single infusion of zoledronic acid 5 mg plus daily subcutaneous teriparatide 20 μg, zoledronic acid alone, or teriparatide alone. BMD increases in the lumbar spine were similar in the teriparatide and combination group at one year, with a more rapid rate of increase in the combination group than in the other two groups at earlier time points. In the hip, the increases in BMD in the combination group were significantly greater than that in the teriparatide alone group at all time points, whilst after one year, total hip BMD values were similar in the combination and zoledronic acid groups, with a higher rate of increase in the combination versus zoledronic acid group at week 13. Serum ß-CTX levels in the combination therapy group showed a rapid decrease that was sustained for 2 months and then increased to above baseline values at one year. Serum P1NP levels showed an increase in the combination therapy group from around 6 months to 1 year. As expected, both markers remained suppressed throughout the duration of the study in women receiving zoledronic acid alone.

Comparison of the results of this study with those of Black *et al.* [20] reveals that the changes in areal BMD in the spine after one year of treatment are similar, but the study by Cosman *et al.* enabled demonstration of a more rapid increase in spine BMD at earlier time points in women receiving combination therapy. Longer-term studies indicate that by two years, the gains in spine BMD are greater after PTH monotherapy than with combination therapy [21, 22]. In the hip, it is clear that either combination therapy or treatment with an anti-resorptive agent alone results in greater increases in BMD than PTH monotherapy in the early stages of treatment, although in longer-term studies the increase with PTH exceeded that achieved with combination therapy or an anti-resorptive agent. Monotherapy with PTH is often associated with a transient decrease in hip BMD, probably as a result of increased cortical porosity [20, 24] and its prevention by concomitant anti-resorptive therapy presumably results from reduced cortical remodeling. Combination anti-resorptive and anabolic treatment may therefore be particularly beneficial in patients at high risk of hip fracture, in whom an increase in cortical porosity early in the course of treatment could expose them to an increased risk. However, the effects of combination therapy on hip fracture risk have not been evaluated and, whereas hip fracture reduction has been demonstrated for several anti-resorptive agents [25–27], this has not been shown with PTH peptides [24, 28].

In the PATH study, both hypercalcemia and hypercalciuria occurred more frequently in both the combination therapy group and the PTH-treated group than in the alendronate group, although this was generally mild. Combination and PTH therapy were also associated with significant increases in the mean serum uric acid level, and three women developed gout (one in the PTH group and two in the combination group) [20]. In men, a higher incidence of hypercalcemia and hypercalciuria was also reported after either combination therapy or PTH therapy alone as compared to treatment with alendronate alone [21]. Finally, in the study of Cosman *et al.* the reported percentages of women with serum calcium levels that were normal at baseline but above the normal range during the study were 13.4% for the combination group, 15% for the teriparatide group and 4% for the zoledronic acid group. Significant hypercalcemia, defined as a serum calcium >2.89 mmol/l, occurred in one woman in the combination group and in two women in the teriparatide group [23].

Anabolic and anti-resorptive therapy

Sequential therapy: anti-resorptive before anabolic therapy

Several studies have indicated that prior bisphosphonate therapy reduces the anabolic effects of PTH peptides. Ettinger *et al.* [29], in a study of postmenopausal women who were switched from either raloxifene or alendronate to teriparatide, reported greater increases in hip and spine BMD during the first 6 months of teriparatide therapy in the group of women who had previously received raloxifene as compared to the group of women who were previously treated with alendronate. After 18 months of teriparatide therapy, the mean increases in spine BMD were 10.2% and 4.1%, respectively. In the total hip, BMD did not change significantly over 18 months in the women who had previously received alendronate, but showed a mean increase of 1.8% in women with prior raloxifene therapy. In postmenopausal women with osteoporosis, the addition of teriparatide to on-going alendronate therapy resulted in significant increases in bone formation markers [30]; significant increases in spine and total hip BMD (9.6% and 2.7% respectively) were also reported after one year of treatment with PTH (1-34) in women previously treated with raloxifene [31]. In postmenopausal women with osteoporosis who had been taking alendronate for at least one year, both daily and cyclic PTH (1-34) treatment for 15 months were associated with significant increases in spine and hip BMD, the increase in spine BMD being significantly greater than in women who continued on alendronate alone [32]. In a nonrandomized, prospective study in postmenopausal women with osteoporosis, Miller *et al.* reported the effects of 12 months teriparatide therapy following previous treatment for at least 24 months with either risedronate or alendronate. A significantly greater increase in the bone formation marker, P1NP, and in spine areal and volumetric BMD was seen in the women who had previously been treated with risedronate as compared to the women who had previously received alendronate [33]. However, none of these studies included a comparator group of treatment-naïve women receiving PTH peptide therapy.

In the European Study of Forsteo (EUROFORS) the effect on BMD of teriparatide therapy was compared in postmenopausal women with established osteoporosis who had or had not received prior anti-resorptive therapy, most commonly alendronate, for a median period of 11 months. Prior anti-resorptive treatment was associated with modest blunting of BMD response in the spine and hip [34] and in a secondary subgroup analysis in which women with prior anti-resorptive treatment were subdivided into four groups (alendronate, etidronate, risedronate and nonbisphosphonate), increases in spine and hip BMD were seen in all groups after 24 months of teriparatide, the largest of which occurred in etidronate pretreated women [35]. The ability of PTH peptide therapy to produce anabolic effects despite prior anti-resorptive therapy has also been demonstrated in postmenopausal women who have been receiving HT. After three years treatment with PTH (1-34), increases in BMD of 13% and 2.7% in the spine and hip, respectively were seen [36], and a significantly lower vertebral fracture rate was reported in the women taking both HT and PTH (1-34) compared to those receiving HT alone [37].

Taken together, these results indicate that some attenuation of the anabolic effect of intermittent PTH therapy occurs in women previously treated with anti-resorptive therapy, particularly more potent agents. In general, blunting of the BMD response appears to be relatively small, but the consequences, if any, on fracture reduction have not been established.

Sequential therapy: anti-resorptive after anabolic therapy

PTH therapy is approved for a maximum duration of 24 months. Following its discontinuation, loss of BMD in the following year has been reported in the total hip and femoral neck [38] and spine [38–40], providing a rationale for anti-resorptive therapy after treatment with PTH is discontinued. In a study of postmenopausal women with osteoporosis who were treated with either PTH (1-84) or placebo for one year and then with alendronate 10 mg/d for the following year, further gains in spine, femoral neck and total body BMD were seen in the women who were previously treated with PTH [41]. Black *et al.* reported that following one year of PTH (1-84) treatment in postmenopausal women, subsequent alendronate treatment for one year maintained or increased the gains in BMD in the spine and hip [39]. Similar results have been reported in women treated with raloxifene following withdrawal of teriparatide [42]. In men treated for two years with teriparatide, bisphosphonate therapy for the subsequent two years was associated with further gains in lumbar spine BMD, whereas a decrease in BMD was seen in men who received no treatment after teriparatide withdrawal [43].

Conclusions

The use of combination anti-resorptive therapy is associated with greater increases in BMD than the use of a single anti-resorptive agent. Furthermore, switching a patient from a less potent to a more potent anti-resorptive agent has been shown to result in greater gains in BMD for that individual. When treatment with strontium ranelate is initiated following bisphosphonate therapy, the BMD response to strontium ranelate is blunted for at least 6 months in the spine and up to two years in the hip. The implications for fracture risk of either combined or sequential anti-resorptive therapy have not been established.

Combined therapy with PTH and anti-resorptive agents produces similar benefits on lumbar spine areal BMD to those seen with PTH monotherapy in the first year of treatment although the rate of increase in BMD is more rapid with combination therapy, at least when zoledronic acid is used. In the hip, combination therapy is superior to PTH monotherapy in the first year of treatment; however, longer treatment periods are associated with greater increases in both spine and hip BMD with PTH monotherapy than with combination therapy. The implications for fracture reduction are unknown; however, protection by combination therapy against the early bone loss in the hip associated with PTH monotherapy might be advantageous.

Acknowledgements

JEC acknowledges support from the Cambridge Biomedical Research Centre and National Institute for Health Research (NIHR).

References

1 Compston J (2012) The use of combination therapy in the treatment of postmenopausal osteoporosis. *Endocrine* **41**: 11–18.

2 Reginster JY, Deroisy R, Dougados M, Jupsin I, Colette J, Roux C (2002) Prevention of early postmenopausal bone loss by strontium ranelate: the randomised, two-year, double-masked, dose-ranging, placebo-controlled PREVOS study. *Osteoporos Int* **13**: 925–31.

3 Meunier PJ, Slosman DO, Delmas PD, *et al.* (2002) Strontium ranelate: dose-dependent effects in established postmenopausal vertebral osteoporosis – a 2-year randomised placebo controlled trial. *J Clin Endocrinol Metab* **87**: 2060–6.

4 Blake GM, Compston JE, Fogelman I (2009) Could strontium ranelate have a synergistic role in the treatment of osteoporosis? *J Bone Miner Res* **24**: 1354–7.

5 Wimalawansa SJ (1995) Combined therapy with estrogen and etidronate has an additive effect on bone mineral density in the hip and vertebrae: four-year randomized study. *Am J Med* **99**: 36–42.

6 Wimalawansa SJ (1998) A four-year randomized controlled trial of hormone replacement and bisphosphonate, alone or in combination, in women with postmenopausal osteoporosis. *Am J Med* **104**: 219–26.

7 Lindsay R, Cosman F, Lobo RA, *et al.* (1999) Addition of alendronate to ongoing hormone replacement therapy in the treatment of osteoporosis: a randomized, controlled clinical trial. *J Clin Endocrinol Metab*; **84**: 3076–81.

8 Bone HG, Greenspan SL, McKeever C, *et al.* (2000) Alendronate and estrogen effects in postmenopausal women with low bone mineral density. Alendronate/Estrogen Study Group. *J Clin Endocrinol Metab* **85**: 720–6.

9 Greenspan SL, Resnick NM, Parker RA (2003) Combination therapy with hormone replacement and alendronate for prevention of bone loss in elderly women. *JAMA* **289**: 2525–33.

10 Harris ST, Eriksen EF, Davidson M, *et al.* (2001) Effect of combined risedronate and hormone replacement therapies on bone mineral density in postmenopausal women. *J Clin Endocrinol Metab* **86**: 1890–7.

11 Tuppurainen M, Härmä K, Komulainen M, *et al.* (2010) Effects of continuous combined hormone replacement therapy and clodronate on bone mineral density in osteoporotic postmenopausal women: a 5-year follow-up. *Maturitas* **66**: 423–30.

12 Johnell O, Scheele WH, Lu Y, Reginster JY, Need AG, Seeman E (2002) Additive effects of raloxifene and alendronate on bone density and biochemical markers of bone remodeling in postmenopausal women with osteoporosis. *J Clin Endocrinol Metab* **87**: 985–92.

13 Watts NB, Notelovitz M, Timmons MC, Addison WA, Wiita B, Downey LJ (1995) Comparison of oral estrogens and estrogens plus androgen on bone mineral density, menopausal symptoms, and lipid-lipoprotein profiles in surgical menopause. *Obstet Gynecol* **85**: 529–37.

14 Meschia M, Brincat M, Barbacini P, Crossignani PG, Albisetti W (1993) A clinical trial on the effects of a combination of elcatonin (carbocalcitonin) and conjugated estrogens on vertebral bone mass in early postmenopausal women. *Calcif Tissue Int* **53**: 17–20.

15 Kendler DL, Roux C, Benhamou CL, *et al.* (2010) Effects of denosumab on bone mineral density and bone turnover in postmenopausal women transitioning from alendronate therapy. *J Bone Miner Res* **25**: 72–81.

16 Middleton ET, Steel SA, Aye M, Doherty SM (2010) The effect of prior bisphosphonate therapy on the subsequent BMD and bone turnover response to strontium ranelate. *J Bone Miner Res* **25**: 455–62.

17 Middleton ET, Steel SA, Aye M, Doherty SM (2012) The effect of prior bisphosphonate therapy on the subsequent therapeutic effects of strontium ranelate over 2 years. *Osteoporos Int* **23**: 295–303.

18 Delmas PD, Vergnaud P, Arlot ME, Pastoureau P, Meunier PJ, Nilssen MH (1995) The anabolic effect of human PTH (1-34) on bone formation is blunted when bone resorption is inhibited by the bisphosphonate tiludronate – is activated resorption a prerequisite for the in vivo effect of PTH on formation in a remodeling system? *Bone* **16**: 603–10.

19 Deal C, Omizo M, Schwartz EN, *et al.* (2005) Combination teriparatide and raloxifene therapy for postmenopausal osteoporosis: results from a 6-month double-blind placebo-controlled trial. *J Bone Miner Res* **20**: 1905–11.

20 Black DM, Greenspan SL, Ensrud KE, *et al.* (2003) The effects of parathyroid hormone and alendronate alone or in combination in postmenopausal osteoporosis. *N Engl J Med* **349**: 1207–15.

21 Finkelstein JS, Hayes A, Hunzelman JL, Wyland JJ, Lee H, Neer RM (2003) The effects of parathyroid hormone, alendronate, or both in men with osteoporosis. *N Engl J Med* **349**: 1216–26.

22 Finkelstein JS, Wyland JJ, Lee H, Neer RM (2010) Effects of teriparatide, alendronate, or both in women with postmenopausal osteoporosis. *J Clin Endocrinol Metab* **95**: 1838–45.

23 Cosman F, Eriksen EF, Recknor C, *et al.* (2011) Effects of intravenous zoledronic acid plus subcutaneous teriparatide [rhPTH(1-34)] in postmenopausal osteoporosis. *J Bone Miner Res* **26**: 503–11.

24 Greenspan SL, Bone HG, Ettinger MP, *et al.* (2007) Treatment of osteoporosis with Parathyroid Hormone Study Group. Effect of recombinant human parathyroid hormone (1-84) on vertebral fracture and bone mineral density in postmenopausal women with osteoporosis: a randomized trial. *Ann Intern Med* **146**: 326–39.

25 Black DM, Cummings SR, Karpf DB, *et al.* (1996) Randomised trial of effect of alendronate on risk of fracture in women with existing vertebral fractures. Fracture Intervention Trial Research Group. *Lancet* **348**: 1535–41.

26 McClung MR, Geusens P, Miller PD, *et al.* (2001) Hip Intervention Program Study Group. Effect of risedronate on the risk of hip fracture in elderly women. Hip Intervention Program Study Group. *N Engl J Med* **344**: 333–40.

27 Black DM, Delmas PD, Eastell R, *et al.*; HORIZON Pivotal Fracture Trial (2007) Once-yearly zoledronic acid for treatment of postmenopausal osteoporosis. *N Engl J Med* **356**: 1809–22.

28 Neer RM, Arnaud CD, Zanchetta JR, *et al.* (2001) Effect of parathyroid hormone (1-34) on fractures and bone mineral density in postmenopausal women with osteoporosis. *N Engl J Med* **344**: 1434–41.

29 Ettinger B, San Martin J, Crans G, Pavo I (2004) Differential effects of teriparatide on BMD after treatment with raloxifene or alendronate. *J Bone Miner Res* **19**: 745–51.

30 Cosman F, Nieves J, Woelfert L, Shen V, Lindsay R (1998) Alendronate does not block the anabolic effect of PTH in postmenopausal osteoporotic women. *J Bone Miner Res* **13**: 1051–5.

31 Cosman F, Wermers RA, Recknor C, *et al.* (2009) Effects of teriparatide in postmenopausal women with osteoporosis on prior alendronate or raloxifene: differences between stopping and continuing the antiresorptive agent. *J Clin Endocrinol Metab* **94**: 3772–80.

32 Cosman F, Nieves J, Zion M, Woelfert L, Luckey M, Lindsay R (2005) Daily and cyclic parathyroid hormone in women receiving alendronate. *N Engl J Med* **353**: 566–75.

33 Miller PD, Delmas PD, Lindsay R, *et al.* (2008) Early responsiveness of women with osteoporosis to teriparatide after therapy with alendronate or risedronate. *J Clin Endocrinol Metab* **93**: 3785–93.

34 Obermayer-Pietsch BM, Marin F, McCloskey EV, *et al.*; EUROFORS Investigators (2008) Effects of two years of daily teriparatide treatment on BMD in postmenopausal women with severe osteoporosis with and without prior antiresorptive treatment. *J Bone Miner Res* **23**: 1591–1600.

35 Boonen S, Marin F, Obermayer-Pietsch B, *et al.*; EUROFORS Investigators (2008) Effects of previous antiresorptive therapy on the bone mineral density response to two years of teriparatide treatment in postmenopausal women with osteoporosis. *J Clin Endocrinol Metab* **93**: 852–60.

36 Lindsay R, Nieves J, Formica C, *et al.* (1997) Randomised controlled study of effect of parathyroid hormone on vertebral-bone mass and fracture incidence among postmenopausal women on oestrogen with osteoporosis. *Lancet* **350**: 550–5.

37 Cosman F, Nieves J, Woelfert L, *et al.* (2001) Parathyroid hormone added to established hormone therapy: effects on vertebral fracture and maintenance of bone mass after parathyroid hormone withdrawal. *J Bone Miner Res* **16**: 925–31.

38 Prince R, Sipos A, Hossain A, *et al.* (2005) Sustained nonvertebral fragility fracture risk reduction after discontinuation of teriparatide treatment. *J Bone Miner Res* **20**: 1507–13.

39 Black DM, Bilezikian JP, Ensrud KE, *et al.* (2005) One year of alendronate after one year of parathyroid hormone (1-84) for osteoporosis. *N Engl J Med* **353**: 555–65.

40 Leder BZ, Neer RM, Wyland JJ, Lee HW, Burnett-Bowie SM, Finkelstein JS (2009) Effects of teriparatide treatment and discontinuation in postmenopausal women and eugonadal men with osteoporosis. *J Clin Endocrinol Metab* **94**: 2915–21.

41 Rittmaster RS, Bolognese M, Ettinger MP, *et al.* (2000) Enhancement of bone mass in osteoporotic women with parathyroid hormone followed by alendronate. *J Clin Endocrinol Metab* **85**: 2129–34.

42 Eastell R, Nickelsen T, Marin F, *et al.* (2009) Sequential treatment of severe postmenopausal osteoporosis after teriparatide: final results of the randomized, controlled European Study of Forsteo (EUROFORS). *J Bone Miner Res* **24**: 726–36.

43 Kurland ES, Heller SL, Diamond B, McMahon DJ, Cosman F, Bilezikian JP (2004) The importance of bisphosphonate therapy in maintaining bone mass in men after therapy with teriparatide [human parathyroid hormone (1-34)]. *Osteoporos Int* **15**: 992–7.

CHAPTER 14

Emerging Therapies

Michael R. McClung[1] *& Cristiano A. F. Zerbini*[2]

[1] Oregon Osteoporosis Center, Portland, OR, USA
[2] Hospital Heliópolis, São Paulo, Brazil

While general measures have important benefits for skeletal health, pharmacological agents are required in adults with osteoporosis to strengthen the skeleton and reduce the serious consequences of skeletal fragility. Treatments for osteoporosis in several drug classes are available that can prevent bone loss and substantially reduce vertebral fracture risk. None of the current therapies, however, restore skeletal mass, structure or strength to normal, young adult levels. Even the most potent treatments reduce hip fracture risk by only 40–50%, and their effect on other nonvertebral fracture risk is much more modest. All our effective therapies are associated with intolerance and side effects, limiting the acceptance of our current drugs by both patients and clinicians. Inconvenient dosing regimens and other factors result in poor adherence to most treatment options, minimizing their effectiveness in daily clinical practice. All of these issues provide opportunities for the development of safer, more effective, and more acceptable pharmacological agents. In this chapter, we will review the current state of new drug development for osteoporosis including some very promising agents as well as some recent disappointments. We will predominantly focus on clinical results rather than provide a detailed review of preclinical data.

New forms of current agents

Estrogen agonist/antagonist (EAAs)

These agents, previously known as selective estrogen receptor modulators (SERMs), behave as estrogen agonists in some tissues, including the skeleton, but block undesired effects of estrogen in reproductive tissues. Raloxifene, the prototype EAA for treating osteoporosis, reduces vertebral fracture risk in postmenopausal women with osteoporosis but has not been shown to reduce the incidence of nonvertebral or hip fracture

Osteoporosis: Diagnosis and Management, First Edition. Edited by Dale W. Stovall.
© 2013 John Wiley & Sons, Ltd. Published 2013 by John Wiley & Sons, Ltd.

[1]. Many EAAs, some more potent inhibitors of bone resorption than raloxifene, have been developed. Several of these agents have been withdrawn from phase II or III trials because of worrisome cystic changes in the uterine endometrium or pelvic floor relaxation. Three agents in this class have completed phase III fracture prevention trials in women with postmenopausal osteoporosis. The clinical responses to both basedoxifene and arzoxifene did not demonstrate advantages compared to raloxifene [2, 3]. Development of both of these agents as osteoporosis treatments was halted. Basedoxifene is still being developed for possible use in combination with estrogen therapy for management of menopausal symptoms. Lasofoxifene therapy reduced the incidence of both vertebral and nonvertebral fracture and the incidence of invasive breast cancer in postmenopausal women with osteoporosis [4]. These data led to registration of lasofoxifene in some European countries, but safety concerns precluded registration in many other countries, including the United States.

Calcitonin

This natural, potent endogenous inhibitor of bone resorption has been an attractive candidate therapy for many years. In its current nasal spray form, bioavailability is variable, effects on bone turnover and bone mineral density are minimal and documentation of fracture risk reduction is weak. Oral formulations of calcitonin induce a modestly greater increase in BMD than nasal calcitonin and have greater effects on bone resorption than does nasal calcitonin [5]. However, the duration of the effect on bone resorption is very limited, abating within hours, well before the next daily dose [6]. This pharmacodynamic response to oral calcitonin therapy is very different from the sustained reduction in bone turnover achieved with current antiresorptive agents. A large phase III placebo-controlled fracture trial demonstrated no effect on vertebral or nonvertebral fracture risk reduction, ending the clinical development of that formulation of oral calcitonin [7].

Bisphosphonates

Orally administered bisphosphonates are the most commonly used treatments for osteoporosis. Because of poor bioavailability and the ability of food and beverages to impair absorption, strict before-breakfast dosing rules are required. Poor compliance, acceptance and persistence with this dosing regimen limit the clinical effectiveness of these treatments in clinical practice. A new formulation of risedronate that contains the chelating agent EDTA and is enteric-coated to prevent dissolution of the tablet until it reached the small bowel was developed to be given after breakfast once weekly [8]. This provides a more convenient dosing regimen for patients and minimizes concern about poor compliance with the usual oral bisphosphonate dosing instructions.

Parathyroid hormone

Two forms of parathyroid hormone, teriparatide (PTH 1-34) and intact (PTH 1-84) are available for treating osteoporosis. Both require daily subcutaneous injection, limiting acceptance by patients. Oral and nasal routes of delivering teriparatide are currently being explored. Compared to the subcutaneous injection of teriparatide, higher peak concentrations, a shorter half-life, and modestly greater 6 month increases in hip and spine BMD were observed using a micro-needle transdermal delivery system [9]. Other PTH molecules including PTH 1–31 and a PTHrP analogue are being studied [10, 11]. Preclinical data raise the possibility that these molecules might have greater anabolic responses as opposed to inducing bone resorption or causing hypercalcemia than do either PTH 1-34 or 1-84 [11]. Daily subcutaneous injections of a synthetic PTHrP analogue therapy induced greater increases in serum markers of bone formation and BMD than did daily teriparatide therapy after six and twelve months [12]. Whether the new delivery methods for teriparatide or the other forms of PTH will improve the acceptance and/or effectiveness of therapy remains to be determined.

New treatment strategies

The development of new targets for treatments derives from recent insights and advances in our understanding of molecular mechanisms of the regulation of bone metabolism. The first of these new treatments, denosumab, effectively exploits the central role of the RANK ligand/RANK/OPG pathway in the genesis of osteoclasts [13]. It is unlikely that a more potent inhibitor of osteoclast activity than denosumab will be developed. Like bisphosphonates, denosumab decreases the number and activity of osteoclasts; communication between osteoclast and osteoblast is reduced, and bone formation decreases. Potent antiresorptive agents can prevent the progression of osteoporosis but cannot restore lost bone mass or repair damaged architecture. Conversely, PTH stimulates bone formation, but the anabolic effect is attenuated by the subsequent increase in bone resorption. To achieve a better skeletal response, new drugs must either inhibit bone resorption without inhibiting bone formation or be truly anabolic agents that induce bone formation without stimulating bone resorption. Both strategies could be achieved by either monotherapy or by combining an agent that stimulates bone formation with an antiresorptive drug. The two most promising classes of emerging osteoporosis treatments, inhibitors of cathepsin K and sclerostin, may prove to be examples of monotherapy that utilize these two treatment mechanisms.

Cathepsin K inhibitors
Role of cathepsin K in bone metabolism

Osteoclasts dissolve bone mineral by creating a local acidic environment, and they digest the organic matrix by secreting proteolytic enzymes. Several cathepsins (lysosomal proteases) are found in many types of cells. They are differentiated by their structure, catalytic mechanism, and the kind of proteins they cleave (cysteine, aspartyl or serine proteases). Cathepsin K (CatK), a lysosomal cysteine protease, is abundantly expressed in osteoclasts along bone resorption surfaces, in both transcytotic vesicles and intracellular lysosomes [14, 15]. CatK is secreted from the osteoclast into the acidic environment of the resorption space and promotes the degradation of type I collagen, the major component (90%) of organic bone matrix, by cleaving the N-telopeptide and the C-terminal telopeptide of type I collagen, resulting in the commonly measured bone resorption biomarkers [16]. CatK can also cleave type I collagen at multiple sites in triple helical domains and noncollagenous bone matrix proteins such as osteocalcin, osteopontin, ostenectin, proteoglycans, and growth factors [16–18]. CatK is also expressed in other cells such as osteoblasts, osteocytes, macrophages and smooth muscle cells of atherosclerotic lesions, synovial fibroblasts and macrophages, white adipose tissue, breast and prostate cancer cells, and thyroid epithelial cells [19]. This wide distribution may explain the implication of CatK in disorders not related to bone metabolism and some of the adverse effects seen with cathepsin K inhibition in clinical trials.

Genetic deficiency of CatK in humans results in pycnodysostosis, a rare autosomal recessive human syndrome of skeletal dysplasia associated with short stature, brachycephaly, wide cranial sutures, osteosclerosis and fragility fractures [20, 21]. The absence of CatK function leads to a lifelong defect in bone resorption causing increased bone mass and bone brittleness (osteopetrosis). Targeted disruption of the CatK gene in mice results in a phenotype similar to pycnodysostosis with an osteosclerotic skeleton characterized by increased trabecular and cortical bone mass [22, 23]. Unlike patients who have pycnodysostosis, CatK−/− mice did not show poor bone quality. Histological examination of these animals has demonstrated normal bone mineralization and normal or increased osteoclast numbers, but a decrease in the osteoclasts' ability to resorb bone matrix. Compared to normal animals, CatK−/− mice have a high rate of bone formation and increased bone strength at the vertebral body and femoral mid-shaft. The increase in bone formation and bone strength might be the result of decreased cleavage by CatK of local osteogenic factors during resorption [24].

Cathepsin K inhibitors

The role of CatK in bone matrix degradation makes it an attractive pharmaceutical target for the treatment of osteoporosis and other diseases associated with high bone turnover. To be used safely without off-target side effects, drugs must specifically inhibit CatK without affecting related enzymes. Several potent, stable, reversible small molecular weight inhibitors of the active form of human CatK have been developed [19, 25]. Because of molecular differences between rodent and human CatK, inhibitors of human CatK cannot be studied in mice or rats. However, because of near homology between human CatK and that of rabbits and nonhuman primates, these animals have been used to study *in vivo* effects. CatK inhibitors have pharmacokinetics properties very different from potent antiresorptive drugs such as bisphosphonates or denosumab. CatK inhibitors do not bind to bone and are not sequestered into bone tissue; it is their concentration in resorption lacunae and lysosomes that is relevant to their action. Serum concentration and concentration in bone are in close relation. CatK inhibitors are metabolized by cytochrome enzymes and may interact with other drugs, but there is no concern about fasting or food effects.

Four CatK inhibitors have been evaluated in both preclinical and clinical studies [19, 25]. Differences in specificity have been observed among these agents. Relacatib (SB-462795) is an oral compound developed by GlaxoSmithKline that nonselectively acts on cathepsins K, L and V. Balicatib (AAE-581, Novartis) is a basic, highly selective nitrile-based CatK inhibitor in enzyme-based assays, but the selectivity is largely lost in whole cell assays due its accumulation in lysosomes (a property called lysosomotropism) where high concentrations exert effects on non-K cathepsins. Odanacatib (MK-822, Merck) is a nonbasic, nonlysosomotropic, nitrile-based molecule that retains its high enzyme selectivity in cell-based assay systems [26]. ONO-5334 (ONO Pharmaceutical) is a potent hydrazine-based nonlysosomotropic inhibitor of CatK with selectivity compared to other cathepsins [27].

Cathepsin K inhibitors in preclinical studies

In ovariectomized monkeys and rabbits, CatK inhibitors caused dose-dependent decreases in the levels of bone resorption markers, serum C-telopeptide (CTX) and urinary N-telopeptide (NTX) of type I collagen, and preservation of areal bone density (BMD) [28–32]. Bone resorption, assessed by histomorphometric analysis, was reduced at both trabecular and cortical sites. Unlike bisphosphonates and RANK ligand inhibitors that decrease osteoclast number and activity, odanacatib treatment increased osteoclast numbers when assessed by histomorphometry, and increased serum levels of tartrate resistant acid phosphatase 5b (TRAP5b), a marker of osteoclast number. Osteoclasts treated with CatK inhibitors and osteoclasts isolated from CatK−/− mice have been shown to maintain normal cell development and functions including differentiation, migration, polarization, survival and secretion [33]. Osteoclasts exposed to odanacatib are capable of beginning the bone resorptive process, but because the degradation of bone matrix is blocked, multiple, very shallow resorption lacunae are produced in comparison to the deeper lacunae observed in untreated cells [33]. Multiple intracellular vesicles with high concentrations of Cat K and incompletely digested collagen appear in osteoclasts after odanacatib treatment. The effects of CatK inhibition on bone formation are complex. Like others resorption inhibitors, relacatib, balicatib and odanacatib inhibit trabecular bone formation in ovariectomized monkeys, but, unlike other agents, endocortical bone formation is maintained [28–30]. In a direct comparison of odanacatib and alendronate treatment of ovariectomized rabbits, both treatments reduced bone resorption and prevented bone loss [31]. However, the reduction in bone formation rate was less with CatK inhibition than with alendronate. Odanacatib and balicatib therapy was associated with increased periostial bone formation in the femur, and increased cortical bone thickness and volume in the hip in estrogen deficient rabbits and monkeys and, with odanacatib, improved bending strength of monkey long bones [29, 32].

These preclinical data document that inhibiting CatK reduces the capability of osteoclasts to resorb bone matrix without reducing osteoclast number or affecting other osteoclast functions and effects. Cytokine signaling from osteoclasts to osteoblasts is maintained. Combined with the release of osteoblast activators from the multiple, shallow resorptive pits and the decreased proteolysis of these growth factors in presence of CatK inhibition, osteoblast activity is maintained on endocortical surfaces and perhaps stimulated on the periosteal surface, resulting in accrual of cortical bone mass and strength. Some CatK inhibitors tested in preclinical studies have advanced into clinical development.

Cathepsin K inhibitors in clinical trials

Clinical trials with ralecatib were discontinued after Phase I because of drug-drug interactions with the commonly prescribed medications acetaminophen, ibuprofen and atorvastatin [34]. Four daily oral doses of balicatib (5, 10, 25 or 50 mg) were evaluated in a Phase II dose-ranging study involving 675 postmenopausal women with low bone mass. At one year, treatment with balicatib 25 mg and 50 mg reduced bone resorption markers (CTX 61%, urinary NTX 55%) without changes in bone formation markers and resulted in dose-related increases in BMD [35]. With the highest dose, significant increases in lumbar spine BMD (4.5%) and hip BMD (2.2%) were observed. Despite these results, the clinical development of balicatib was discontinued after one year, due to skin-related adverse events including rashes and scleroderma-like lesions similar to morphea [36]. The dermatologic toxicities of balicatib might be due to inhibition of CatK in skin or to the lysosomotropism described above, causing off-target inhibition of cathepsins B, L and S that are expressed in skin fibroblasts, leading to a reduction of dermal matrix turnover [37].

In a multicenter, randomized, double-blind Phase II trial, 285 postmenopausal women with osteoporosis were randomized to receive placebo, alendronate 70 mg weekly, or one of three regimens of oral ONO-5334 (50 mg twice daily, 100 mg once daily or 300 mg once daily) [38]. After twelve months of therapy, ONO-5334 reduced indices of bone resorption (CTX and NTX) but had very modest effects on bone formation markers. The 300 mg daily dose reduced bone resorption markers comparable to alendronate, but the effects on bone formation markers BSAP and P1NP were less than that observed with alendronate (Figure 14.1). Levels of TRAP5b were reduced by alendronate but increased by the CatK inhibitor. Compared to placebo, treatment for one year with ONO-5334 300 mg daily resulted in significant increases in the BMD of the lumbar spine (5.1 %), total hip (3%) and femoral neck (2.6%), comparable to the alendronate responses. No clinically relevant safety concerns were noted, and no difference was detected in the rate of skin adverse events among the study groups.

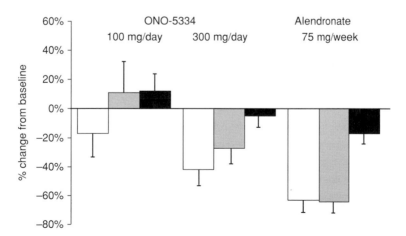

Figure 14.1 Changes from baseline (%) in serum CTX (white), serum P1NP (grey) and serum TRAP5b (black) after 12 months treatment with ONO-5334 100 mg daily or 300 mg daily and alendronate 70 mg weekly. (*Source*: Eastell R, Nagase S, Ohyama M *et al.* (2011) [38]).

Odanacatib is the most extensively studied CatK inhibitor in clinical trials. In regards to this agent, the results of two Phase 1 clinical trials that enrolled healthy postmenopausal women for a ≤ 3 weeks course of odanacatib in a daily (n = 30) or weekly (n = 49) dosing regimen have been published [39]. After 21 days of treatment with odanacatib, serum CTX and urinary NTX were reduced to 62% of baseline levels with weekly doses of at least 50 mg. Odanacatib has a long half-life (66–93 hours) allowing once weekly administration. A Phase II randomized, multicenter, placebo-controlled trial enrolled 399 postmenopausal women with low BMD (T-score ≤ −2.0 and ≥−3,5) who were allocated to one of the following weekly odanacatib treatments: 3, 10, 25 and 50 mg [40]. The primary end-point was the lumbar spine BMD percentage change from baseline at month 12. Secondary end-points included changes in BMD at other skeletal sites and time points and evaluation of bone turnover markers. After 12 months of treatment, a dose dependent increase at the lumbar spine and femoral neck was observed. At the highest weekly dose (50 mg), BMD at the lumbar spine and total hip progressively increased over 24 months to 5.7% and 4.1% versus placebo, respectively. Urinary NTX was quickly reduced; persistent reductions were observed at 12 and 24 months (58% and 52% versus placebo, respectively) with odanacatib 50 mg weekly. Small initial reductions in bone formation markers were observed (20% for BSAP and 30% for P1NP), but levels then gradually returned toward baseline. Histomorphometry from biopsies of 32 patients showed no remarkable differences in the activation frequency or bone formation rate between odanacatib-treated and placebo-treated patients [40].

This study was extended by enrolling 189 patients of the 280 participants who completed the initial 24 months of the study [41, 42]. Participants who received odanacatib 50 mg once a week continuously for five years showed almost linear increases in BMD from baseline at the lumbar spine (11.9%), total hip (8.5%) (Figure 14.2). This pattern of BMD response differs from the response seen with alendronate therapy where BMD appeared to plateau beyond three years of treatment [43]. In participants continuously treated, urinary NTX values remained well below baseline (50% at 3 years; 55.6% at 5 years). After year two, bone formation markers remained close to baseline levels. The levels of TRAP5b remained above baseline during the five years of odanacatib treatment but were not significantly different from those in the placebo group, confirming maintenance of osteoclast survival despite the decrease in bone resorption.

After two years, therapy was withdrawn in a group of participants that had received odanacatib 50 mg weekly [41, 42] (Figure 14.2). Markers of both bone resorption and formation quickly rose above baseline values, returning to baseline 12–24 months after therapy was discontinued.

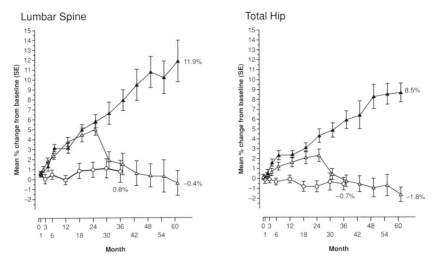

Figure 14.2 Changes in BMD of lumbar spine and total hip with odanacatib 50 mg weekly (closed circles) or placebo (open squares). (*Source*: Langdahl B, Binkley N, Bone H *et al.* (2012) [42]).

BMD values decreased to levels seen in the placebo group 12 months after withdrawing treatment. This rapid reversibility following odanacatib discontinuation is similar to that seen with other nonbisphosphonate antiresorptive treatments [44, 45]. The increased number of active osteoclasts and the intracellular CatK retention induced by CatK inhibitors may explain the rapid return of bone turnover markers to and above pretreatment levels after discontinuation of treatment.

Safety and tolerability were evaluated during the first 3 years of the study while a placebo group was available for comparison [41]. During these years, all doses of odanacatib were well tolerated. During year three (but not earlier), more subjects reported noncomplicated urinary tract infections with odanacatib (n = 12) compared to placebo (n = 3). Most cases had dysuria treated empirically without confirmation of infection. The incidence of skin and pulmonary events were similar in the treatment and placebo groups, and morphea-like skin lesions were not reported through 5 years of therapy.

An international, multicenter randomized, placebo-controlled Phase III event-driven fracture outcome trial evaluated the effects of treatment with odanacatib 50 mg weekly on the incidence of hip and spine fracture in more than 16 000 postmenopausal women with osteoporosis [46]. This study was recently discontinued early because of "robust effectiveness" [47]. Subjects in the Phase II and Phase III studies will be followed for several years to evaluate long-term effects of odanacatib therapy.

Summary

Preclinical data document that inhibiting CatK reduces the capability of osteoclasts to resorb bone matrix without reducing osteoclast number, activity or survival and does not affect other osteoclast functions. Cytokine signaling from osteoclasts to osteoblasts is maintained. Combined with the release of osteoblast activators from the multiple, shallow resorptive pits and the decreased proteolysis of these growth factors in presence of CatK inhibition, osteoblast activity is maintained on endocortical surfaces and perhaps stimulated on the periosteal surface, resulting in accrual of cortical bone mass and strength.

The clinical observations to date are consistent with preclinical data. Bone resorption is reduced while osteoclast numbers and overall bone formation are not decreased. While not true anabolic (bone formation stimulating) agents, CatK inhibitors may be "indirect anabolic" drugs by significantly reducing bone resorption while sparing bone formation.

Anti-sclerostin therapy

To achieve restoration of normal skeletal mass, reconstitute disordered architecture, and to return bone strength to normal, activation of osteoblastic bone formation is required. Studies of rare patients with genetic forms of high bone mass have provided molecular mechanisms that could be therapeutic targets to augment bone mass. Although patients with osteopetrosis have high bone mass due to osteoclast dysfunction, their bones are brittle and of poor quality. In contrast, patients with sclerosteosis or Van Buchem disease have very high bone mass, acquired during childhood, with normal or improved bone quality and increased bone strength [48]. Unraveling the genetic abnormality in these patients led to the discovery of sclerostin, a protein expressed almost exclusively by skeletal osteocytes, that functions as an endogenous inhibitor of osteoblast activity by inhibiting Wnt-signaling, the major activating pathway in osteoblasts. More recently, other genetic disorders have documented the importance of the Wnt-signaling pathway in skeletal development. LRP5 binding to the Wnt receptor up-regulates the pathway. Activating mutations of the LRP5 gene increase osteoblast number and function resulting in high bone mass of good quality [49]. Inactivating mutations decrease Wnt-signaling and are associated with the osteoporosis-pseudoglioma syndrome characterized by low bone mass [50]. Sclerostin deficiency in mice was associated with increased bone formation in both trabecular and cortical bone, high bone mass and substantially stronger skeletons [51]. These observations suggest that inhibiting sclerostin might "uninhibit" osteoblast activity, providing a molecular mechanism to achieve an anabolic skeletal response.

Inhibiting sclerostin activity with an anti-sclerostin antibody in aged, ovariectomized rats induced anabolic responses on trabecular, endocortical, intracortical and periosteal bone surfaces [52]. Trabecular and cortical bone thickness was increased, and cortical porosity was reduced. Treatment for five weeks not only restored skeletal abnormalities induced by ovariectomy but resulted in bone mass and bone strength that exceeded the sham-operated control animals.

In gonad-intact female Cynomolgus monkeys, treatment with a humanized sclerostin-neutralizing antibody once monthly for two months transiently increased markers of bone formation, increased BMD in the lumbar spine, femoral neck, proximal tibia and distal radius [53]. Anabolic responses on all skeletal surfaces were observed. Substantial increase in lumbar spine bone strength occurred, and a strong correlation between bone mineral content (measured by quantitative CT) and peak load was observed in both the lumbar spine and femoral diaphysis.

Patients with sclerosteosis and Van Buchem syndrome experience increased bone formation during years of growth as well as after skeletal maturation, resulting in skeletal abnormalities such as enlargement of jaw and skull and bony narrowing of neural foramina and canals. It is unknown if inhibiting sclerostin activity in adults could, or will result in skeletal overgrowth. No such problems were observed after short-term anti-sclerostin therapy in animals.

In the only clinical study available, single doses of a humanized anti-sclerostin antibody (romosozumab [AMG 785/CDP7851]) were administered to healthy men and postmenopausal women between 45 and 59 years of age who did not have osteoporosis [54]. Subjects received placebo or 0.1–10 mg/kg of romosozumab given as a single subcutaneous dose or 1 or 5 mg/kg in one intravenous dose. Study participants were followed for up to 85 days after dosing. Nonlinear pharmacokinetics were observed with apparent clearance of the antibody decreasing with increasing dose. Serum levels achieved with 1 or 5 mg/kg per day subcutaneously were 50–70% of values resulting from the same dose given intravenously, and detectable levels of antibody persisted for more than two months after the highest doses were given.

In response to romosozumab, serum markers of bone formation exhibited a dose-dependent increase. Serum P1NP increased by 184% and 167% from baseline with the 10 mg/Kg SC and 5 mg/Kg IV doses, respectively (Figure 14.3a). Values reached maximum levels about 30 days after subcutaneous dosing and after 15–30 days following IV administration and returned to baseline approximately two months after dosing. Serum CTX, a marker of bone resorption, was reduced in a dose-dependent manner. With the 10 mg/kg SQ and 5 mg/kg IV doses, values decreased by 50–60% within 1 to 2 weeks and then gradually returned to baseline. BMD of the

(a)

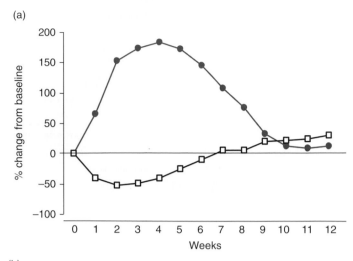

(b)

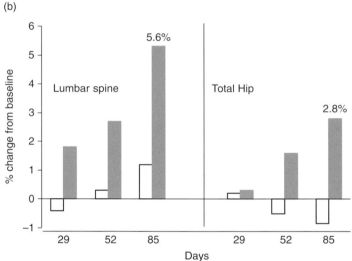

Figure 14.3 Changes in serum CTX and serum P1NP (a) and in BMD of lumbar spine and total hip (b), of after single subcutaneous dose of romosozumab 10 mg/Kg (closed circles and gray bar) or placebo (open squares and white bar). (*Source*: Padhi D, Jang G, Stouch B *et al.* (2011) [54]).

lumbar spine and hip region increased progressively over the 85 days of follow-up, rising, compared to baseline, by 5.3% and 2.8%, respectively at the end of the study (Figure 14.3b).

Mild injection site reactions were observed in some study participants, more frequently with higher doses. One subject experienced a transient elevation in hepatic function tests. Six subjects (11%) who received the study drug developed antibodies against romosozumab, including two subjects who had neutralizing antibody.

On the basis of these results, a phase II dose-ranging study was conducted. In postmenopausal women with low bone mass, responses to subcutaneous dosing with romosozumab were compared to placebo and open-label alendronate or teriparatide. With romosozumab, markers of bone formation increased and resorption markers decreased but returned to baseline during the first 12 months of treatment. BMD responses after treatment with romosozumab were greater than with alendronate or teriparatide [55]. Response to treatment for a second year will be evaluated. Two Phase III studies will compare the anti-fracture efficacy of romosozumab with teriparatide and alendronate in postmenopausal women with osteoporosis (ClinicalTrials.gov identifiers: NCT01631214 and (AMG 785/CDP7851).

Inhibiting sclerostin induces a pure anabolic response, not accompanied by an increase in bone resorption. In preclinical models, severe osteoporosis was reversed – even "cured". If this occurs in humans, anti-sclerostin therapy could be used to treat patients until they no longer have osteoporosis or even until they have normal bone strength. Early clinical data are encouraging. Studies in progress will reveal how long the anabolic effect will be sustained. Theoretical concerns about inducing bone overgrowth and off-target effects will be evaluated in large, long-term studies.

Conclusions

Potent antiresorptive agents are available for the treatment of osteoporosis. It is unlikely that more effective antiresorptive drugs will or can be developed. The unmet need in our field is to have anabolic therapies that protect patients from both spine and nonvertebral fractures. Inhibitors of CatK and of sclerostin are interesting prospects for the next generation of osteoporosis drugs.

References

1 Ettinger B, Black DM, Mitlak BH, *et al.* (1999) Reduction of vertebral fracture risk in postmenopausal women with osteoporosis treated with raloxifene: results from a 3-year randomized clinical trial. Multiple Outcomes of Raloxifene Evaluation (MORE) Investigators. *JAMA* **282**(7): 637–45.

2 Silverman SL, Christiansen C, Genant HK, *et al.* (2008) Efficacy of bazedoxifene in reducing new vertebral fracture risk in postmenopausal women with osteoporosis: results from a 3-year, randomized, placebo-, and active-controlled clinical trial. *J Bone Miner Res* **23**(12): 1923–34.

3 Cummings SR, McClung M, Reginster JY, *et al.* (2011) Arzoxifene for prevention of fractures and invasive breast cancer in postmenopausal women. *J Bone Miner Res* **26**(2): 397–404.

4 Cummings SR, Ensrud K, Delmas PD, *et al.* (2010) Lasofoxifene in postmenopausal women with osteoporosis. *N Engl J Med* **362**(8): 686–96.

5 Binkley N, Bolognese M, Sidorowicz-Bialynicka A, *et al.* (2012) A phase 3 trial of the efficacy and safety of oral recombinant calcitonin: The ORACAL trial. *J Bone Miner Res* **27**(8): 1821–9.

6 Henriksen K, Bay-Jensen AC, Christiansen C, Karsdal MA (2010) Oral salmon calcitonin-pharmacology in osteoporosis. *Expert Opin Biol Ther* **10**(11): 1617–29.

7 ClinicalTrials.gov. *A study to evaluate oral salmon calcitonin in the treatment of osteoporosis in postmenopausal women taking calcium and vitamin D.* http://clinicaltrial.gov/ct2/show/NCT00525798?term=calcitonin&rank=11. (accessed September 1, 2012).

8 McClung MR, Miller PD, Brown J, *et al.* (2012) Efficacy and safety of a novel delayed-release risedronate 35 mg once-a-week tablet in the treatment of postmenopausal osteoporosis. *Osteoporos Int* **23**(1): 267–76.

9 Cosman F, Lane NE, Bolognese MA, *et al.* (2010) Effect of transdermal teriparatide administration on bone mineral density in postmenopausal women. *J Clin Endocrinol Metab* **95**(1): 151–8.

10 Nemeth EF (2008) ZT-031, a cyclized analog of parathyroid hormone (1–31) for the potential treatment of osteoporosis. *IDrugs* **11**(11): 827–40.

11 Wysolmerski JJ (2012) Parathyroid hormone-related protein: an update. *J Clin Endocrinol Metab* **97**(9): 2947–56.

12 Hattersly G and Radius Health Investigators (2012) Bone anabolic efficacy and safety of BA-58, a novel analog of hPTHrP: results from a Phase 2 clinical trial in post-menopausal women with osteoporosis. Abstract OR08-1, Annual Meeting of The Endocrine Society.

13 Lacey DL, Boyle WJ, Simonet WS (2012) Bench to bedside: elucidation of the OPG-RANK-RANKL pathway and the development of denosumab. *Nat Rev Drug Discov* **11**(5): 401–19.

14 Vaaraniemi J, Halleen JM, Kaarlonen K, *et al.* (2004) Intracellular machinery for matrix degradation in bone-resorbing osteoclasts. *J Bone Miner Res* **19**(9): 1432–40.

15 Rieman DJ, McClung HA, Dodds RA, *et al.* (2001) Biosynthesis and processing of cathepsin K in cultured human osteoclasts. *Bone* **28**(3): 282–9.

16 Garnero P, Borel O, Byrjalsen I, *et al.* (1998) The collagenolytic activity of cathepsin K is unique among mammalian proteinases. *J Biol Chem* **273**(48): 32347–52.

17 Bossard MJ, Tomaszek TA, Thompson SK, *et al.* (1996) Proteolytic activity of human osteoclast cathepsin K: expression, purification, activation, and substrate identification. *J Biol Chem* **271**(21): 12517–24.

18 Fuller K, Lawrence KM, Ross JL, *et al.* (2008) Cathepsin K inhibitors prevent matrix-derived growth factor degradation by human osteoclasts. *Bone* **42**(1): 200–11.

19 Brömme D, Lecaille F (2009) Cathepsin K inhibitors for osteoporosis and potential off-target effects. *Expert Opin Investig Drugs* **18**(5): 585–600.

20 Gelb BD, Shi GP, Chapman HA, *et al.* (1996) Pycnodysostosis, a lysosomal disease caused by cathepsin K deficiency. *Science* **273**(5279): 1236–8.

21 Schilling AF, Mulhausen C, Lehmann W, *et al.* (2007) High bone mineral density in pycnodysostotic patients with a novel mutation in the propeptide of cathepsin K. *Osteoporos Int* **18**(5): 659–69.

22 Gowen M, Lazner F, Dodds R, *et al.* (1999) Cathepsin K knockout mice develop osteopetrosis due to a deficit in matrix degradation but not demineralization. *J Bone Miner Res* **14**(10): 1654–63.

23 Pennypacker B, Shea M, Liu Q, *et al.* (2009) Bone density, strength, and formation in adult cathepsin K (−/−) mice. *Bone* **44**(2): 199–207.

24 Fuller K, Lawrence KM, Ross JL, *et al.* (2008) Cathepsin K inhibitors prevent matrix-derived growth factor degradation by human osteoclasts. *Bone* **42**(1): 200–11.

25 Rodan SB, Duong LT (2008) Cathepsin K – a new molecular target for osteoporosis. *IBMS BoneKEy* **5**: 16–24.

26 Gauthier JY, Chauret N, Cromlish W, *et al.* (2008) The discovery of odanacatib (MK-0822), a selective inhibitor of cathepsin K. *Bioorg Med Chem Lett* **18**(3): 923–98.

27 Ochi Y, Yamada H, Mori H, *et al.* (2011) Effects of ONO-5334, a novel orally-active inhibitor of cathepsin K, on bone metabolism. *Bone* **49**(6): 1351–6.

28 Stroup GB, Kumar S, Jerome CP (2009) Treatment with a potent cathepsin K inhibitor preserves cortical and trabecular bone mass in ovariectomized monkeys. *Calcif Tissue Int* **85**(4): 344–55.

29 Jerome C, Missbach M, Gamse R (2011) Balicatib, a cathepsin K inhibitor, stimulates periosteal bone formation in monkeys. *Osteoporos Int* **22**(12): 3001–11.

30 Masarachia PJ, Pennypacker BL, Pickarski M, *et al.* (2012) Odanacatib reduces bone turnover and increases bone mass in the lumbar spine of skeletally mature ovariectomized rhesus monkeys. *J Bone Miner Res* **27**(3): 509–23.

31 Pennypacker BL, Duong le T, Cusick TE, *et al.* (2011) Cathepsin K inhibitors prevent bone loss in estrogen-deficient rabbits. *J Bone Miner Res* **26**(2): 252–62.

32 Cusick T, Chen CM, Pennypacker BL, *et al.* (2012) Odanacatib treatment increases hip bone mass and cortical thickness by preserving endocortical bone formation and stimulating periosteal bone formation in the ovariectomized adult rhesus monkey. *J Bone Miner Res* **27**(3): 524–37.

33 Leung P, Pickarski M, Zhuo Y, *et al.* (2011) The effects of the cathepsin K inhibitor odanacatib on osteoclastic bone resorption and vesicular trafficking. *Bone* **49**(4): 623–35.

34 ClinicalTrials.gov. Study to determine the effects of doses of relacatib on the metabolism of acetaminophen, ibuprofen and atorvastatin. http://clinicaltrials.gov/ct2/show/NCT00411190?term=relacatib&rank=1. Accessed September 1, 2012.

35 Costa AG, Cusano NE, Silva BC, *et al.* (2011) Cathepsin K: its skeletal actions and role as a therapeutic target in osteoporosis. *Nat Rev Rheumatol* **7**(8): 447–56.

36 Rünger TM, Adami S, Benhamou CL, *et al.* (2012) Morphea-like skin reactions in patients treated with the cathepsin K inhibitor balicatib. *J Am Acad Dermatol* **66**(3): e89–96. Epub 2011 May 14.

37 Falgueyret JP, Desmarais S, Oballa R, *et al.* (2005) Lysosomotropism of basic cathepsin K inhibitors contributes to increased cellular potencies against off-target cathepsins and reduced functional selectivity. *J Med Chem* **48**(24): 7535–43.

38 Eastell R, Nagase S, Ohyama M, *et al.* (2011) Safety and efficacy of the cathepsin K inhibitor ONO-5334 in postmenopausal osteoporosis: the OCEAN study. *J Bone Miner Res* **26**(6), 1303–12.

39 Stoch SA, Zajic S, Stone J, *et al.* (2009) Effect of the cathepsin K inhibitor odanacatib on bone resorption biomarkers in healthy postmenopausal women: two double-blind, randomized, placebo-controlled phase I studies. *Clin Pharmacol Ther* **86**(2): 175–82.

40 Bone HG, McClung MR, Roux C, *et al.* (2010) Odanacatib, a cathepsin-K inhibitor for osteoporosis: a two-year study in postmenopausal women with low bone density. *J Bone Miner Res* **25**(5): 937–47.

41 Eisman JA, Bone HG, Hosking DJ, *et al.* (2011) Odanacatib in the treatment of postmenopausal women with low bone mineral density: three-year continued therapy and resolution of effect. *J Bone Miner Res* **26**(2): 242–51.

42 Langdahl B, Binkley N, Bone H, *et al.* (2012) Odanacatib in the treatment of post-menopausal women with low bone mineral density: 5 years of continued therapy in a phase 2 study. *J Bone Miner Res* **27**(11): 2231–2416.

43 Black DM, Schwartz AV, Ensrud KE, *et al.* (2006) Effects of continuing or stopping alendronate after 5 years of treatment: the Fracture Intervention Trial Long-term Extension (FLEX): a randomized trial. *JAMA* **296**(24): 2927–38.

44 Wasnich RD, Bagger YZ, Hosking DJ, *et al.* (2004) Changes in bone density and turnover after alendronate or estrogen withdrawal. *Menopause* **11**(6 Pt 1): 622–30.

45 Miller PD, Bolognese MA, Lewiecki EM, *et al.* (2008) Effect of denosumab on bone density and turnover in postmenopausal women with low bone mass after long-term continued, discontinued, and restarting of therapy: a randomized blinded phase 2 clinical trial. *Bone* **43**(2): 222–9.

46 ClinicalTrials.gov. *A study of MK0822 in postmenopausal women with osteoporosis to assess fracture risk.* http://clinicaltrials.gov/ct2/show/NCT00529373?term=odanacatib&rank=6 (accessed September 1, 2012).

47 HuffPost Healthy Living (2012) *Odanacatib: osteoporosis drug reduces fracture risk In trial.* http://www.huffingtonpost.com/2012/07/12/odanacatib-osteoporosis-drug-fracture-bone_n_1666631.html. (accessed, September 1, 2012)

48 Gardner JC, van Bezooijen RL, Mervis B (2005) Bone mineral density in sclerosteosis; affected individuals and gene carriers. *J Clin Endocrinol Metab* **90**(12): 6392–5.

49 Little RD, Carulli JP, Del Mastro RG, *et al.* A mutation in the LDL receptor-related protein 5 gene results in the autosomal dominant high bone-mass trait. *Am J Hum Genet* **70**(1): 11–19.

50 Tüysüz B, Bursalı A, Alp Z, *et al.* (2012) Osteoporosis-pseudoglioma syndrome: three novel mutations in the LRP5 gene and response to bisphosphonate treatment. *Horm Res Paediatr* **77**(2): 115–20.

51 Li X, Ominsky MS, Warmington KS, *et al.* (2009) Sclerostin antibody treatment increases bone formation, bone mass, and bone strength in a rat model of post-menopausal osteoporosis. *J Bone Miner Res* **24**(4): 578–88.

52 Li X, Ominsky MS, Niu QT, *et al.* (2008) Targeted deletion of the sclerostin gene in mice results in increased bone formation and bone strength. *J Bone Miner Res* **23**(6): 860–9.

53 Ominsky MS, Vlasseros F, Jolette J, *et al.* (2010) Two doses of sclerostin antibody in cynomolgus monkeys increases bone formation, bone mineral density, and bone strength. *J Bone Miner Res* **25**(5): 948–59.

54 Padhi D, Jang G, Stouch B, *et al.* (2011) Single-dose, placebo-controlled, randomized study of AMG 785, a sclerostin monoclonal antibody. *J Bone Miner Res* **26**(1): 19–26.

55 McClung MR, Grauer A, Boonen S, *et al.* (2012) Inhibition of sclerostin with romosozumab (AMG 785/CDP7851) in postmenopausal women with low bone mineral density: phase 2 trial results. *American Society for Bone and Mineral Research* Abstract 1025, Vol 27, Supplement 1: S8.

CHAPTER 15

Monitoring Therapy for Osteoporosis

E. Michael Lewiecki
New Mexico Clinical Research & Osteoporosis Center, Inc, Albuquerque, NM, USA

Introduction

Approved pharmacological therapies for the treatment of osteoporosis reduce fracture risk in randomized placebo-controlled clinical trials (RCTs) with postmenopausal women at high risk for fracture. This benefit of treatment has been observed for compounds that include alendronate [1–3], risedronate [4–6], ibandronate [7], zoledronate [8, 9], salmon calcitonin [10], raloxifene [11], teriparatide [12], recombinant human parathyroid hormone (1-84) [13], and strontium ranelate [14, 15]. Estrogen, administered as monotherapy [16] or combined with medroxyprogesterone acetate [17], reduces the incidence of fractures in postmenopausal women not selected for high baseline fracture risk. It is less clear, however, whether individual patients treated with these drugs in the clinical practice setting achieve that same level of benefit as groups of clinical trial subjects, and whether the balance of benefit and risk with long-term therapy is the same as reported for the relatively short duration of RCTs. The application of RCT data to clinical practice patients is confounded by differences between patients and clinical trial subjects that include age, comorbidities, concomitant medications, disease-state education, and adherence to therapy. Patients with indications for the treatment of osteoporosis commonly do not qualify for participation in RCTs that are conducted to assess the efficacy and safety of drugs to reduce fracture risk [18]. RCTs for drugs to treat osteoporosis typically maintain a placebo-group for 3–4 years and involve several thousand subjects; following approval and use in clinical practice, many more individuals (hundreds of thousands or millions) may be exposed to the same drugs and treated for a longer duration of time. These differences lead to uncertainties regarding the effectiveness and safety of osteoporosis treatment in individual patients. It is therefore desirable and necessary to monitor patients being treated for osteoporosis. Monitoring can provide some evidence that the treatment is effective and that adverse effects of therapy have not developed. It provides opportunities to periodically assess the balance of benefit and risk, reassure the patient that taking the medication is worth the trouble and the cost, and perhaps help to improve adherence to therapy.

The goal of osteoporosis therapy is to reduce fracture risk. This can be accomplished by improving bone strength, preventing falls, and by minimizing the force applied to a bone if a fall occurs. The ideal outcome of treatment is no fracture. There is no test that can directly measure bone strength in a living human and no drug that can totally eliminate all fractures. In monitoring the treatment of osteoporosis, we must rely on indirect measures that are correlated with bone strength and recognize that a fracture on therapy, while undesirable, does not necessarily represent a failure of treatment. Fractures are stochastic events that can occur in any patient when the force applied to a bone exceeds its strength. Properties associated with a useful clinical tool to monitor therapy include general availability, good precision (reproducibility of measurements), responsiveness to therapy, correlation with reduction in fracture risk, low exposure to ionizing irradiation, and low cost [19]. This chapter reviews the use of two types of measurements to monitor osteoporosis therapy in clinical practice – bone mineral density (BMD) and bone turnover markers (BTMs) – and provides a strategy for evaluating patients who are not responding to therapy as expected.

Bone density testing

Technologies for measuring bone density include dual-energy X-ray absorptiometry (DXA), peripheral DXA (pDXA), quantitative ultrasound (QUS), quantitative computed tomography (QCT), and peripheral QCT (pQCT). DXA, which measures areal BMD (g/cm^2) is the technology most often used to monitor therapy [20] and is the most versatile of these clinical tools (Table 15.1) because of its utility for diagnostic classification according to criteria established by the World Health Organization (WHO) [21], assessment of fracture risk with or without a fracture risk algorithm, such as FRAX [22], and inclusion in treatment guidelines, such as those of the National Osteoporosis Foundation [23]. The best skeletal site to monitor by DXA is the lumbar spine, which has a favorable combination of response to therapy and good precision; when lumbar spine cannot be used (e.g., when structural abnormalities, such as severe osteoarthritis or scoliosis, are present), then the total hip is usually the best alternative. The use of BMD testing to monitor therapy requires adherence to quality standards, including precision assessment and calculation of the "least

Table 15.1 Bone density testing technologies.

Technology	Measurement (units)	Monitor	Diagnose	Predict fracture risk	Input for FRAX
DXA	aBMD (g/cm^2)	Yes	Yes	Yes	Yes
pDXA	aBMD (g/cm^2)	Limited	Yes	Yes	No
QUS	SOS (m/sec), BUA (dB/MHz)	No	No	Limited	No
QCT	vBMD (mg/cm^3)	Yes	No	Yes	No
pQCT	vBMD (mg/cm^3)	Limited	No	No	No

DXA is the BMD testing technology most often used for monitoring; it provides the greatest versatility for other clinical applications as well. The use of pDXA for monitoring is generally limited to conditions, such as primary hyperthyroidism, that mainly have adverse effects on cortical bone. QUS is not practical for monitoring because measured changes are generally too slow to be clinically useful. Although QCT and pQCT can be used for monitoring, their application for this purpose is limited by the higher cost, limited availability, and greater ionizing radiation than DXA. The diagnosis of osteoporosis according to the WHO criteria and input for FRAX requires a DXA-based measurement.

aBMD, areal bone mineral density; BUA, broadband ultrasound attenuation; DXA, dual-energy X-ray absorptiometry; FRAX, World Health Organization fracture risk algorithm; pDXA, peripheral dual-energy X-ray absorptiometry; pQCT, peripheral dual-energy X-ray absorptiometry; QCT, dual-energy X-ray absorptiometry; QUS, quantitative ultrasound; SOS, speed of sound; vBMD, volumetric bone mineral density; WHO, World Health Organization.

significant change" (LSC), the smallest change in BMD that is statistically significant, usually with a 95% level of confidence [24]. Precision assessment is typically conducted by measuring BMD in 15 patients 3 times or 30 patients 2 times each with repositioning of the patient after each scan. This is, in essence, a test of the technologist's ability to correctly reposition the patient with each scan in order to measure the same region of interest in each skeletal site in a reproducible fashion. Without calculation of the LSC, it is not possible to distinguish a genuine change in the patient's BMD from a measurement error that has to clinical or statistical significance. It is important to recognize that the LSC supplied by the DXA manufacturer, which may appear on the DXA printout, is not the same as a calculated LSC and cannot be used for comparing serial DXA studies in patients. In order to obtain a quantitative comparison of serial BMD studies, each study must be with the same well-calibrated instrument by a skilled technologist. Serial BMD measurements using different instruments, even with similar or identical models of the same manufacturer, cannot be quantitatively compared unless cross-calibration has been done according to standardized procedures [25].

Most drugs used to treat osteoporosis increase BMD in clinical trials, with variability in the BMD response depending on the drug and patient factors. With bisphosphonates, the drugs most often used to treat osteoporosis, the greatest BMD increase is typically seen in the first year after starting therapy, followed by a slower rate of BMD increase and then a plateau. There is a correlation between BMD increase with treatment and reduction in fracture risk. A meta-analysis analysis of 13 placebo-controlled RCTs showed that larger BMD increases were associated with greater reductions in vertebral fracture risk [26], with small BMD increases associated with substantial reductions in fracture risk. Statistical modeling of clinical trial data predicted that an increase in lumbar spine BMD of 8% would reduce vertebral fracture risk by 54%, with 41% of vertebral fracture risk reduction explained by the BMD increase. Another meta-analysis of 12 clinical trials using different statistical methods also reported a correlation between BMD increase with therapy and reduction in vertebral fracture risk, although the increase in BMD explained only a small portion of the fracture risk reduction [27]. A meta-analysis of 18 placebo-controlled RCTs of antiresorptive drugs in women with postmenopausal osteoporosis found that larger changes in BMD at the spine and hip were associated with greater reductions in the risk of nonvertebral fractures [28]. A recent study evaluating BMD change with denosumab and fracture incidence found a strong correlation between BMD increases and fracture risk reduction [29], suggesting that some previous studies may have underestimated the strength of this relationship.

There is heterogeneity of BMD response to therapy in clinical practice, with one study finding that about 10% of patients treated with a bisphosphonate had a statistically significant decrease in BMD; subsequent evaluation revealed previously unrecognized clinically relevant contributing factors in about 50% of these [30]. This suggests that there is benefit in using BMD testing to monitor treated patients, and that evaluation of these patients may lead to changes in management and perhaps improved clinical outcomes.

QUS measures the speed of sound (SOS) and broadband ultrasound attenuation (BUA) at peripheral skeletal sites with instruments that are portable, less expensive than DXA, and use no ionizing radiation [31]. QUS parameters with validated instruments are correlated with fracture risk [32], but QUS cannot be used to diagnose osteoporosis according to the WHO criteria, cannot be used to monitor therapy [33], and cannot be used as input for FRAX. QCT and pQCT measure volumetric BMD (mg/cm^2) in trabecular and cortical bone. Trabecular BMD of the lumbar spine measured by QCT is validated for monitoring treatment-related BMD changes [34]. QCT is more expensive, less widely available, and exposes the patient to a higher dose of ionizing radiation compared with DXA. It cannot be used for diagnostic classification with the WHO criteria and cannot provide input for FRAX. High resolution magnetic resonance imaging (HR-MRI) and high resolution peripheral QCT (HR-pQCT) at peripheral skeletal sites are used to evaluate trabecular microarchitecture in the research setting, but have no established role in clinical practice at this time [35, 36].

Bone turnover markers

BTMs are biochemical by-products (e.g., enzymes, fragments of collagen) of bone remodeling that are released into the systemic circulation and measured in blood or urine. They are customarily classified as markers of bone resorption or bone formation. Bone resorption markers include N-terminal telopeptide of type 1 collagen (NTX), C-terminal telopeptide of type 1 collagen (CTX), deoxypyridinoline (DPD), and pyridinoline (PYD); these are protein fragments resulting from the degradation of type 1 collagen beneath the surface of bone resorbing osteoclasts. NTX, CTX, DPD, and PYD provide measures of osteoclast activity, while another BTM, tartrate resistant acid phosphatase isoform 5b (TRACP 5b), is correlated with the number of osteoclasts rather than their bone resorbing activity. Bone formation markers, such as bone specific alkaline phosphatase (BSAP), procollagen type 1 N-propeptide (P1NP), and osteocalcin (OC) are proteins secreted by osteoblasts or byproducts of type I collagen synthesis. BTMs have been helpful in defining the pathophysiology of osteoporosis and understanding the mechanism of action of drugs used to treat osteoporosis. Women with postmenopausal osteoporosis typically have high bone remodeling, as reflected by high levels of BTMs. Women with elevated BTM levels have reduced BMD [37], accelerated rates of bone loss [38], and increased fracture risk [39], compared with women with lower BTM levels. A decrease in BTM levels with antiresorptive therapy is predictive of a subsequent increase in BMD [40] and reduction in fracture risk [28, 41–43]. Anabolic therapy with teriparatide is associated with an increase in BTM levels that is predictive of a subsequent increase in BMD [44].

When pharmacological therapy for osteoporosis is followed by the expected change in BTMs (i.e., decreased with antiresorptive therapy, increased with anabolic therapy), it provides reassurance that medication has been taken as prescribed and absorbed, with enough drug reaching bone to have the expected effect on bone remodeling and reduction in fracture risk. The absence of the expected BTM response suggests the need for further evaluation and reassessment of treatment [45]. The use of BTMs to monitor therapy is a component of some evidence-based clinical

Table 15.2 Comparison of bone mineral density (BMD) and bone turnover markers (BTMs) in monitoring therapy for osteoporosis.

Parameter	BMD	BTMs
Signal (expected change with treatment)	6–8%	20–300%
Noise (variability, expressed as LSC)	3%	30–60%
Signal/noise ratio (approximate)	2–3	1–5
Time to significant change	1–3 years	1–3 months

BTMs are biochemical by-products of bone remodeling that can be measured in the serum or urine. These are commercially available laboratory testing that are potentially clinically useful in assessing the effect of therapy on bone resorption and formation. While the variability of BTM measurements is much higher than with BMD, the expected changes in response to therapy are much higher, so that the "signal to noise ratio" for both tests is acceptable for appropriate clinical applications.
LSC, least significant change
(*Source*: Adapted from [46, 51]).

practice guidelines [23, 46, 47]. Since BTMs changes occur sooner than measurable changes in BMD, their use provides a more rapid assessment of respond to therapy than BMD (Table 15.2). This may be particularly useful when there are concerns that a patient may not respond as expected, as with a patient with a gastrointestinal disorder that might impair absorption of an oral bisphosphonate, or when poor adherence to therapy is a concern. BTMs may be helpful in evaluating a patient who is losing BMD despite therapy, in evaluating premenopausal women with low BMD, and perhaps as an aid in selecting a particular drug. A BTM cannot be used to diagnose osteoporosis and is not validated as a risk factor for FRAX input.

Limitations in the use of BTMs to monitor therapy include preanalytical and analytical variability, lack of well-established reference values, and uncertainties in selecting the optimal BTM to measure for the drug used and the clinical circumstances of the patient. Preanalytical sources of variability that cannot be controlled include age, sex, menopausal status, fractures, pregnancy, lactation, comorbidities, drugs, and immobility, while those that are controllable include time of day, fasting status, and exercise [48]. Analytical variability is associated with specimen processing and type of assay. Populations for establishing BTM reference ranges may vary according to demographics, procedures for specimen collection and processing, and the type of BTM. Determination of the significance of apparent changes in BTM levels requires knowledge of the LSC, just as for comparing serial BMD measurement. Some guidelines suggest calculation of the LSC [23], while others recommend an imputed LSC of about 30% for serum BTMs and about 50–60% for urine BTMs [46]. A favorable response to antiresorptive therapy is suggested by a reduction of BTM level to the lower portion of the healthy premenopausal reference range and/or a decrease in the pretreatment BTM level that is at least equal to the LSC. When a patient is prescribed teriparatide, an increase in a marker of bone formation is consistent with the expected anabolic effect of therapy.

The use of BTMs to monitor therapy is complimentary to BMD testing. Measurement of BTM levels may be particularly useful when is it is desirable to have a more rapid assessment of therapeutic effect than the 1–2 years typically required for a significant change in BMD to occur. The best BTM to use may in part depend on what is available and affordable, as well as the familiarity of the physician with a specific BTM. The International Osteoporosis Foundation (IOF) and the International Federation of Clinical Chemistry and Laboratory Medicine (IFCC) have recommended that CTX and P1NP be the reference markers for bone resorption and formation, respectively, in clinical trials [49]. By doing so, it is hoped that stronger evidence for the use of these BTMs in clinical practice can be obtained.

Monitoring for adherence and safety

Although monitoring osteoporosis therapy usually focuses on demonstration of effectiveness by measuring surrogates of bone strength, monitoring for adherence and safety is equally important. Much of this can be accomplished by a focused medical history, and sometimes by laboratory testing or imaging. A few of many possible examples follow. Incorrect administration of an oral bisphosphonate with only a sip of water or failure to remain upright for the specified amount of time after dosing could increase the risk of adverse upper gastrointestinal effects. Asking the patient to describe the method of drug administration can help to identify this potential safety concern. If there is concern that therapy might cause or exacerbate impaired renal function, then a serum creatinine and estimated glomerular filtration rate can be measured. A patient on long-term bisphosphonate therapy who develops unexplained pain in the lateral thigh may have an incomplete atypical femur fracture that could be identified by X-ray, nuclear imaging, or MRI.

Monitoring patients on a bisphosphonate "drug holiday"

With increasing concerns regarding the long-term efficacy and safety of bisphosphonates, it may be appropriate to withhold therapy for an undefined period in patients at low risk for fracture who has been treated for at least 3–5 years. Due to the long skeletal retention time of bisphosphonates, these patients may continue to benefit from the antiresorptive effects and fracture risk reduction of their bisphosphonate therapy, while reducing the potential risks of long-term therapy, such as atypical femur fractures. However, with advancing age, loss of BMD, and increasing bone remodeling, fracture risk will rise with time and may again require treatment [50]. Despite the absence of evidence-based guidelines on starting and stopping a drug holiday, it is appropriate to monitor patients on a drug holiday to assess a waning of antiresorptive effect, loss of BMD, and increasing fracture risk. If there is a significant rise in BTMs or significant decrease in BMD that is associated with an estimation of fracture risk that meets the threshold for treatment [23], it may be time to end the drug holiday.

Evaluation of suboptimal responders

A patient who does not respond as expected to therapy should be evaluated for contributing factors (Table 15.3). This may involve laboratory testing that is similar to that done to evaluate patients for secondary causes of osteoporosis prior to starting therapy. In addition, adherence to therapy and adequacy of calcium and vitamin D intake should be determined. And finally, the patient should be thoroughly assessed for the development of any disease or condition associated with adverse skeletal effects that may not have been previously identified. Those that are correctable should be addressed, and a change in treatment should be considered [45].

Table 15.3 Consideration of factors contributing to suboptimal response to therapy.

Category	Examples	Evaluation
Initiation	Prescription never filled	Medical history, pharmacy data
Compliance	Not taking medication correctly	Medical history
Persistence	Not taking medication long enough to benefit	Medical history
Calcium	Inadequate intake, poor absorption	Medical history, 24-hour urinary calcium
Vitamin D	Inadequate intake, poor absorption	Medical history, serum 25-hydroxyvitamin D
Comorbidities	Primary hyperparathyroidism, excessive thyroid replacement	Serum calcium, thyroid stimulating hormone
Medications	Glucocorticoids, aromatase inhibitor	Medical history

The evaluation of patients who do not respond to therapy as expected should be customized according to clinical circumstances. This table provides categories and examples of factors that could be responsible for a suboptimal response. Most of these can be identified by medical history or easily available laboratory tests.

Summary

All patients being treated for osteoporosis should be monitored to assess both the effectiveness and safety of their prescribed therapy. The clinical tools that are available to monitor patients for effectiveness are BMD testing and BTMs. Safety concerns can be addressed by a focused medical history and physical examination, with appropriate laboratory testing and imaging as indicated. Patients who are not responding as expected, have adverse effects of therapy, or are at high risk for adverse effects, should be thoroughly evaluated for potential contributing factors. Patient management decisions must consider the balance of benefit and risk with continuing or changing treatment.

References

1 Liberman UA, Weiss SR, Broll J, Minne H, Quan H, Bell NH, *et al.* (1995) Effect of oral alendronate on bone mineral density and the incidence of fractures in postmenopausal osteoporosis. *N Engl J Med* **333**: 1437–43.

2 Black DM, Cummings SR, Karpf DB, Cauley JA, Thompson DE, Nevitt MC, *et al.* (1996) Randomised trial of effect of alendronate on risk of fracture in women with existing vertebral fractures. *Lancet* **348**: 1535–41.

3 Cummings SR, Black DM, Thompson DE, Applegate WB, Barrett-Connor E, Musliner TA, *et al.* (1998) Effect of alendronate on risk of fracture in women with low bone density but without vertebral fractures: Results from the fracture intervention trial. *JAMA* **280**(24): 2077–82.

4 McClung MR, Geusens P, Miller PD, Zippel H, Bensen WG, Roux C, *et al.* (2001) Effect of risedronate on the risk of hip fracture in elderly women. *N Engl J Med* **344**: 333–40.

5 Reginster J-Y, Minne HW, Sorensen OH, Hooper M, Roux C, Brandi ML, *et al.* (2000) Randomized trial of the effects of risedronate on vertebral fractures in women with established postmenopausal osteoporosis. *Osteoporos Int* **11**: 83–91.

6 Harris ST, Watts NB, Genant HK, McKeever CD, Hangartner T, Keller M, *et al.* (1999) Effects of risedronate treatment on vertebral and nonvertebral fractures in women with postmenopausal osteoporosis: a randomized controlled trial. Vertebral Efficacy With Risedronate Therapy (VERT) Study Group. *JAMA* **282**(14): 1344–52.

7 Chesnut III CH, Skag A, Christiansen C, Recker R, Stakkestad JA, Hoiseth A, *et al.* (2004) Effects of oral ibandronate administered daily or intermittently on fracture risk in postmenopausal osteoporosis. *J Bone Miner Res* **19**(8): 1241–9.

8 Black DM, Delmas PD, Eastell R, Reid IR, Boonen S, Cauley JA, *et al.* (2007) Once-yearly zoledronic acid for treatment of postmenopausal osteoporosis. *N Engl J Med* **356**(18): 1809–22.

9 Lyles KW, Colon-Emeric CS, Magaziner JS, Adachi JD, Pieper CF, Mautalen C, *et al.* (2007) Zoledronic acid and clinical fractures and mortality after hip fracture. *N Engl J Med* **357**(18): 1799–1809.

10 Chesnut III CH, Silverman S, Andriano K, Genant H, Gimona A, Harris S, *et al.* (2000) A randomized trial of nasal spray salmon calcitonin in postmenopausal women

with established osteoporosis: the prevent recurrence of osteoporotic fractures study. PROOF Study Group. *Am J Med* **109**(4): 267–76.

11 Ettinger B, Black DM, Mitlak BH, Knickerbocker RK, Nickelsen T, Genant HK, *et al.* (1999) Reduction of vertebral fracture risk in postmenopausal women with osteoporosis treated with raloxifene – Results from a 3-year randomized clinical trial. *JAMA* **282**(7): 637–45.

12 Neer RM, Arnaud CD, Zanchetta JR, Prince R, Gaich GA, Reginster J-Y, *et al.* (2001) Effect of parathyroid hormone (1-34) on fractures and bone mineral density in postmenopausal women with osteoporosis. *N Engl J Med* **344**: 1434–41.

13 Greenspan SL, Bone HG, Ettinger MP, Hanley DA, Lindsay R, Zanchetta JR, *et al.* (2007) Effect of recombinant human parathyroid hormone (1-84) on vertebral fracture and bone mineral density in postmenopausal women with osteoporosis: a randomized trial. *Ann Intern Med* **146**(5): 326–9.

14 Reginster JY, Seeman E, De Vernejoul MC, Adami S, Compston J, Phenekos C, *et al.* (2005) Strontium ranelate reduces the risk of nonvertebral fractures in postmenopausal women with osteoporosis: Treatment of Peripheral Osteoporosis (TROPOS) study. *J Clin Endocrinol Metab* **90**(5): 2816–22.

15 Meunier PJ, Roux C, Seeman E, Ortolani S, Badurski JE, Spector TD, *et al.* (2004) The effects of strontium ranelate on the risk of vertebral fracture in women with postmenopausal osteoporosis. *N Engl J Med* **350**(5): 459–68.

16 Anderson GL, Limacher M, Assaf AR, Bassford T, Beresford SA, Black H, *et al.* (2004) Effects of conjugated equine estrogen in postmenopausal women with hysterectomy: the Women's Health Initiative randomized controlled trial. *JAMA* **291**(14): 1701–12.

17 Writing Group for the Women's Health Initiative Investigators (2002) Risks and benefits of estrogen plus progestin in healthy postmenopausal women. *JAMA* **288**: 321–33.

18 Dowd R, Recker RR, Heaney RP (2000) Study subjects and ordinary patients. *Osteoporosis International* **11**(6): 533–6.

19 Lewiecki EM (2010) Monitoring pharmacological therapy for osteoporosis. *Rev Endocr Metab Disord* **11**(4): 261–73.

20 Baim S, Binkley N, Bilezikian JP, Kendler DL, Hans DB, Lewiecki EM, *et al.* (2008) Official Positions of the International Society for Clinical Densitometry and executive summary of the 2007 ISCD Position Development Conference. *J Clin Densitom* **11**(1): 75–91.

21 WHO Study Group on Assessment of Fracture Risk and its Application to Screening for Postmenopausal Osteoporosis (1994) *Assessment of Fracture Risk and Its Application to Screening for Postmenopausal Osteoporosis*. Geneva: World Health Organization; 1994.

22 Kanis JA, on behalf of the World Health Organization Scientific Group (2007) Assessment of osteoporosis at the primary health-care level. Technical Report. World Health Organization Collaborating Centre for Metabolic Bone Diseases, University of Sheffield, UK. Printed by the University of Sheffield.

23 National Osteoporosis Foundation (2008) *Clinician's Guide to Prevention and Treatment of Osteoporosis*. Washington, DC: National Osteoporosis Foundation.

24 Lewiecki EM, Binkley N, Petak SM (2006) DXA quality matters. *J Clin Densitom* **9**(4): 388–92.

25 Shepherd JA, Lu Y, Wilson K, Fuerst T, Genant H, Hangartner TN, *et al.* (2006) Cross-calibration and minimum precision standards for dual-energy x-ray absorptiometry: The 2005 ISCD official positions. *J Clin Densitom* **9**(1): 31–6.

26 Wasnich RD, Miller PD (2000) Antifracture efficacy of antiresorptive agents are related to changes in bone density. *J Clin Endocrinol Metab* **85**(1): 231–6.

27 Cummings SR, Karpf DB, Harris F, Genant HK, Ensrud K, LaCroix AZ, *et al.* (2002) Improvement in spine bone density and reduction in risk of vertebral fractures during treatment with antiresorptive drugs. *Am J Med* **112**: 281–9.

28 Hochberg MC, Greenspan S, Wasnich RD, Miller P, Thompson DE, Ross PD (2002) Changes in bone density and turnover explain the reductions in incidence of nonvertebral fractures that occur during treatment with antiresorptive agents. *J Clin Endocrinol Metab* **87**(4): 1586–92.

29 Austin M, Yang YC, Vittinghoff E, Adami S, Boonen S, Bauer DC, *et al.* (2012) Relationship between bone mineral density changes with denosumab treatment and risk reduction for vertebral and nonvertebral fractures. *J Bone Miner Res* **27**(3): 687–93.

30 Lewiecki EM, Rudolph LA (2002) How common is loss of bone mineral density in elderly clinical practice patients receiving oral bisphosphonate therapy for osteoporosis? *J Bone Miner Res* **17**(Suppl 2): S367.

31 Lewiecki EM, Richmond B, Miller PD (2006) Uses and misuses of quantitative ultrasonography in managing osteoporosis. *Cleve Clin J Med* **73**(8): 742–52.

32 Moayyeri A, Adams JE, Adler RA, Krieg MA, Hans D, Compston J, *et al.* (2012) Quantitative ultrasound of the heel and fracture risk assessment: an updated meta-analysis. *Osteoporos Int* **23**(1): 143–53.

33 Krieg MA, Barkmann R, Gonnelli S, Stewart A, Bauer DC, Del Rio BL, *et al.* (2008) Quantitative ultrasound in the management of osteoporosis: the 2007 ISCD Official Positions. *J Clin Densitom* **11**(1): 163–87.

34 Engelke K, Adams JE, Armbrecht G, Augat P, Bogado CE, Bouxsein ML, *et al.* (2008) Clinical use of quantitative computed tomography and peripheral quantitative computed tomography in the management of osteoporosis in adults: the 2007 ISCD Official Positions. *J Clin Densitom* **11**(1): 123–62.

35 Majumdar S, Link TM, Augat P, Lin JC, Newitt D, Lane NE, *et al.* (1999) Trabecular bone architecture in the distal radius using magnetic resonance imaging in subjects with fractures of the proximal femur. Magnetic Resonance Science Center and Osteoporosis and Arthritis Research Group. *Osteoporos Int* **10**(3): 231–9.

36 Boutroy S, Van RB, Sornay-Rendu E, Munoz F, Bouxsein ML, Delmas PD (2008) Finite element analysis based on in vivo HR-pQCT images of the distal radius is associated with wrist fracture in postmenopausal women. *J Bone Miner Res* **23**(3): 392–9.

37 Garnero P, Sornay-Rendu E, Chapuy M-C, Delmas PD (1996) Increased bone turnover in late postmenopausal women is a major determinant of osteoporosis. *J Bone Miner Res* **11**: 337–49.

38 Ross PD, Knowlton W (1998) Rapid bone loss is associated with increased levels of biochemical markers. *J Bone Miner Res* **13**(2): 297–302.

39 Gerdhem P, Ivaska KK, Alatalo SL, Halleen JM, Hellman J, Isaksson A, *et al.* (2004) Biochemical markers of bone metabolism and prediction of fracture in elderly women. *J Bone Miner Res* **19**(3): 386–93.

40 Greenspan SL, Parker RA, Ferguson L, Rosen HN, Maitland-Ramsey L, Karpf DB (1998) Early changes in biochemical markers of bone turnover predict the long-term response to alendronate therapy in representative elderly women: a randomized clinical trial. *J Bone Miner Res* **13**: 1431–8.

41 Eastell R, Barton I, Hannon RA, Chines A, Garnero P, Delmas PD (2003) Relationship of early changes in bone resorption to the reduction in fracture risk with risedronate. *J Bone Miner Res* **18**: 1051–6.

42 Bauer DC, Black DM, Garnero P, Hochberg M, Ott S, Orloff J, *et al.* (2004) Change in bone turnover and hip, non-spine, and vertebral fracture in alendronate-treated women: the fracture intervention trial. *J Bone Miner Res* **19**(8): 1250–8.

43 Sarkar S, Reginster JY, Crans GG, Diez-Perez A, Pinette KV, Delmas PD (2004) Relationship between changes in biochemical markers of bone turnover and BMD to predict vertebral fracture risk. *J Bone Miner Res* **19**(3): 394–401.

44 Chen P, Satterwhite JH, Licata AA, Lewiecki EM, Sipos AA, Misurski DM, *et al.* (2005) Early changes in biochemical markers of bone formation predict BMD response to teriparatide in postmenopausal women with osteoporosis. *J Bone Miner Res* **20**(6): 962–70.

45 Lewiecki EM, Watts NB (2008) Assessing response to osteoporosis therapy. *Osteoporos Int* **19**(10): 1363–8.

46 Bergmann P, Body JJ, Boonen S, Boutsen Y, Devogelaer JP, Goemaere S, *et al.* (2009) Evidence-based guidelines for the use of biochemical markers of bone turnover in the selection and monitoring of bisphosphonate treatment in osteoporosis: a consensus document of the Belgian Bone Club. *Int J Clin Pract* **63**(1): 19–26.

47 Brown JP, Albert C, Nassar BA, Adachi JD, Cole D, Davison KS, *et al.* (2009) Bone turnover markers in the management of postmenopausal osteoporosis. *Clin Biochem* **42**(10–11): 929–42.

48 Hannon R, Eastell R (2000) Preanalytical variability of biochemical markers of bone turnover. *Osteoporos Int* **11**(Suppl 6): S30–S44.

49 Vasikaran S, Cooper C, Eastell R, Griesmacher A, Morris HA, Trenti T, *et al.* (2011) International Osteoporosis Foundation and International Federation of Clinical Chemistry and Laboratory Medicine Position on bone marker standards in osteoporosis. *Clin Chem Lab Med* **49**(8): 1271–4.

50 Bonnick SL (2011) Going on a drug holiday? *J Clin Densitom* **14**(4): 377–83.

51 Miller PD, Baran DT, Bilezikian JP, Greenspan SL, Lindsay R, Riggs BL, *et al.* (1999) Practical clinical application of biochemical markers of bone turnover: Consensus of an expert panel. *J Clin Densitom* **2**(3): 323–42.

CHAPTER 16

Persistence and Compliance with Medications to Prevent Fractures: Epidemiology, Etiology, and Management Issues

John T. Schousboe

Park Nicollet Health Services *and* University of Minnesota, Minneapolis, MN, USA

Introduction

Optimal reduction of the risk of osteoporotic fractures often requires the use of fracture prevention medications for prolonged periods of time. Many individuals being advised by their physicians to take medications to prevent future adverse health events either do not fill even the first prescription, stop taking them prematurely, or do not take them at the appropriate times in the correct dosage and manner; thereby either eliminating or significantly limiting their effectiveness [1]. In this chapter we will review the medical literature regarding the epidemiology, consequences, and etiology of nonpersistence and noncompliance with fracture prevention medications; and describe interventions to improve both the persistence and compliance with fracture prevention medication.

For the purpose of this chapter, the term "adherence" refers to the collection of ways in which patients' follow recommended instructions for use of medications [2]. As previously discussed by other authors and for the purposes of this chapter, we define *primary nonadherence* as the scenario in which a prescription from a health care provider is never redeemed at a pharmacy. *Secondary nonadherence* is defined by the scenario in which a prescribed medication is filled at least once but is either stopped altogether prematurely (called *nonpersistence*) or the medication is taken at the wrong time intervals or wrong manner (*noncompliance*) [3].

Osteoporosis: Diagnosis and Management, First Edition. Edited by Dale W. Stovall.
© 2013 John Wiley & Sons, Ltd. Published 2013 by John Wiley & Sons, Ltd.

Measurement of medication persistence and adherence

The easiest way to measure medication persistence and adherence is patient self-report. However, patients tend to overestimate the degree to which they are adherent with their medications, possibly because they fear being labeled as noncompliant. Carefully worded questions that remove this social desirability bias allow for the use of self-report to assess whether or not a person has discontinued medication (has become nonpersistent); however, due to recall bias, self-report is still a poor method to quantify the degree of medication noncompliance.

In addition to self-report, a very common method used to measure non-adherence is the use of pharmacy claims data. Pharmacy claims records typically have information regarding the date a prescription was filled, the dose per tablet, prescribing instructions (how many tablets are pre-scribed to be taken at a time, how often, and under what specific circum-stances if any apply) and the number of tablets that were dispensed. From these data, the date that the person would be expected to have used up their medication, if taken consistently as prescribed, can be calculated. The actual date that the person has taken all of the tablets is assumed to be the date of the next refill. The number of days the prescription was *expected* to last can be divided by the number of days it *actually* lasted. This ratio is called the *Percent Days Covered (PDC)*, and represents the proportion of days in between the two fills of medication that the patient could have taken the medication in the prescribed manner. Most studies somewhat arbitrar-ily define full compliance with a medication as the time periods during which the PDC was ≥80%.

At some point, if a medication is not refilled beyond the expected date, it is likely that the person has stopped taking the medication altogether (become nonpersistent). Generally, a person is considered to have become nonpersistent when this gap is 1.5 to 2 times as long as the expected time period between refills of the medication.

Epidemiology of medication nonadherence

Strikingly, the time course of medication nonadherence is similar across chronic conditions, particularly if the condition is asymptomatic in the present time and medication is being advised to reduce the risk of adverse health events that may occur in the future [1]. In the United States, 15–22% of all prescriptions are never filled [4–6]. Among individuals who do fill their first prescription of a new therapy, about 30% of them do not fill it a second time, and by one year about 50% of those who filled the first prescription have become nonpersistent [7]. Non-persistence with oral medications to prevent osteoporotic fracture, or to treat hypertension, hyperlipidemia, or diabetes mellitus is remarkably similar, with only 30% to 55% remaining on the medication one year after its initiation.[1] However, among bisphosphonate users, up to 60% restart medication (usually a different medication than the first one) after becoming nonpersistent with the first medication [8].

Adherence with weekly oral bisphosphonates has been shown to be modestly better than with daily bisphosphonates [9, 10], but it remains controversial as to whether or not adherence with oral monthly bisphosphonate therapy is better than with weekly therapy [11, 12]. Surveys generally show that patients would prefer once yearly intravenous therapy over oral bisphosphonate therapy [13]. However, the only study that has evaluated persistence with IV zoledronic acid in the context of clinical practice reported that only 36% of those who had received an initial infusion returned one year later and agreed to receive a second infusion [14].

There are no specific characteristics of patients that have consistently been shown to be associated with nonadherence. Age [9, 15–23], gender [6, 24, 25], race [26–31] and health claims for previous fractures [15, 18, 20, 21, 32] have not been consistently linked to nonadherence. Having had a bone density test [20, 33] and accurate knowledge of the results of that test [34–37] are associated with persistence to fracture prevention medication.

Cognitive impairment adversely affects adherence to oral medications used to treat a variety of chronic illnesses [38–42]. Although the affect of depression on adherence to fracture prevention medication has not been reported, depression has been shown to adversely affect adherence to medications used to treat diabetes mellitus [43–46], HIV [47], and hypercholesterolemia [48]. With these two exceptions, comorbidity has not been consistently shown to adversely affect medication adherence [40, 49–52].

Consequences of nonpersistence and noncompliance with fracture prevention medications

A recent meta-analysis based on 27 studies of pharmacy utilization databases estimated hazard ratios of incident clinical fractures to be 1.28 and 1.32, respectively in those with poor compliance or poor persistence compared to those with high compliance and persistence [53]. Among patients with documented osteoporosis at the femoral neck (T-score ≤ -2.5), Rabenda and colleagues noted a linear 4% increase in the incidence of hip for every 10% decrease in compliance (assessed as percent days covered from pharmacy claims) [54]. Landfeldt and colleagues showed that patients who were persistent with fracture prevention medication for 1 month to 1 year, 1 to 2 years, and 2 to 3 years respectively had hazard ratios for hospitalization due to acute fracture of 0.86, 0.67, and 0.59 compared to untreated individuals [24]. Costs attributable to fractures and wasted medication are associated with noncompliance [55]. Two studies have documented increases in *total* medical costs associated with poor compliance with fracture prevention medications ranging from 3.5% to 18% depending on the study population [56, 57].

Etiology of nonadherence to fracture prevention medication

Given the pervasive nature and consequences of osteoporosis medication nonadherence, understanding the etiology of the phenomenon is critical to craft practical management strategies that may mitigate the problem. While side effects are the most commonly reported reason for stopping medication [58, 59], they account for only a portion of the phenomenon of poor medication adherence.

Several common themes have emerged from focus group studies of patients being treated for osteoporosis, hypertension, epilepsy, diabetes, and other chronic diseases. Included are the fact that most patients need to be convinced that they have a health problem that requires a solution, that nonmedicinal solutions that are not as effective as proposed medications, and that the proposed medication is safe. Ambivalence regarding use of medications is very common. While the majority of patients in one survey study agreed with the statement "modern medicines have improved people's health," [60] many worry about the risk of harm from medications [61–65], sometimes linking such risks to perceptions that medications are artificial and foreign to the human body (Table 16.1) [61–66]. Some describe feeling a sense of loss of control when agreeing to take medication [65–68], and dislike the sense that that their health status depends on taking medication [62–67, 69]. Taking medication can also challenge a person's social identity in part by forcing them to accept that they do have an illness or health condition that requires management and the accompanying sense of vulnerability [62–64, 67, 69]. Many patients perceive that physicians are too quick to suggest medication as a solution to a medical problem and overprescribe medications [61, 63–65].

Dowell and Hudson found a range of beliefs about medications in their focus group study that could be categorized into three groups (Figure 16.1) [70]. "Believers" in medications were more likely to have faith in their physicians' recommendations to take medication and accept their illness.

Table 16.1 Qualitative studies of patients' medication concerns.

Study/citation/ diagnoses	Direct harm*	Dependence	Loss of social identity	Loss of control over health management	Artificiality of meds	Lack of understanding how they work	Physician overuse or misuse of medication
				Fear/concern			
Unson et al., 2003 osteoporosis [61]	X				X	X	X
Britten, 1994, general practice [62]	X	X	X		X		
Conrad, 1985, epilepsy [67]		X	X	X			
Adams, 1997, asthma [69]		X	X				
Lin et al., 2003, depression [63]	X	X	X		X		X
Donovan, 1992, rheumatoid arthritis [66]		X		X	X	X	
Benson & Britten, 2002, hypertension [64]	X	X	X		X		X
Horne, 1999, renal failure or MI [65]	X	X		X	X	X	X

*Especially with long-term or continuous use.

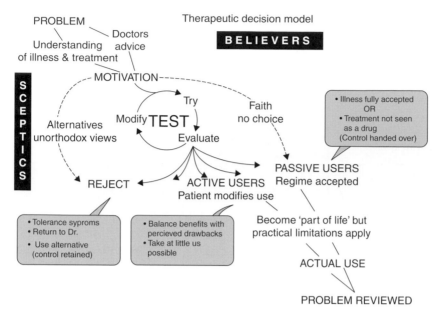

Figure 16.1 Therapeutic decision model regarding medication use. (*Source*: Dowell J, Hudson H (1997) [70]).

"Skeptics" were more likely to distrust medications and embrace non-medicinal remedies. A third group of "active medication users" were likely to actively consider perceived benefits and drawbacks to taking medication, and were prone to alter the use of the medication to limit their exposure. Sale and colleagues have recently reported that about half of all patients found the decision as to whether or not to take fracture prevention medication a difficult one and weighed carefully the perceived risks and benefits of the medication (similar to the "active medication users" in Dowell and Hudson's study) [71]. Half of this subset chose not to start fracture prevention medication.

Several explanatory conceptual frameworks incorporating these concepts for medication nonadherence have been proposed over the last few decades, most of which were based on social cognition theories such as the Health Belief Model [72–74]. The Extended Health Belief Model posits medication adherence as a decision-making process whereby the patient weighs the perceived benefits of undertaking the medication, the perceived barriers to carrying out medication use behavior, and whether or not they perceive they have the ability to successfully take the medication in the context of their daily lives (medication use self-efficacy) (Figure 16.2) [75–77]. Whether or not the problem is of sufficient magnitude to warrant intervention depends on the perceived susceptibility to the

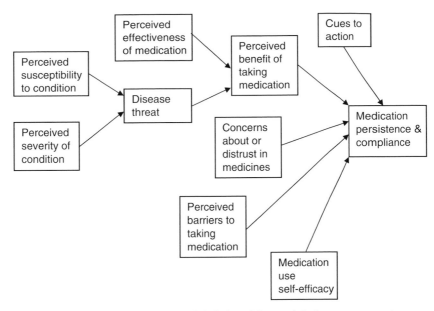

Figure 16.2 Modified extended health belief model to explain fracture prevention medication use behavior.

problem, and the perceived severity of the condition should it occur. However, a patient also needs to have the confidence that they can successfully take the medication in the context of their daily lives (medication use self-efficacy), and the skills to actually do so. Five of six studies that than have evaluated the association between medication beliefs and fracture prevention medication use behavior have postulated an additional predictor of medication use behavior, *concerns about* or *distrust in medications.* Concerns about or distrust in medications is a construct separate from actually experienced side effects.

Perceived benefits from taking fracture prevention medication

Other than the experience of actual side effects, the perceived benefit from taking fracture prevention medication is perhaps the strongest predictor of overall adherence and specifically persistence with fracture prevention medication. Cline and colleagues showed that perceived benefits of taking an antiresorptive drug, as measured by the Osteoporosis Health Belief Scale, were modestly associated with self-reported use of the antiresorptive agent (odds ratio 1.34) [78]. Similarly, McHorney and colleagues documented those in the lowest tertile of drug effectiveness beliefs were far more likely to be noncompliant with fracture prevention medication compared to those in the top tertile (odds ratio 5.70) [79]. Yood and colleagues showed that patients with strong effectiveness beliefs compared to those with weak effectiveness beliefs in fracture prevention medication had an odds ratio of 2.04 of filling an initial prescription for a fracture prevention medication (primary adherence) [80].

Schousboe and colleagues subsumed perceived effectiveness under the concept of *perceived necessity of medication* [81, 82], postulating that perceived necessity would reflect belief not only in the effectiveness of the medication, but that better nonmedicinal alternatives were not available. Among 686 surveyed patients with medical record evidence of at least one prescription for bisphosphonate therapy, the odds ratio of self-reported nonpersistence was 0.54 for each standard deviation increase in perceived need for fracture prevention medication [81]. However, perceived need for medication was not associated with self reported noncompliance (missing doses).

Perceived susceptibility to and severity of fractures

Three studies have found that perceived susceptibility to fractures is associated with fracture prevention medication adherence as assessed via both self-report [78, 82] and pharmacy claims [83]. Two of these studies have also documented an association between perceived severity (health effects) of fractures and fracture prevention medication adherence [82, 83].

Concerns about or distrust in medication

Yood and colleagues found that those with a strong distrust for medications were only half as likely to fill a prescription for a fracture prevention medication at least once (primary nonadherence) [80]. Other studies have documented a modest association of concerns about medications with self-reported nonpersistence [84], and with noncompliance assessed by pharmacy claims [79] or self-report [84].

Barriers to medication utilization
Medication costs

Financial out of pocket cost can be an important barrier to prescription drug utilization, at least among low income populations [85]. Cost has been cited by some patients as a reason they stopped taking fracture prevention medication [37, 86], and the extent of prescription drug coverage is associated with use of fracture prevention medication [9, 27, 87–92]. Medication utilization decreases when out of pocket drug costs increase through either elimination of prescription drug coverage [93–95], or increases in medication co-pays or co-insurance [96–100].

Regimen complexity

Concomitant prescription for multiple additional medications is associated with lower persistence with fracture prevention and other medications in some [20, 21], but not all studies [101–104]. Regimen complexity, defined as the number of medication doses per day one has to take, has been consistently associated with poor medication compliance [31, 105–108].

Social support

Social support is in general associated with better health status [109, 110]. Emotional and informational social support have been shown to be associated with compliance to a wide variety of health behaviors, including keeping physician appointments, dietary compliance, blood glucose monitoring among those with diabetes, and medication compliance. Instrumental social support, defined as actions by others that directly facilitate one's use of medications (such as putting medications out or giving reminders to take medication) has been the most consistently associated with compliance. This may be particularly important to sustain compliance among the cognitively impaired or frail elderly.

Medication use self-efficacy

Self-efficacy, defined as the belief that one is capable of action that can result in favorable outcomes, has been linked to better health status and specifically to a sense of personal behavioral control, more optimistic outcomes expectations, higher motivation to act, and greater effort to achieve the target behavior or outcome [111]. Among patients with osteoporosis who are being treated with fracture prevention medications, two studies have documented a positive association between medication use self-efficacy and fracture prevention medication adherence [84, 112]. In Schousboe's study, those in the lowest quartile of medication use self-efficacy were more likely to be nonpersistent, but there was little difference in persistence among those with self-efficacy greater than the lower quartile. In contrast, those in the highest quartile of self-efficacy had an odds ratio of 0.09 for noncompliance compared to those in the lowest quartile [84]. These findings suggest that a mild level of self-efficacy is necessary for the patient to maintain an active prescription for the medication, but that compliance improves further with higher levels of self-efficacy.

Physician–patient relationship

In spite of a patient's access to medical information through friends, relatives, medical advocacy groups, and the internet; the physician actually prescribing the medication typically is in command of more knowledge and expertise than the patient [113, 114]. Hence, in view of being unable to fully independently confirm or refute information the physician provides, the patient's *trust in the physician* may have a significant association with acceptance of and adherence to medication recommended by that physician [115–117]. This is conceptualized by Hall to consist of trust in the physician's competence, that the physician puts the patient's interests first, that the physician is not following an agenda contrary to those interests, that the physician is honest, and that the physician will honor the patient's confidentiality [118].

Few studies have specifically examined the association between the patient's trust in their physician and medication use behavior. Piette and colleagues found that patients with type 2 diabetes who were troubled by the cost of their medications were more likely to adhere to them if they had a high level of trust in their physician [119]. Wroth and colleagues found that a patient's lack of trust that their physician could help them and patient perceptions that the physician was not concerned about them were associated with self-reported nonpersistence [120].

Among patients with osteoporosis, Yood and colleagues found that trust in the physician was nearly significantly associated with primary adherence to fracture prevention medication (p-value = 0.67), but that this possible relationship disappeared when adjusted for medication effectiveness beliefs and distrust of medications [80]. Schousboe and colleagues noted that trust in the physician was indirectly associated with self-reported bisphosphonate persistence and compliance; that a higher level of trust in physician was associated with higher perceived necessity of fracture prevention medication and lower concerns about that medication, and that these in turn were associated with persistence and compliance (Figure 16.3) [121].

The concept of trust in the physician has been thought by some authors to include patient perceptions of how well the physician communicates with them, and patient satisfaction with the physician's decision making style. Open affiliative communication refers to patient perceptions that the physician is disclosing all relevant information about the target disease and medication proposed to treat it, listens to the patient's concerns carefully, and addresses all of the patient's questions and concerns [122]. Physician decision making style has been conceptualized as falling into one of three categories; the physician takes full charge of the medical decisions to be made, the patient takes full charge and tells the physician what they want done, or a middle category where the patient and physician share the decision making and come to a consensus as to what to do [123, 124]. In the path analysis of Schousboe *et al.*, physician open communication from

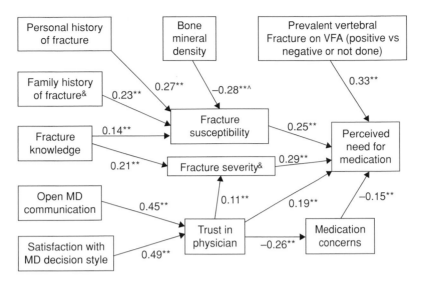

*p-value of association <0.05   **p-value of association <0.01
^Per one unit increase of worst T-score of lumbar spine, total hip, femoral neck, or forearm
&Family history of fracture effect on fracture severity 0.19 (p-value = 0.06)

Figure 16.3 Predictors of perceived need for fracture prevention medication. (*Source*: Schousboe JT *et al.* (2011) [82]).

the patient's perception and patient satisfaction with the decision making style of the physician were not associated with perceived necessity of medication and concerns about medication independent of trust, but were strongly associated with trust in the physician (Figure 16.3) [121]. Hence, open communication and patient satisfaction with the physician's decision making style may be necessary for patients to trust their physician, and the effects of these two variables on medication use behavior may be indirect through trust in the physician primarily and through medication beliefs secondarily.

A recent survey study suggests that patients and physicians view the level of fracture risk at which fracture prevention medication is appropriate quite differently. While the median 10-year risk of hip fracture at which physicians thought fracture prevention medication should be prescribed was 10%, the median 10-year risk of hip fracture at which patients though fracture prevention medication should be taken was 50% [125]. Although physicians and patients rank-ordered the severity of osteoporosis as a disease compared to other chronic conditions (such as hypertension, breast cancer, diabetes and arthritis) similarly, it remains unclear if the patients in this study had the same understanding of the quality of life consequences of osteoporotic fractures as the physicians.

Interventions to improve medication adherence

Many interventions to improve adherence to medication to treat chronic conditions have been tried. The taxonomy of these interventions are complex (Table 16.2), but can be characterized as: a) educational efforts in regards to the medication and the target condition, delivered as written material or orally in person, or both; b) involving patients more actively in their care, such as improving their skills and actions in monitoring their blood sugar and blood pressure; c) improving their social support by engaging spouses and family members; c) follow-up phone call reminders, automated or manual; or d) helping patients organize their medications to fit their day to day task requirements and lifestyle, including use of pill organizers.[126, 127]

Simple interventions employing only one of the interventions listed above typically have failed to improve adherence. Successful interventions have usually combined in-depth educational efforts with simplified medication regimens and follow-up (often by telephone) to assess and encourage adherence to the medication regimen.[128] With few exceptions [129], the magnitude of success of these intervention studies to improve adherence to fracture prevention medications has at best been modest [127, 130].

Eleven investigations of interventions to improve adherence to fracture prevention medication have been published to date, and the findings of these studies are quite similar to what has been reported regarding medication adherence in other chronic diseases (Table 16.2). Formal education about osteoporosis and the consequences of fractures, delivered either as written material or orally at the time of fracture prevention medication has failed in two studies to improve persistence based on either pharmacy claims [131] or self-reported adherence [132]. Follow-up phone calls from a nurse by itself was unsuccessful at improving persistence with fracture prevention medication one year after the initial prescription [133]. Follow-up monthly reminders to patients prescribed once monthly ibandronate was associated with better adherence than with once weekly alendronate, but it remains unclear if the improved adherence was attributable to the longer dosing interval or the reminder phone calls [134]. However, nurse follow-up visits in person did improve compliance with raloxifene (PDC 68%) compared with no intervention (PDC 42%) [135]. Similarly, follow-up phone calls combined with management by an osteoporosis specialty clinic did improve persistence at one year (assessed by pharmacy claims) to 69%, compared to 45% for a control group sent back to usual care with their primary care physician [136].

Some have postulated that demonstrating the positive biologic effect of fracture prevention medication by showing a reduction in markers of bone

Table 16.2 Interventional studies to improve adherence to fracture prevention medications.

Reference/study	Study design	Patient population/setting	*Type of intervention	Results
Shu, 2009 [131]	Cluster RCT (prescribing physicians randomized) both physician & patient education vs. usual care	Blue Cross Blue Shield of New Jersey Insurees (1867 patients nested in 436 providers)	1	Negative; median PDC (pharmacy claims) 74% intervention group 73% control group
Guilera, 2006 [132]	Cluster RCT (prescribing physicians randomized) review of educational leaflet vs. no intervention	745 Women age ≥50 years prescribed Raloxifene	1	Negative; by Moriskey scale 56% of intervention group & 62% of control group highly adherent
Cooper, 2006 [134]	RCT; Ibandronate + education + monthly phone reminders Vs. Alendronate	1103 United Kingdom patients with osteoporosis recruited from primary care practices	2	Positive: persistence at 6 months (pharmacy claims) Ibandronate+ patient support: 56.6% Alendronate: 38.6%
Schousboe, 2005 [133]	RCT; Nurse education plus phone calls every 3 months vs. usual care	310 postmenopausal women in one clinical U.S. clinic	2	Negative; nurse group vs. usual care initiating Rx: odds ratio 1.10 still on Rx 1 year later: odds ratio 0.95
Waalen, 2009 [136]	RCT; education plus monthly follow-up phone calls	235 women age 60 and older with newly diagnosed osteoporosis at U.S. Staff Model HMO	3	Positive; by pharmacy claims 69% of intervention on Rx 1 year later 45% of control group on Rx 1 year later
Clowes, 2004 [135]	RCT: (1) Nurse follow-up 3 monthly visits vs. (2) Nurse follow-up visits + bone markers (BTMs) vs. (3) No intervention	75 post-menopausal women age 50 to 80 recruited at academic metabolic bone disease center in U.K.	4	Positive for nurse education & follow-up PDC ≥ 75% (pharmacy claims): no monitoring (control): 42% nurse education & follow-up only: 68% nurse education, follow-up, BTMs: 63%

(continued)

Table 16.2 (*Continued*)

Reference/study	Study design	Patient population/setting	*Type of intervention	Results
Delmas, 2007 [137]	RCT: (1) Intervention: bone marker Test feedback at 3 and 6 months + education (2) Control: education alone	2382 postmenopausal women age 65 to 80 years with new diagnosis osteoporosis prescribed risedronate; 171 centers worldwide	4	Negative: persistence at 1 year (electronic pill cap monitoring) bone marker feedback group 80% control group 77%
Silverman, 2012 [138]	RCT four groups: (1) Education + BTM feed back; (2) Education alone;(3) BTM feedback alone; (4) No intervention	240 postmenopausal women with T-score <−2.0 from two U.S. health care delivery groups	4	Negative; adjusted odds ratios of persistence vs. control: education alone 0.95; BTM feedback alone 1.09;education + BMT feedback 1.18
Cook, 2007 [142]	Observational cohort: nurse counseling with motivational interviewing for subset to be at high risk for nonadherence; Comparison to historical controls	402 individuals prescribed risedronate by 57 practitioners (94% female, age range 30 to 94 years) 260 judged to be at high risk for nonadherence recieved intervention	5	Positive: cohort persistence at 3 months 77%; at 6 months 69% For national control group prescribed risedronate: persistence at 3 months 67%; at 6 months 40%

Solomon, 2011 [143]	RCT: Intervention; telephone-based counseling using motivational interviewing Control; mailed educational materials	2097 participants recruited from state-run pharmacy benefits program in U.S. for low-income adults age 65 & older 1046 intervention, 1041 controls	5	Borderline positive: median PDC over 1 year: intervention 49%, control 41% (p-value for difference = 0.07)
Lai, 2011 [146]	RCT: Intervention; pharmacist education & monthly counseling phone calls. Control; no intervention	198 with new diagnosis of osteoporosis (T-score $\leq$ −2.5) in Malaysia 100 intervention, 98 control	6	Negative (pharmacy claims) persistence at 1 year: intervention 87%, control 89%

*Types of Interventions.
1. Education only at time of visit.
2. Education only, at time of visit and with follow-up educational phone calls.
3. Specialty care management plus education follow-up educational phone calls.
4. Use of bone markers plus education.
5. Psychologically based counseling (motivational interviewing or cognitive behavioral).
6. Pharmacist education, review of medications, and monthly phone calls.

turnover within the first three months of therapy may improve compliance and persistence. Three studies of the effect of feedback to patients regarding the changes in bone turnover markers have been done to date, and all showed no effect of the bone marker information on medication compliance or persistence [135, 137, 138]. Those with no change in bone turnover markers are much more likely to be noncompliant and/or nonpersistent with fracture prevention medication, but the changes in bone turnover markers appear to be an indicator of, rather than a direct influence on medication use behavior [137].

All of the intervention studies described above applied interventions to groups of patients regardless of the specific barriers or concerns that patients may have and that vary from individual to individual [139]. Counseling using motivational interviewing techniques is designed to elicit from patients their specific goals and what barriers or concerns they have regarding use of medication to achieve those goals, and then to attempt to address and/or resolve those barriers and concerns [140, 141]. Among 402 patients who were prescribed risedronate, Cook and colleagues counseled 260 patients, who were considered to be at high risk for nonadherence, using motivational interviewing and cognitive-behavior techniques. Persistence among the total cohort at 3 and 6 months, respectively, was 77% and 69%. In contrast, for a historical control group prescribed risedronate persistence at 3 and 6 months, respectively, was 67% and 40% [142]. However, a randomized controlled trial of 2097 patients prescribed a fracture prevention medication found that follow-up counseling using motivational interviewing techniques delivered by telephone only marginally improved persistence one year after the initial prescription (49% for the intervention group and 41% for the control group) [143].

Pharmacist-led education and counseling regarding the importance of medication adherence has been used to successfully improve medication adherence in other conditions such as HIV [144] and hypercholesterolemia [145]. Only one study of a pharmacist-led intervention to improve adherence to fracture prevention medication has been reported thus far. This study employed initial pharmacist education at the start of fracture prevention therapy followed by monthly counseling phone calls from the pharmacist. No benefit from the pharmacist intervention was noted in this study, but persistence at one year was very high in both the intervention group (87%) and the control group (89%) [146].

Summary

Nonadherence to fracture prevention medication remains a substantial barrier to efforts to reduce the societal burden of osteoporotic fractures along with their associated costs and loss of quality of life. Efforts to reduce nonadherence to fracture prevention medication thus far have at best been only modestly successful. A long path of research and inquiry may be required to better characterize and understand this phenomenon in order to develop interventions that reduce nonadherence with better success than what has been achieved to date.

References

1 Yeaw J, *et al.* (2009) Comparing adherence and persistence across 6 chronic medication classes. *Journal of Managed Care Pharmacy* **15**(9): 728–40.
2 World Health Organization (2003) Adherence to Long-Term Therapies: Evidence for Action 2003 [cited March 27, 2012]; available from: www.who.int/chp/knowledge/publications/adherence_report/en/.
3 Cramer JA, *et al.* (2008) Medication compliance and persistence: terminology and definitions. *Value in Health* **11**(1): 44–7.
4 Shah NR, *et al.* (2009) Factors associated with first-fill adherence rates for diabetic medications: a cohort study. *Journal of General Internal Medicine* **24**(2): 233–7.
5 Shah NR, *et al.* (2009) Predictors of first-fill adherence for patients with hypertension. *Am J Hypertens* **22**(4): 392–6.
6 Fischer MA, *et al.* (2010) Primary medication non-adherence: analysis of 195,930 electronic prescriptions. *Journal of General Internal Medicine* **25**(4): 284–90.
7 Kothawala P, *et al.* (2007) Systematic review and meta-analysis of real-world adherence to drug therapy for osteoporosis. *Mayo Clin Proc* **82**(12): 1493–1501.
8 Burden AM, *et al.* (2012) Bisphosphonate prescribing, persistence and cumulative exposure in Ontario, Canada. *Osteoporos Int* **23**(3): 1075–82.
9 Recker RR, Gallagher R, MacCosbe PE (2005) Effect of dosing frequency on bisphosphonate medication adherence in a large longitudinal cohort of women. *Mayo Clin Proc* **80**(7): 856–61.
10 Ettinger MP, Gallagher R, MacCosbe PE (2006) Medication persistence with weekly versus daily doses of orally administered bisphosphonates. *Endocr Pract* **12**(5): 522–8.
11 Weiss TW, *et al.* (2007) Persistence across weekly and monthly bisphosphonates: analysis of US retail pharmacy prescription refills. *Curr Med Res Opin* **23**(9): 2193–2203.
12 Rossini M, *et al.* (2009) Once-monthly oral ibandronate in postmenopausal osteoporosis: translation and updated review. *Clinical Therapeutics* **31**(7): 1497–1510.
13 Hadji P, *et al.* (2012) Quality of life and health status with zoledronic acid and generic alendronate-a secondary analysis of the Rapid Onset and Sustained Efficacy (ROSE) study in postmenopausal women with low bone mass. *Osteoporos Int* **23**(7): 2043–51.
14 Lee Y-K, *et al.* (2012) Persistence with intravenous zoledronate in elderly patients with osteoporosis. *Osteoporosis International* **23**(9): 2329–33.
15 Papaioannou A, *et al.* (2003) Adherence to bisphosphonates and hormone replacement therapy in a tertiary care setting of patients in the CANDOO database. *Osteoporos Int* **14**(10): 808–13.

16 Briesacher BA, *et al.* (2008) Comparison of drug adherence rates among patients with seven different medical conditions. *Pharmacotherapy* **28**(4): 437–43.

17 Jones TJ, Petrella RJ, Crilly R (2008) Determinants of persistence with weekly bisphosphonates in patients with osteoporosis. *J Rheumatol* **35**(9): 1865–73.

18 McCombs JS, *et al.* (2004) Compliance with drug therapies for the treatment and prevention of osteoporosis. *Maturitas* **48**(3): 271–87.

19 Penning-van Beest FJ, *et al.* (2008) Determinants of non-compliance with bisphosphonates in women with postmenopausal osteoporosis. *Curr Med Res Opin* **24**(5): 1337–44.

20 Solomon DH, *et al.* (2005) Compliance with osteoporosis medications. *Arch Intern Med* **165**(20): 2414–19.

21 Lo JC, *et al.* (2006) Persistence with weekly alendronate therapy among postmenopausal women. *Osteoporos Int* **17**(6): 922–8.

22 Downey TW, *et al.* (2006) Adherence and persistence associated with the pharmacologic treatment of osteoporosis in a managed care setting. *South Med J* **99**(6): 570–5.

23 Carr AJ, Thompson PW, Cooper C (2006) Factors associated with adherence and persistence to bisphosphonate therapy in osteoporosis: a cross-sectional survey. *Osteoporos Int* **17**(11): 1638–44.

24 Landfeldt E, *et al.* (2012) Adherence to treatment of primary osteoporosis and its association to fractures – the Swedish Adherence Register Analysis (SARA). *Osteoporos Int* **23**(2): 433–43.

25 Devine J, *et al.* (2012) A retrospective analysis of extended-interval dosing and the impact on bisphosphonate compliance in the US Military Health System. *Osteoporos Int* **23**(4): 1415–24.

26 Benner JS, *et al.* (2002) Long-term persistence in use of statin therapy in elderly patients. *JAMA* **288**(4): 455–61.

27 Ellis JJ, *et al.* (2004) Suboptimal statin adherence and discontinuation in primary and secondary prevention populations. *J Gen Intern Med* **19**(6): 638–45.

28 Monane M, *et al.* (1996) Compliance with antihypertensive therapy among elderly Medicaid enrollees: the roles of age, gender, and race. *Am J Public Health* **86**(12): 1805–8.

29 Ellis J (1998) Prospective memory and medicine taking, in LB. Myers, K Midence (eds.), *Adherence to Treatment in Medical Conditions*. Amsterdam: Harwood Academic Publishers, pp. 113–31.

30 Monane M, *et al.* (1997) The effects of initial drug choice and comorbidity on antihypertensive therapy compliance: results from a population-based study in the elderly. *Am J Hypertens* **10**(7 Pt 1): 697–704.

31 Eisen SA, *et al.* (1990) The effect of prescribed daily dose frequency on patient medication compliance. *Arch Intern Med* **150**(9): 1881–4.

32 Zambon A, *et al.* (2008) Discontinuity and failures of therapy with bisphosphonates: joint assessment of predictors with multi-state models. *Pharmacoepidemiol Drug Saf* **17**(3): 260–9.

33 Pressman A, *et al.* (2001) Initiation of osteoporosis treatment after bone mineral density testing. *Osteoporos Int* **12**(5): 337–42.

34 Solomon DH, Levin E, Helfgott SM (2000) Patterns of medication use before and after bone densitometry: factors associated with appropriate treatment. *J Rheumatol* **27**(6): 1496–1500.

35 Rubin SM, Cummings SR (1992) Results of bone densitometry affect women's decisions about taking measures to prevent fractures. *Ann Intern Med* **116**(12 Pt 1): 990–5.

36 Silverman SL, *et al.* (1997) Effect of bone density information on decisions about hormone replacement therapy: a randomized trial. *Obstet Gynecol* **89**(3): 321–5.

37 Pickney CS, Arnason JA (2005) Correlation between patient recall of bone densitometry results and subsequent treatment adherence. *Osteoporos Int* **16**(9): 1156–60.

38 Gould ON, McDonald-Miszcak L, King B (1997) Metacognition and medication adherence: how do older adults remember? *Experimental Aging Research* **23**: 315–42.

39 Rosen MI, *et al.* (2003) Neuropsychological correlates of suboptimal adherence to metformin. *J Behav Med.* **26**(4): 349–60.

40 Gray SL, Mahoney JE, Blough DK (2001) Medication adherence in elderly patients receiving home health services following hospital discharge. *Ann Pharmacother* **35**(5): 539–45.

41 Salas M, *et al.* (2001) Impaired cognitive function and compliance with anti-hypertensive drugs in elderly: the Rotterdam Study. *Clin Pharmacol Ther* **70**(6): 561–6.

42 Kiortsis DN, *et al.* (2000) Factors associated with low compliance with lipid-lowering drugs in hyperlipidemic patients. *J Clin Pharm Ther* **25**(6): 445–51.

43 Kilbourne AM, *et al.* (2005) How does depression influence diabetes medication adherence in older patients? *Am J Geriatr Psychiatry* **13**(3): 202–10.

44 Lerman I *et al.* (2004) Psychosocial factors associated with poor diabetes self-care management in a specialized center in Mexico City. *Biomed Pharmacother* **58**(10): 566–70.

45 Lin EH, *et al.* (2004) Relationship of depression and diabetes self-care, medication adherence, and preventive care. *Diabetes Care* **27**(9): 2154–60.

46 Park H, *et al.* (2004) Individuals with type 2 diabetes and depressive symptoms exhibited lower adherence with self-care. *J Clin Epidemiol* **57**(9): 978–84.

47 van Servellen G, *et al.* (2002) Individual and system level factors associated with treatment nonadherence in human immunodeficiency virus-infected men and women. *AIDS Patient Care STDS* **16**(6): 269–81.

48 Stilley CS, *et al.* (2004) Psychological and cognitive function: predictors of adherence with cholesterol lowering treatment. *Ann Behav Med* **27**(2): 117–24.

49 McLane CG, Zyzanski SJ, Flocke SA (1995) Factors associated with medication non-compliance in rural elderly hypertensive patients. *Am J Hypertens* **8**(2): 206–9.

50 McElnay JC, *et al.* (1997) Self-reported medication non-compliance in the elderly. *Eur J Clin Pharmacol* **53**(3–4): 171–8.

51 Coons SJ, *et al.* (1994) Predictors of medication noncompliance in a sample of older adults. *Clin Ther* **16**(1): 110–17.

52 Hulka BS, *et al.* (1976) Communication, compliance, and concordance between physicians and patients with prescribed medications. *Am J Public Health* **66**(9): 847–53.

53 Ross S, *et al.* (2011) A meta-analysis of osteoporotic fracture risk with medication nonadherence. *Value in Health* **14**(4): 571–81.

54 Rabenda V, *et al.* (2008) Adherence to bisphosphonates therapy and hip fracture risk in osteoporotic women. *Osteoporos Int* **19**(6): 811–18.

55 Sheehy O, *et al.*, Adherence to weekly oral bisphosphonate therapy: cost of wasted drugs and fractures. *Osteoporosis International* **20**(9): 1583–94.

56 Halpern R, *et al.* (2011) The association of adherence to osteoporosis therapies with fracture, all-cause medical costs, and all-cause hospitalizations: a retrospective claims analysis of female health plan enrollees with osteoporosis. *Journal of Managed Care Pharmacy* **17**(1): 25–39.

57 Sunyecz JA, *et al.* (2008) Impact of compliance and persistence with bisphosphonate therapy on health care costs and utilization. *Osteoporos Int* **19**(10): 1421–9.

58 Tosteson AN, *et al.* (2003) Early discontinuation of treatment for osteoporosis. *Am J Med* **115**(3): 209–16.

59 Hamilton B, McCoy K, Taggart H (2003) Tolerability and compliance with risedronate in clinical practice. *Osteoporos Int* **14**(3): 259–62.

60 Britten N, Ukoumunne OC, Boulton MG (2002) Patients' attitudes to medicines and expectations for prescriptions. *Health Expect* **5**(3): 256–69.

61 Unson CG, *et al.* (2003) Nonadherence and osteoporosis treatment preferences of older women: a qualitative study. *J Women's Health (Larchmt)* **12**(10): 1037–45.

62 Britten N (1994) Patients' ideas about medicines: a qualitative study in a general practice population. *Br J Gen Pract* **44**(387): 465–8.

63 Lin EH, *et al.* (2003) Enhancing adherence to prevent depression relapse in primary care. *Gen Hosp Psychiatry* **25**(5): 303–10.

64 Benson J, Britten N (2002) Patients' decisions about whether or not to take antihypertensive drugs: qualitative study. *BMJ* **325**(7369): 873.

65 Horne R, Weinman J, Hankins M (1999) The Beliefs about Medications Questionnaire: the development of a new method for assessing the cognitive representation about medication. *Psychol Health* **14**: 1–24.

66 Donovan JL, Blake DR (1992) Patient non-compliance: deviance or reasoned decision-making? *Soc Sci Med* **34**(5): 507–13.

67 Conrad P (1985) The meaning of medications: another look at compliance. *Soc Sci Med* **20**(1): 29–37.

68 Shoemaker SJ, *et al.* (2011) The medication experience: Preliminary evidence of its value for patient education and counseling on chronic medications. *Patient Education and Counseling* **83**(3): 443–50.

69 Adams S, Pill R, Jones A (1997) Medication, chronic illness and identity: the perspective of people with asthma. *Soc Sci Med* **45**(2): 189–201.

70 Dowell J, Hudson H (1997) A qualitative study of medication-taking behaviour in primary care. *Fam Pract* **14**(5): 369–75.

71 Sale JEM, *et al.* (2011) Decision to take osteoporosis medication in patients who have had a fracture and are "high" risk for future fracture: a qualitative study. *BMC Musculoskeletal Disorders*, **12**: 92.

72 Becker MH, *et al.* (1977) The Health Belief Model and prediction of dietary compliance: a field experiment. *J Health Soc Behav* **18**(4): 348–66.

73 Janz N, Becker M (1984) The Health Belief Model: a decade later. *Health Education Quarterly* **11**(1): 1–47.

74 Sheeran P, Abraham C (1995) The Health Belief Model, in M Connor, P Norman (eds.), *Predicting Health Behavior*. Philadelphia: Open University Press, pp. 23–61.

75 Buglar ME, White KM, Robinson NG (2010) The role of self-efficacy in dental patients' brushing and flossing: testing an extended Health Belief Model. *Patient Education & Counseling* **78**(2): 269–72.

76 Bylund CL, *et al.* (2011) Using the Extended Health Belief Model to understand siblings' perceptions of risk for hereditary hemochromatosis. *Patient Education & Counseling* **82**(1): 36–41.

77 Gillibrand R, Stevenson J (2006) The extended health belief model applied to the experience of diabetes in young people. *Br J Health Psychol* **11**(Pt 1): 155–69.

78 Cline RR, *et al.* (2005) Osteoporosis beliefs and antiresorptive medication use. *Maturitas* **50**(3): 196–208.

79 McHorney CA, *et al.* (2007) The impact of osteoporosis medication beliefs and side-effect experiences on non-adherence to oral bisphosphonates. *Curr Med Res Opin* **23**(12): 3137–52.

80 Yood RA, *et al.* (2008) Patient decision to initiate therapy for osteoporosis: the influence of knowledge and beliefs. *Journal of General Internal Medicine* **23**(11): 1815–21.

81 Schousboe JT, *et al.* (2010) Association of medication attitudes with non-persistence and non-compliance with medication to prevent fractures. *Osteoporos Int* **21**(11): 1899–1909.

82 Schousboe JT, *et al.* (2011) Predictors of patients' perceived need for medication to prevent fracture. *Medical Care* **49**(3): 273–80.

83 Solomon DH, *et al.* (2011) Predictors of very low adherence with medications for osteoporosis: towards development of a clinical prediction rule. *Osteoporos Int* **22**(6): 1737–43.

84 Schousboe JT, *et al.* (2010) Association of medication attitudes with non-persistence and non-compliance with medication to prevent fractures. *Osteoporos Int* **21**(11): 1899–1909.

85 Stuart B, Grana J (1998) Ability to pay and the decision to medicate. *Med Care* **36**(2): 202–11.

86 Rossini M, *et al.* (2006) Determinants of adherence to osteoporosis treatment in clinical practice. *Osteoporos Int* **17**(6): 914–21.

87 Cadarette SM, *et al.* (2012) Osteoporosis medication prescribing in British Columbia and Ontario: impact of public drug coverage. *Osteoporos Int* **23**(4): 1475–80.

88 Adams AS, Soumerai SB, Ross-Degnan D (2001) Use of antihypertensive drugs by Medicare enrollees: does type of drug coverage matter? *Health Aff (Millwood)* **20**(1): 276–86.

89 Blustein J (2000) Drug coverage and drug purchases by Medicare beneficiaries with hypertension. *Health Aff (Millwood)* **19**(2): 219–30.

90 Babazono A, *et al.* (2005) Effects of the increase in co-payments from 20 to 30 percent on the compliance rate of patients with hypertension or diabetes mellitus in the employed health insurance system. *Int J Technol Assess Health Care* **21**(2): 228–33.

91 Federman AD, *et al.* (2001) Supplemental insurance and use of effective cardiovascular drugs among elderly medicare beneficiaries with coronary heart disease. *JAMA* **286**(14): 1732–9.

92 Blais L, *et al.* (2003) Impact of a cost sharing drug insurance plan on drug utilization among individuals receiving social assistance. *Health Policy* **64**(2): 163–72.

93 Christian-Herman J, Emons M, George D (2004) Effects of generic-only drug coverage in a Medicare HMO. *Health Aff (Millwood)* Suppl Web Exclusives: W4-455-68.

94 Soumerai SB, *et al.*, Effects of a limit on Medicaid drug-reimbursement benefits on the use of psychotropic agents and acute mental health services by patients with schizophrenia. *N Engl J Med* **331**(10): 650–5.

95 Soumerai SB, *et al.* (1987) Payment restrictions for prescription drugs under Medicaid. Effects on therapy, cost, and equity. **317**(9): 550–6.

96 Goldman DP, *et al.* (2004) Pharmacy benefits and the use of drugs by the chronically ill. *JAMA* **291**(19): 2344–50.

97 Huskamp HA, *et al.* (2005) Impact of 3-tier formularies on drug treatment of attention-deficit/hyperactivity disorder in children. *Arch Gen Psychiatry* **62**(4): 435–41.

98 Ozminkowski RJ, *et al.* (2004) The use of disease-modifying new drugs for multiple sclerosis treatment in private-sector health plans. *Clin Ther* **26**(8): 1341–54.

99 Roblin DW, *et al.* (2005) Effect of increased cost-sharing on oral hypoglycemic use in five managed care organizations: how much is too much? *Med Care* **43**(10): 951–9.

100 Tamblyn R, *et al.* (2001) Adverse events associated with prescription drug cost-sharing among poor and elderly persons. *JAMA* **285**(4): 421–9.

101 Zafran N, *et al.* (2005) Incidence and causes for failure of treatment of women with proven osteoporosis. *Osteoporos Int* **16**(11): 1375–83.

102 Venturini F. *et al.* (1999) Compliance with sulfonylureas in a health maintenance organization: a pharmacy record-based study. *Ann Pharmacother* **33**(3): 281–8.

103 Kogut SJ, *et al.* (2004) Nonadherence as a predictor of antidiabetic drug therapy intensification (augmentation). *Pharmacoepidemiol Drug Saf* **13**(9): 591–8.

104 Grant RW, *et al.* (2003) Polypharmacy and medication adherence in patients with type 2 diabetes. *Diabetes Care* **26**(5): 1408–12.

105 Claxton AJ, Cramer J, Pierce C (2001) A systematic review of the associations between dose regimens and medication compliance. *Clin Ther* **23**(8): 1296–1310.

106 Greenberg RN (1984) Overview of patient compliance with medication dosing: a literature review. *Clin Ther* **6**(5): 592–9.

107 Paes AH, Bakker A, Soe-Agnie CJ (1997) Impact of dosage frequency on patient compliance. *Diabetes Care* **20**(10): 1512–17.

108 Ammassari A, *et al.* (2002) Correlates and predictors of adherence to highly active antiretroviral therapy: overview of published literature. *J Acquir Immune Defic Syndr* **31**(Suppl 3): S123–7.

109 Berkman L, Glass T (2000) Social integration, social networks, social support, and health, in L Berkman, I Kawachi (eds.), *Social Epidemiology*, New York: Oxford University Press.

110 House JS, Landis KR, Umberson D (1988) Social relationships and health. *Science* **241**(4865): 540–5.

111 Bandura A (1989), Human agency in social cognitive theory. *Am Psychol* **44**(9): 1175–84.

112 Resnick B, Wehren L, Orwig D (2003) Reliability and validity of the self-efficacy and outcome expectations for osteoporosis medication adherence scales. *Orthop Nurs* **22**(2): 139–47.

113 Bloom G, Standing H, Lloyd R (2008) Markets, information asymmetry and health care: towards new social contracts. *Soc Sci Med* **66**(10): 2076–87.

114 Blomqvist A (1991) The doctor as double agent: information asymmetry, health insurance, and medical care **10**(4): 411–32.

115 Anderson LA, Dedrick RF (1990) Development of the Trust in Physician scale: a measure to assess interpersonal trust in patient-physician relationships. *Psychol Rep* **67**(3 Pt 2): 1091–1100.

116 Thom DH, *et al.* (1999) Further validation and reliability testing of the Trust in Physician Scale. The Stanford Trust Study Physicians. *Med Care* **37**(5): 510–17.

117 Thorne SE, Robinson CA (1988) Reciprocal trust in health care relationships. *J Adv Nurs* **13**(6): 782–9.

118 Hall MA, *et al.* (2001) Trust in physicians and medical institutions: what is it, can it be measured, and does it matter? *Milbank Q* **79**(4): 613–39.

119 Piette JD, *et al.* (2005) The role of patient-physician trust in moderating medication nonadherence due to cost pressures. *Arch Intern Med* **165**(15): 1749–55.

120 Wroth TH, Pathman DE (2006) Primary medication adherence in a rural population: the role of the patient-physician relationship and satisfaction with care. *J Am Board Fam Med* **19**(5): 478–86.

121 Schousboe JT, *et al.* (2011) Predictors of patients' perceived need for medication to prevent fracture. *Med Care* **49**(3): 273–80.

122 Buller M, Buller D (1987) Physicians' communication style and patient satisfaction. *Journal of Health and Social Behavior* **28**: 375–88.

123 Charles C, Gafni A, Whelan T (1999) Decision-making in the physician-patient encounter: revisiting the shared treatment decision-making model. *Soc Sci Med* **49**(5): 651–61.

124 Charles C, Whelan T, Gafni A (1999) What do we mean by partnership in making decisions about treatment? *BMJ* **319**(7212): 780–2.

125 Douglas F, *et al.* (2012) Differing perceptions of intervention thresholds for fracture risk: a survey of patients and doctors. *Osteoporos Int* **23**(8): 2135–40.

126 Haynes RB, *et al.* (2008) Interventions for enhancing medication adherence. *Cochrane Database of Systematic Reviews*, **2008**(2). doi:10.1002/14651858.CD000011.pub3

127 McDonald HP, Garg AX, Haynes RB (2002) Interventions to enhance patient adherence to medication prescriptions: scientific review. *JAMA* **288**(22): 2868–79.

128 Banning M (2009) A review of interventions used to improve adherence to medication in older people. *International Journal of Nursing Studies* **46**(11): 1505–15.

129 Lee JK, Grace KA, Taylor AJ (2006) Effect of a pharmacy care program on medication adherence and persistence, blood pressure, and low-density lipoprotein cholesterol – A randomized controlled trial. *JAMA* **296**(21): 2563–71.

130 George J, Elliott RA, Stewart DC (2008) A systematic review of interventions to improve medication taking in elderly patients prescribed multiple medications. *Drugs & Aging* **25**(4): 307–24.

131 Shu AD-H, *et al.* (2009) Adherence to osteoporosis medications after patient and physician brief education: post hoc analysis of a randomized controlled trial. *American Journal of Managed Care* **15**(7): 417–24.

132 Guilera M, *et al.* (2006) Does an educational leaflet improve self-reported adherence to therapy in osteoporosis? The OPTIMA study. *Osteoporos Int* **17**(5): 664–71.

133 Schousboe JT, *et al.* (2005) Education and phone follow-up in post-menopausal women at risk for osteoporosis: effects on calcium intake, exercise frequency, and medication use. *Dis Manage Health Outcomes* **13**(6): 395–404.

134 Cooper A, Drake J, Brankin E (2006) Treatment persistence with once-monthly ibandronate and patient support vs. once-weekly alendronate: results from the PERSIST study. *Int J Clin Pract* **60**(8): 896–905.

135 Clowes JA, Peel NF, Eastell R (2004) The impact of monitoring on adherence and persistence with antiresorptive treatment for postmenopausal osteoporosis: a randomized controlled trial. *J Clin Endocrinol Metab* **89**(3): 1117–23.

136 Waalen J, *et al.* (2009) A telephone-based intervention for increasing the use of osteoporosis medication: a randomized controlled trial. *Am J Manag Care* **15**(8): e60–70.

137 Delmas PD, *et al.* (2007) Effect of monitoring bone turnover markers on persistence with risedronate treatment of postmenopausal osteoporosis. *J Clin Endocrinol Metab* **92**(4): 1296–1304.

138 Silverman SL, *et al.* (2012) Impact of bone turnover markers and/or educational information on persistence to oral bisphosphonate therapy: a community setting-based trial. *Osteoporos Int* **23**(3): 1069–74.

139 Touchette DR, Shapiro NL (2008) Medication compliance, adherence, and persistence: Current status of behavioral and educational interventions to improve outcomes. *Journal of Managed Care Pharmacy* **14**(6): S2–S10.

140 Miller WR (1996) Motivational interviewing: research, practice, and puzzles. *Addict Behav* **21**(6): 835–42.

141 Rollnick S, Miller WR, Butler CC (2007) *Motivational Interviewing in Health Care: Helping Patients Change Behavior (Applications of Motivational Interviewing)*. New York: The Guilford Press.

142 Cook PF, Emiliozzi S, McCabe MM (2007) Telephone counseling to improve osteoporosis treatment adherence: an effectiveness study in community practice settings. *Am J Med Qual* **22**(6): 445–56.

143 Solomon DH, *et al.* (2012) Osteoporosis telephonic intervention to improve medication regimen adherence: a large, pragmatic, randomized controlled trial. *Archives of Internal Medicine* **172**(6): 477–83.

144 Saberi P, *et al.* (2012) The impact of HIV clinical pharmacists on HIV treatment outcomes: a systematic review. *Patient Preference and Adherence*, **6**: 297–332.

145 Taitel M, *et al.* (2012) The impact of pharmacist face-to-face counseling to improve medication adherence among patients initiating statin therapy. *Patient Preference and Adherence* **6**: 323–9.

146 Lai PS, *et al.* (2011) Effects of pharmaceutical care on adherence and persistence to bisphosphonates in postmenopausal osteoporotic women. *J Clin Pharm Ther* **36**(5): 557–67.

A Clinician's Approach to the Patient

Robert Lindsay
Helen Hayes Hospital *and* Columbia Unversity, New York, NY, USA

Introduction

This chapter focuses on the approach to the patient. More specifically, it is a clinician's view of the disease process, its diagnosis, and how one might utilize the available data to manage patients with osteoporosis. The reader is encouraged to refer back to the various chapters in the text to amplify or perhaps refute the opinions expressed in this section. All clinicians can appreciate the fact that all too often it is difficult to determine exactly "what is evidencebased medicine" (e.g., see the discussion below on clinical trial design) for the patient(s) that they see clinically. Management of the individual patient, therefore, requires a combination of both one's experience and a careful study of the available data. The development of the absolute risk assessment tool (FRAX) has significantly aided the process of identifying those individuals whose fracture risk is high enough to justify the use of medications, especially for those who have not yet fractured. Among those individuals who are asymptomatic, compliance with a treatment program is often difficult, especially so if the patient experiences side effects or reads articles appearing in the popular press describing side effects.

The disease

The diagnosis of osteoporosis is still often made after the occurrence of a clinical fracture, especially in older individuals, and most commonly in women. The fractures that are commonly associated with this diagnosis include hip fractures, vertebral fractures and wrist fractures. The clinical community has classically defined these fractures as "minimal" or "low" trauma fractures, and that is indeed true. Hip fractures occur mostly after a fall from a standing height. Sixty percent of vertebral compression

Osteoporosis: Diagnosis and Management, First Edition. Edited by Dale W. Stovall.
© 2013 John Wiley & Sons, Ltd. Published 2013 by John Wiley & Sons, Ltd.

fractures do not come to clinical attention and are assumed to occur spontaneously (and perhaps even gradually) often with minimal or no remembered trauma. While wrist fractures have a somewhat different epidemiology, they are included in this disease process as they also occur mostly from a fall and are assumed to occur more commonly in younger women because of differences in the pattern of falling rather than differences in skeletal pathology. More specifically, younger individuals tend to fall forward using their wrist to protect themselves; whereas older individuals tend to fall to the side and land on their hip. However, fractures with similar epidemiological data occur at many other skeletal sites, and many could easily be classified as "osteoporosis-related" fractures. In addition, as discussed below, a person with osteoporosis who is subjected to significant trauma is much more likely to fracture than an individual with a normal skeleton. Yet such fractures are usually dismissed as "traumatic" even when observed in an individual likely to have a prejudiced skeleton.

Consider a 75-year-old Caucasian woman, with no chronic morbidity, and who is involved in a road traffic accident that results in a fracture of her humerus. She will be seen in the Emergency Department, probably subsequently by an orthopedic surgeon, and treatment will be appropriately directed toward repair of her fracture. She is unlikely to be referred to determine if she has underlying osteoporosis, because the fracture is labeled as "traumatic." Yet, as a 75-year-old Caucasian female, she is a prime candidate for osteoporosis, and that, plus the fracture, places her in a high risk category for further fractures; and therefore, she is an individual who should be evaluated for osteoporosis and if necessary, treated. This is the fate of many older individuals for whom society (medical and social) have pigeon-holed into the traumatic fracture category and dismissed, or more likely, never considered for a potentially underlying skeletal problem. Fortunately, the introduction, in health care systems, of a fracture liaison service is beginning to change that. This service provides individuals who have had a fracture over the age of 50 to get advice and direction, related to the possible presence of low bone mass. However, there is still a long way to go and we clinicians need to change the mind set that says: "I really had a bad injury ... Anyone would have broken a bone. It was a bad fall and the ground was very hard; therefore, I cannot have osteoporosis!" That is especially so when the Healthcare Provider agrees and does not push the issue.

However, that is only part of the picture, and although by itself it does a significant disservice to the management of osteoporosis, there are other issues. The disease we call osteoporosis is defined as a BMD that falls below the range expected for a young healthy peer population (a T-score of -2.5 or below). There are a number of problems with that definition. First, the test we use clinically does not measure density, but the attenuation of x-rays by calcium in its path divided by the area of the bone it sees. Nonetheless the test is a useful predictor of fracture risk, and the lower the result, the higher the fracture risk. The creation of a definition of osteoporosis is; therefore, somewhat arbitrary and in some ways similar to the diagnoses of hypertension and hypercholesterolemia.

All of these definitions define the abnormality as a test result that is outside the normal range for young healthy adults. Using that type of parameter to define a disease can give the false impression that someone who falls into the normal range is at low risk while those with the diagnosis are at high risk and must always be offered intervention designed to lower the risk. Each is indeed a measure of risk, but one that is a gradient of risk and the cut-point obfuscates that. Indeed, many, if not most of the fractures that can be considered a consequence of "osteoporosis" in fact occur in persons with a BMD within the lower section of the normal range for young adults (previously labeled "osteopenia," now defined as "low bone mass"). The problem is that that word, osteopenia (which represents a large population of individuals whose BMD falls between −1 and −2.5) has been construed as a disease (i.e., a polysyllabic, classically derived noun must be a disease!). In fact, only a modest number of those in the "osteopenic" range are in fact at increased risk for fracture. It is finding those at risk from the large population of people with BMD's in the low bone mass range that is daunting. Perhaps also because we use negative numbers for those below the average value for the normal range, and perhaps also because of marketing, many individuals who do not need intervention, have received pharmacologic treatment. The clinical utility of risk assessment is discussed below and in detail in Chapter 4.

Risk assessment includes more than BMD of course, and the introduction of tools to aid the clinician is an attempt to find the "high risk for fracture" individuals in order to recommend intervention. Several have been developed but the most widely recognized is FRAX developed under the aegis of the World Health Organization. All, however, have limitations and mostly do little better than could be done with the knowledge of gender, age, height and weight (or BMI), and BMD. FRAX is available as part of the output of some DXA instruments and thus has come into more common use than any other. The limitations of FRAX are described elegantly by Dr Hamdy in this text. However, it does lead to a discussion about changing the "diagnosis" of osteoporosis. Instead of a BMD diagnosis, maybe it should be both a fracture diagnosis (there would need to be a general agreement about the fractures that should be included) and also a fracture risk diagnosis. If nothing else, that change would serve to place the clinician's focus on the unfavorable outcome of the disease. The problem is that clinical trials of the available therapeutic agents have been recruited using a BMD cut-point, with the addition of only vertebral fractures (which usually allows a higher BMD for entry), and doubt has been expressed about whether we can assume that the medications will work if we move to a risk diagnosis.

Treatment and evidence

Treatment of osteoporosis is generally felt to be guided by "evidence" obtained through the clinical trials required for registration in different countries. However, these provide only limited guidance to physicians. First, they are usually of 3 years' duration, usually, but not always enrolling 5000 to 15 000 individuals, and are sometimes followed by a variety of strategies to try to provide some information about the prolonged use of the agents. Since the initial clinical trials are conducted to show efficacy, they are designed in fashions that provide the maximal opportunity to do just that. Subjects are generally healthier than the patients seen in practice with fewer comorbidities and fewer concomitant medications. Indeed it is a truism that many if not most patients seen in practice have features that would exclude them from the clinical trials. In addition, exclusions from trials often include illegal drug use, excessive alcohol use, steroid use (for studies of postmenopausal osteoporosis), prior treatment with osteoporosis-directed medications, and the investigators' belief that the subject could not complete the study. The continuation beyond 3 years' reverses the order of endpoints with safety becoming prime area of concern. However, true safety is often not discovered until well into the marketing era when large numbers of individuals have been treated for long periods in the "real world." Treatment of osteoporosis implies long-term use of drugs, and with only 3 years of trial data, adverse events may appear with long-term use. Whether the benefits are greater than the perceived risk is then often a discussion in the popular press, and the appearance of adverse events can lead to product liability law suits. This has led to a recommendation that certain drugs be used for around 5 years and then consideration given to introduction of the "drug holiday," although that itself leads to more confusion.

The approach to the patient

Osteoporosis is a disease that is misunderstood by many clinicians. Its importance is purely in its relationship to fracture risk. Bone density, or rather what we equate to bone density, that is the results obtained from dual energy absorptiometry, is a reasonable assessment of fracture risk, but one that is insufficient by itself upon which to always make a decision to treat or not. It is easy to decide not to treat a patient when their BMD at both the spine and hip are above a T-score of −1 (and there is no interference with the measurement as can occur especially in the spine). It is also fairly easy to decide to treat a patient who has suffered a vertebral or hip fracture or who's T-score at one or both skeletal sites is below −3. The clinical problem relates to dealing with those patients who fall in the gray zone (i.e., those with a T score below −1 and above −2.5). For the purposes of this chapter, I have elected to extended the gray zone to include patients with a T-score above −3 (as I will explain below), and to those who present with a fracture such as the one suffered by the patient outlined above.

The need for therapy in a patient who has had a fracture seems obvious. All female patients who present with a fracture after menopause should be counseled about osteoporosis, and evaluated or referred for evaluation if appropriate. The only fractures that one can exclude in this regard are those of the fingers, toes, skull, and facial bones. Ankle fractures form a special group, since their relationship to increasing age, bone density and osteoporosis can be debated. In clinical practice, I tend to include those fractures as it is not easy to explain to patients why they should be excluded. In dealing with patients who have had a fracture, I always obtain a BMD of the hip and spine, and some biochemical investigations (see below). Occasionally I may use the FRAX tool with all its limitations to estimate risk, and assist the decision making process. That is especially true if I feel that treatment is not warranted. In this scenario, calculation of an individual's risk for fracture with FRAX can often support that conclusion. There are some clinicians who feel that fractures of the hip, spine and perhaps wrist; by themselves justify a diagnosis of osteoporosis without the measurement of BMD, and it is hard to argue against that. However, the outcome of interest in treating individual patients is stability or improvement in BMD, so I always obtain BMD before intervention.

Individuals who are asymptomatic, postmenopausal and have been referred for a DXA measurement create more of a problem. For those with a T-score between −1 and −2.5 I recommend that one revert to FRAX to assist in clinical decision making. Remember that BMD is heavily affected by body size (i.e., DXA has difficulty indistinguishing small bones from bad bones). For those with a T-score below −2.5 there is a clinician reflex to treat. The argument is that those below this cut-point have a diagnosis of osteoporosis, and we have effective medicines to treat this disease and thus we should! However there is no measurable change in risk in going from −2.49 to −2.51 and to treat one and not the other is clinically wrong. On the other hand, treating (or not treating) both may be wrong as well. What we are interested in is fracture risk and I see value in treating DXA results as a continuum of risk that we should evaluate in the context of the patient sitting in the office. Consequently, I still calculate the FRAX fracture risk even when the diagnosis of osteoporosis is made by DXA. I use a T-score of −3 as the BMD cut-point at which, irrespective of age and presence (or not) of other risk factors, treatment should be considered.

The next clinical problem is the postmenopausal woman who has never had a bone density measurement. The guidelines generally say that BMD screening should be done around age 65 years, and that the BMD only be measured in younger women if they can be shown to be at risk. But by definition, all postmenopausal women are at risk, and many other factors can contribute to that risk including age, low body weight, cigarette and excessive alcohol use, and comorbidities and medications (see Chapters 5–7). At what level of "risk" should we consider the use of DXA? There is little guidance here. In general for patients who express their concern and state their willingness to deal with the problem, I will consider DXA evaluation. If no such interest is stated, then I would not refer for DXA. If I had a clinical suspicion, I might perform a FRAX evaluation (sans BMD) and use that as a guide for DXA or not.

As noted above, Dr Hamdy elegantly addresses the limitations of FRAX, and clinicians should understand those. However, the ready availability of FRAX as part of the report from most DXA machine reports, makes it convenient for opening a discussion with patients. The original National Osteoporosis Foundation guidelines suggested that those with a 10-year risk of an osteoporosis-related fracture of greater than 20% or a hip fracture risk of 3% should be considered for intervention. These fracture risk cut-points should be viewed only as a guide and not a dictate. If one has a patient with a 3.5% risk of hip fracture and 17% risk of any fracture, treatment will at best offer the patient a hip fracture risk reduction to 2.1% and an all fracture risk reduction to about 13% (absolute risk reductions of 1.4% and 4% respectively). These effects on absolute risk have to be weighed against the adverse effects of medicines and the likelihood that individual patients will take less then 100% of the prescribed medication, a feature that is known to reduce effectiveness. The higher the risk score obtained the greater the benefit, and thus the greater the difference in benefit versus risk.

Treating patients for osteoporosis

It is a sine qua non that patients who are interested in reducing their risk of fractures need to evaluate their lifestyle and diet before resorting to therapeutic intervention. These issues are well outlined in Chapter 12. The importance of stressing physical activity as a prerequisite for healthy aging, and fall prevention cannot be overemphasized (recall that FRAX does not include fall risk or frailty). Changing a lifetime of sedentary living, however, has its own challenges. I provide only two rules: (1) find something to do that you like, and (2) try to make it a social occasion. Both are a response to many years of trying to improve exercise patterns in persons over the age of 50 years after many years of inactivity. It is not easy, and exercise only works if you do it! Exercise will not rebuild the skeleton, but it may retard bone loss and it certainly improves the functioning and well-being of the organism. As I often tell patients, signing a check to join a health club is not exercise.

Diet is also important. The roles of calcium and vitamin D are well outlined in Chapter 12 by Dr Holick, a world-renowned expert in this area. Total calcium intake should be 1000–1500 mg/day on average, preferably from dietary sources. Dietary calcium calculators are available on the web (e.g., NOF.org and NYSOPEP.org). There is debate about the safety of higher calcium intake especially from supplements, and since there is no added benefit to calcium economy, there is little reason to increase intake above 1500 mg/day. For most individuals, vitamin D is difficult to obtain from dietary sources and the contribution from synthesis in the skin continues to decline as sun exposure declines and the use of high SPF sun screen becomes ubiquitous. Consequently most older adults need some vitamin D and we recommend 1000 to 2000 i.u. per day of cholecalciferol (i.e., within the intake boundaries recommended by the Institute of Medicine). In patients with malabsorption this may be insufficient, but further increments in intake require some monitoring of serum 25(OH)D levels. There is little argument for the use of the active hormone 1,25(OH)2D in most cases of osteoporosis, except when renal function is prejudiced.

Deciding the medication to use in a particular patient can be a daunting task. There are no head to head studies with fracture prevention as the outcome, for any of the available therapeutic agents. Due to differences in study design, the population studied, etc., the data from clinical trials cannot be easily compared. In general most of the patients seen clinically would not qualify for inclusion in most of these clinical trials for a variety of reasons; including comorbidities, the use of other therapeutic agents, and too severe disease (or not severe enough!). Only one clinical trial has evaluated fractures in men as the primary outcome.

To obtain approval by regulatory approval for marketing in many countries, osteoporosis medications must show a reduction in vertebral fracture risk. Once on the market, other dosing regimens may be tested against the original using surrogate markers (usually BMD by DXA) as the outcome measure. In men approval also has classically been obtained (with one exception), after approval for women, using surrogate outcomes. Thus the indication for men is "to increase BMD" and not to reduce fracture risk, the assumption being made by clinicians that the fracture benefit will be similar to that observed in women if BMD responses are similar.

From clinical trial data, in addition to vertebral fracture prevention, alendronate is approved for prevention of nonvertebral fractures and hip fracture; risedronate is approved for nonvertebral fracture prevention; ibandronate only for vertebral fracture prevention; and zoledronic acid for hip and nonvertebral fractures. Raloxifene, and perhaps calcitonin, reduce only vertebral fracture risk. Denosumab reduces hip and nonvertebral fracture risk although the mechanism is separate from the bisphosphonate mechanism. All of those agents are classified as "antiresorptive" indicating that their primary effect is inhibition of osteoclast recruitment (denosumab) or action (bisphosphonates). Most are associated with observed increases in BMD, especially in the spine. Biopsies do not confirm, by and large, increased bone tissue and it is assumed that the increase seen with DXA is due to increase in the mineral component of the bone. I use the clinical trial fracture data as a guide to match treatment to patient. In this regard, I tend to use raloxifene in younger postmenopausal patients with vertebral fracture risk. Because of the DVT and death from stroke seen in one clinical trial, I stop raloxifene roughly around age 70 and change to an agent that gives more all round fracture protection. The reduction in risk of estrogen receptor positive breast cancer seen with raloxifene is often the tipping point.

At present only one "anabolic" agent is available, teriparatide [(1-34)rhPTH]. While there are clear increments in bone tissue, especially in the spine, the fracture data cannot be compared with the antiresorptive agents in any way. The teriparatide clinical trial was terminated early when osteosarcoma was reported in a lifetime toxicology study in rats. To date only 3 malignancies have been seen in humans treated with teriparatide and a cause and effect relationship is impossible to determine. A recent population based study involving some 1500 subjects with osteosarcoma found none who had been exposed to teriparatide. Perhaps the difference is in the biological response to teriparatide. With continued exposure to the high doses, rats continue to make more and more bone, eventually eliminating the marrow space (and marked extramedullary hematopoiesis is seen). In humans at 20 mcg/day there is an early response in bone formation, a more delayed increase in remodeling and a gradual decline in drug effect such that by 2–3 years there is no evidence of stimulation of formation or resorption either looking at biochemistry or on examination of bone biopsies. The concern about osteosarcoma led to the restrictions in the label – no more than 2 years of use in any lifespan, and prohibited in patients at increased risk of osteosarcoma. The cost and route of administration (daily subcutaneous) limit the use of teriparatide to those at high risk of fracture, something that is often difficult to define, and can be seen differently by the payors than the prescriber. In general I use teriparatide in those patients presenting with fracture, particularly vertebral fracture, and those with BMD in the spine below a T-score of −3. I may use teriparatide for only one year (rather than the 2 years it is approved for) saving the second year in case it is needed again. Teriparatide treatment must be followed by an antiresorptive agent or the effects dissipate (see Chapter 11). Usually the antiresorptive agent of choice is either a bisphosphonate or denosumab.

Biochemical markers have become somewhat more reliable and I use them to detect an early response to treatment especially if I feel that the patient will need reassurance. I use serum C-Telopeptide drawn in the morning with the patient fasting, before initiating treatment and 1–3 months after initiating treatment. When giving teriparatide I use osteocalcin as the early indicator of increased bone formation, obtained in the same fashion. I repeat the patient's BMD (preferably on the same machine and by the same technician as prior measurements) one year after initiating treatment and thereafter revert to every second year, although often I repeat the BMD even less frequently.

The duration of treatment causes problems, since the issues of osteonecrosis of the jaw and atypical fractures seem to increase after several years of treatment with bisphosphonates and denosumab, although the risks seem to be much less than the fracture benefits that accrue. A recent publication from the FDA recommended 5 years of treatment to be followed by a drug holiday, except for those remaining at high risk. In regards to bisphosphonates, their long skeletal half-life means some continued pharmacologic effect for months or even years. Without formal guidance, this is again a place I find biochemical markers helpful to follow the waning effect of the drug. When I am convinced that much of the drug effect is gone I re-initiate a discussion about therapeutic options.

Secondary osteoporosis

Hardly a week goes by without the description of something that might be harmful to the skeleton. These are well described in Chapters 5–7. Removal of the offending agent or limiting the effects is the place to start, but often that is something that may not be possible. Thereafter patient management follows a similar course as for postmenopausal osteoporosis. Clinically, steroid therapy remains the major insult to the skeleton, with data suggesting there is no real safe dose.

Osteoporosis in men

Men are at about one-half of the lifetime risk of osteoporosis compared to women, but usually do not appreciate their risk. Seeking secondary causes is important in men, especially those with fractures under age 70 years of age. With the exception of raloxifene the therapeutic approach is similar to that in women.

Summary

Osteoporosis remains an important clinical problem, and one that will continue to increase as baby-boomers age. However, detection and management of the disease are still inadequate as we continue to fail to recognize those individuals with fractures who might have this underlying skeletal problem. The realization that bone density is a useful risk assessment tool is important, but what one needs to realize that bone density is but one part of the overall picture, and it must be placed in context with the patient that is being evaluated. While several medicines are available currently, more may be coming along, and the medical profession has an outstanding opportunity to make fracture a much less important feature of aging.

Index

Osteoporosis: Diagnosis and Management, First Edition. Edited by Dale W. Stovall.
© 2013 John Wiley & Sons, Ltd. Published 2013 by John Wiley & Sons, Ltd.

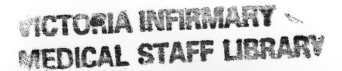